The elderly in modern society

SOCIAL POLICY IN MODERN BRITAIN

General Editor: Jo Campling

POVERTY AND STATE SUPPORT   *Peter Alcock*
HEALTH POLICY AND THE NATIONAL HEALTH SERVICE   *Judy Allsop*
HOUSING AND SOCIAL JUSTICE   *Gill Burke*
THE VOLUNTARY SECTOR IN BRITISH SOCIAL SERVICES   *Maria Brenton*
EDUCATION AS SOCIAL POLICY   *Janet Finch*
WORK AND INEQUALITY   *Susan Lonsdale*
THE PERSONAL SOCIAL SERVICES   *Adrian Webb and Gerald Wistow*
FOUNDATIONS OF THE WELFARE STATE   *Pat Thane*
THE ELDERLY IN MODERN SOCIETY   *Anthea Tinker*
SOCIAL RESPONSES TO HANDICAP   *Eda Topliss*

THE ELDERLY IN MODERN SOCIETY

Anthea Tinker

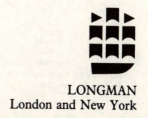

LONGMAN
London and New York

LONGMAN GROUP LIMITED

Longman House
Burnt Mill, Harlow, Essex, UK

Published in the United States of America by
Longman Inc., New York

First published 1981
Second edition 1984

BRITISH LIBRARY CATALOGUING IN PUBLICATION DATA

Tinker, Anthea
   The elderly in modern society. – 2nd ed
   – (Social policy in modern Britain)
   1. Old age assistance – Great Britain
   I. Title   II. Series
   362.6'0941   HV1481.G5

   ISBN 0-582-29649-8

LIBRARY OF CONGRESS CATALOGING IN PUBLICATION DATA

Tinker, Anthea.
   The elderly in modern society.

   (Social policy in modern Britain)
   Bibliography: p.
   Includes index.
   1. Old age assistance – Great Britain. 2. Aged–
Services for – Great Britain.   I. Title.   II. Series.
HV1481.G52T5 1984   362.6'0941   83-25568
ISBN 0-582-29649-8

Set in 10/11 pt Linocomp Plantin
Printed in Hong Kong by
Astros Printing Ltd

CONTENTS

Editor's preface   ix
Author's preface to the first edition   x
Author's preface to the second edition   xi
List of abbreviations   xii
Acknowledgements   xiii

PART ONE. THE BACKGROUND

1. Introduction   2
2. A picture of the elderly   5
3. General review of the literature   19

PART TWO. NEEDS AND HOW THEY ARE MET

4. A critical narrative of the main developments in
   social services   30
5. The financial and employment position   41
6. Health   58
7. Housing   80
8. Personal and other social services   99
9. Community care – the family   119
10. Community care – support from the wider community   133

PART THREE. ASSESSMENT

11. The contribution of the elderly   154
12. Some general problems   173
13. The topic in perspective   187
14. Developments since 1980   194

PART FOUR. DOCUMENTS

Documents 1–53   262

Table of Statutes and Commissions   353
Bibliography   355
Index   360

To the beloved memory of my grandparents.

EDITOR'S PREFACE

This series, written by practising teachers in universities and polytechnics, is produced for students who are required to study social policy and administration, either as social science undergraduates or on the various professional courses. The books provide studies focusing on essential topics in social policy and include new areas of discussion and research, to give students the opportunity to explore ideas and act as a basis of seminar work and further study. Each book combines an analysis of the selected theme, a critical narrative of the main developments and an assessment putting the topic into perspective as defined in the title. The supporting documents and comprehensive bibliography are an important aspect of the series.

Conventional footnotes are avoided and the following system of references is used. A superior numeral in the text refers the reader to the corresponding entry in the list of references at the end of each chapter. A select bibliography is found at the end of the book. A number in square brackets, preceded by 'doc', e.g. [doc 6, 8] refers the reader to the corresponding items in the section of documents which follows the main text.

In *The Elderly in Modern Society*, Anthea Tinker has brought together for the first time the literature and research evidence from many sources about this important group of people. Viewing the topic in the widest perspective, it provides basic information on the development of the services together with a more theoretical approach, redefining concepts like community care in relation to the elderly and their needs, and identifying likely issues for the future. It will be invaluable for students and indeed professionals in a variety of disciplines.

Jo Campling

AUTHOR'S PREFACE

Many people, academic, professional and the elderly themselves, have influenced my thinking on this subject. I have quoted some of them and express my gratitude to them for allowing me to do so.

I am particularly grateful to the following. To Mrs Joan Clegg, formerly Senior Lecturer in Social Policy at the City University, who encouraged my early research. The material for this book was collected while I was at the City University, and I am grateful to everyone there for their help. To the staff and students of the University of London, Department of Extra-Mural Studies (particularly the Social Work Course) with whom I discussed many of these ideas. To Mrs Carole Austin and Mrs Jenny Wren who typed the script. But most of all, to my husband, Eric, for his practical help without which this book would not have been written.

I alone, of course, am responsible for the views expressed, which do not necessarily reflect those of the Department of the Environment, and for any errors.

Anthea Tinker
January 1980

AUTHOR'S PREFACE TO THE SECOND EDITION

Since writing this book a number of events have taken place. These include changes in legislation, a Government White Paper, *Growing Older*, and the World Assembly on Ageing. At the same time much of the research which was in progress when I wrote this book has been completed.

In this new edition I update some of the original material and add a new chapter discussing some of the important new developments in policy and practice which have occurred in the last three and a half years.

I renew my thanks to my husband and again say that my views are not necessarily those of the Department of the Environment.

Anthea Tinker
July 1983

LIST OF ABBREVIATIONS

BASW	British Association of Social Workers
BMA	British Medical Association
CAB	Citizens' Advice Bureau
CIPFA	Chartered Institute of Public Finance and Accountancy
COI	Central Office of Information
CPA	Centre for Policy on Ageing
CPRS	Central Policy Review Staff
CSO	Central Statistical Office
DOE	Department of the Environment
DHSS	Department of Health and Social Security
ECA	Exceptional Circumstances Addition
ENP	Exceptional Needs Payment
EOC	Equal Opportunities Commission
FES	*Family Expenditure Survey*
GHS	*General Household Survey*
GP	General Practitioner
HIP	Housing Investment Programme
HMSO	Her Majesty's Stationery Office
MHLG	Ministry of Housing and Local Government
MOH	Ministry of Health
MPNI	Ministry of Pensions and National Insurance
NAB	National Assistance Board
NCSS	National Council of Social Service
NCCOP	National Corporation for the Care of Old People
NDHS	*National Dwelling and Housing Survey*
NOPWC	National Old People's Welfare Council
NHS	National Health Service
OPCS	Office of Population, Censuses and Surveys
SBC	Supplementary Benefits Commission
WO	Welsh Office

ACKNOWLEDGEMENTS

We are grateful to the following for permission to reproduce copyright material:

Age Concern England for extracts from pages 3, 4 and 6 of 'On the Place of the Retired Elderly in Modern Society' from the *Manifesto* (1975); Mr Hugh Faulkner for an extract from his letter in *The Times* 5th December, 1972; The Controller of Her Majesty's Stationery Office for a figure from *Population Trends* No. 15, 1979, table 2 by Harris from *Handicapped and Impaired in Great Britain*, part of table 3 from *National Dwelling and Housing Survey*, 1978 and table 1.2 from *Social Trends*, No. 13, 1982; Office of Population Censuses and Surveys table 10.44, p 214 from *General Household Survey 1980*, HMSO, 1983; Syndication International Ltd for an extract from a letter to *Woman's Own*, 23rd September, 1978.

ACKNOWLEDGMENTS

We are grateful to the following for permission to reproduce copyright material:

...

Part one
THE BACKGROUND

Chapter one
INTRODUCTION

This book is intended both for students of social administration and for all who are concerned about the elderly. Many students, particularly postgraduates and those engaged in professional training, either choose, or find they have to take, a course in social administration. Social science students, social workers, town planners, the medical and allied professions, together with those working for voluntary bodies such as the Citizens' Advice Bureaux (CAB), all share an interest in this relatively new subject.

Social administration is a hybrid subject which owes its origins to the other social sciences. Although it has developed considerably since Donnison and Chapman wrote in 1965 there is still a good deal of truth in their description: 'We are concerned with an ill-defined but recognizable territory: the development of collective action for the advancement of social welfare. Our job is to identify and clarify problems within this territory, to throw light upon them – drawing light from any discipline that appears to be relevant – and to contribute when we can to the solution of these problems.'[1]

Because it is this 'synthesis – an interdisciplinary way of studying certain social institutions, problems and processes in society' it can draw on the theory of other disciplines, such as sociology and government. It has the advantage of looking at a subject from many perspectives. The problem lies always in deciding in what depth to consider each aspect. In this book, for example, decisions had to be made continually about how far to explore such issues as the social implications of the family, the medical aspects of health, the architectural aspects of design and the political theories of decision making. But to bring together these aspects, even though not always in great depth, and to relate them is the function and the fascination of social administration.

This book also reflects the current state of social administration in another way. The study of the subject has gone on in parallel with the growth of the welfare state, through the expansion and extension of the statutory and voluntary social services. Probably as a result of this, social administration has tended to concentrate on two major facets:

1. A study of social pathology;
2. An evaluation of provision by the statutory and voluntary services.

Policy makers and researchers have paid much less attention to alternative systems of providing care. As R. Parker demonstrates, not only does the market (e.g. private health insurance) have a considerable role to play but the involvement of family and neighbourly help has in the past been largely ignored. However, in the last 10 years more attention has been given to examining the wider aspects of the supply of social services. Researchers have looked beyond the conventional suppliers of services (statutory and voluntary bodies) to the more ill-defined area of what is provided by family, friends and neighbours.

The elderly are particularly interesting to study. Not only are they one of the largest of what are labelled 'special groups' but they are also the group to which in due time most people will belong. Unlike deviant groups such as offenders, or people with particular physical characteristics such as the disabled, the elderly represent a cross-section of ordinary people whose sole common denominator is their age. Because they are such a large group and because most people will in time reach old age it is a matter of self-interest to consider their role in, and contribution to, society as well as their problems.

This book attempts to present some of the evidence about the elderly in society, neither assuming that they necessarily have the same characteristics as younger age groups nor assuming that they present no problems. There are widely contrasting images of this group. Senior citizen or silly old woman? Consumers of large amounts of social services or the proud minority who prefer to suffer cold or poverty and not ask for help? A golden age or one which is 'sans everything'? This book is intended to bring together existing evidence about the elderly and how they live. It is not written from a particular political or other stance and its aim is to give the facts and summarise both research and the views of others. For those who have extended essays or a thesis to prepare it gives ample references and points to other sources of information.

The outline of the book is as follows. Part one provides background material in two parts. A picture is presented of the elderly, giving basic data about who they are. This brings out some of the reasons why the elderly represent one of the most important challenges in social policy. Alongside this demographic background there is a discussion about how society sees ageing. Then follows a review of the literature which shows that what has been written falls into a number of different categories.

Part two seeks to outline the major general developments in policy, first with a broad brush and then in detail for individual services with a concentration on statutory provision. This is followed by evidence about informal networks of care.

In Part three an assessment is made of the elderly in society. First there is a discussion about the contribution of the elderly both to their own welfare and to that of others. Then there is an examination of some of the general problems. These include variations in services, take-up of benefits and questions of need and evaluation. Finally, the topic is considered in perspective and similarities and differences with other groups discussed. A new chapter deals with developments since 1980.

Part four comprises the documents which relate to the text.

REFERENCES

1. DONNISON, D. V. and CHAPMAN, V., *Social Policy and Adminis-tration*, Allen and Unwin, 1965, p. 26.

Chapter two
A PICTURE OF THE ELDERLY

INTRODUCTION

One of the concerns of social policy is with particular groups. It is important, therefore, that they should be defined with some accuracy. The disabled have different levels of impairment which can be measured and their social handicap assessed. Offenders can be categorised by type of crime and by kind of sentence. Ethnic minorities can be divided into groups by country of birth, country of parents' birth and by the colour of their skin.

In contrast to this the elderly are the whole of a generation of people who have reached a certain age. *Our Future Selves* is the apt title of one book on the elderly.[1] They are not a deviant group or one small special section of the population. They are ordinary people who happen to have reached a particular age. This cannot be emphasised too much, particularly to professionals who are, as a result of their training and experience at work, concerned primarily with the abnormal.

PROBLEMS OF DEFINITION

The most commonly accepted definition of the elderly is those over retirement age, i.e. 60 for a woman and 65 for a man. However, sometimes in research and in statistics, 65 is used for both sexes and the move towards equal opportunities may lead to this becoming more usual practice (see also Ch. 12).

However, the lack of a generally agreed definition creates difficulty for those who wish to compare research data. Document 9 summarises some of the important surveys of elderly people and shows the variations. What is particularly interesting is the distinction that is increasingly being made in medical and social studies between the young elderly and the old elderly. For example Hodkinson confirms that it is the elderly over 75 with whom the geriatrician is mostly concerned.[2] Two studies which came out in 1978, *The Elderly at Home*[3] and *Beyond Three Score and Ten*,[4] both made comparisons between elderly people under 75 and those above that age.

If the elderly are such a varied collection of people, why are they then labelled as one group? One of the main reasons is that retirement marks a watershed. Becoming 60 for a woman and 65 for a man usually means the end of employment and the beginning of entitlement to a pension. In a pre-industrial society and for the self-employed the definition may be less satisfactory. People may go on working for as long as they are physically capable and, if they continue in their job, their status remains that of a worker. But for most people now retirement brings an end to that particular role.

THE FOLLY OF GENERALISING

Few people would attribute the same characteristics to a 30 year old as they would to a 60 year old. Why then should the 60s and 90s be classed together as one group? It is very easy to assume that all the elderly want this or feel that. It might be more realistic to generalise if people were divided according to how old they appeared in behaviour, attitudes and thought. 'As old as you feel' is one approach and if to act old is to be set in one's ways, to lack flexibility of thought and to look generally old-fashioned, then there are many people in their 20s and 30s who would qualify.

Social class, family support, physical and mental disability, religion and work patterns vary among the elderly as much as they do among the rest of the population. It is therefore only reasonable to expect that the demands of this group on society, their expectations of it and their contributions to it will be as varied as those of the rest of the population.

The Director of Age Concern once rightly rounded on a speaker at a conference who described this group rather patronisingly as 'old dears'. He pointed out that some may well be the exact opposite of 'old dears'. It seems unlikely that someone who is awkward and finds difficulty in making friends will suddenly become the life and soul of the bingo sessions on reaching the magic age of retirement. And why the association between bingo and old age? Just as some teenagers enjoy chess while others opt for pop music, so the leisure pursuits of the elderly are likely to be just as varied.

HOW SOCIETY SEES AGEING

It is difficult to make comparisons with attitudes in past years since so little is known except what is recorded in fiction. Was there a time when old people in this country were looked on as founts of all knowledge and repositories of great wisdom? Even if there was, there are a number of reasons why this should not be so now. Old people, at least until this century, were not as numerous as they are now. Children were much less likely to have had a grandparent alive and so the latter had a scarcity value. They were also likely to have had comparatively greater skills and knowledge, since these then changed little from generation to generation. Today the rapid increase in knowledge and changes in technology make it difficult for one generation to keep up with the next. This is especially so in specialist subjects.

Shakespeare painted a depressing picture of old age in *As You Like It* and one commentator on social policy took the final two words of one speech *Sans Everything* as the title of her book.[5] But anyone concerned with social policy needs to be aware of the physical changes which actually happen to the elderly because attitudes and social policy are often the result of what are perceived to be these changes.

The physical changes that come with age are varied and do not necessarily develop at the same time in each old person. It is important to have some understanding of these physical and mental changes, and to know what is normal and what is abnormal. A growing number of books (e.g. Hooker[6] and Keddie[7]) are attempting to provide some of this background information for professionals, relatives and friends who want to understand what is happening to the elderly people with whom they have contact.

Keddie, a consultant psychiatrist, argues that: 'Positive thinking is needed here. Unfortunately many of the public still feel that little can be done for an elderly man or woman who is ill – it is assumed that the old person's condition is simply due to his age. In fact, most old people, who are unwell, are suffering from a treatable disease of one sort or another.'[8] Hodkinson, a geriatrician, has taken a similar view: 'As a group, elderly patients have tended to have been under-investigated in the past on the basis that accurate diagnosis was unnecessary as nothing useful could be achieved at their age. Geriatric experience has shown this view to be totally inappropriate and that much treatable disease can be found among elderly patients who are comprehensively investigated.'[9] In what way then does society view this ageing process, and what bearing has this on social policy? There is little doubt that in a society that seems geared to youth there is great emphasis on remaining young. Advice on appearance, particularly hair and skin, is not confined to women. And when people are old the terms often used to describe them, such as members of 'evergreen' clubs, seem to deny the process of ageing.

Will more attention now be focused on the elderly, since their numbers have increased so rapidly? A distinguished social scientist has claimed that since the 1960s the fortunes of teenagers have been the focus of discussion and research, but that the elderly are about to come into their own [doc 1]. Yet society does not always find it easy to come to terms with this group. Hobman in an article in *Social Work Today* discussed some of the issues [doc 2]. Some, like Comfort, would argue that the whole concept of ageism is itself part of the prejudice against the elderly [doc 3].

The sociological concept of disengagement also must be noted. This is the theory that the individual, recognising the inevitability of death, starts a process of advance adjustment to it. At the extreme he is 'portrayed as happily withdrawing from a variety of roles as citizen, worker, parent, and in turning in on himself'. But this view is now strongly challenged as neither necessarily happening nor being desirable. For example Professor J. C. Brocklehurst addressing the British Association of Social Workers (BASW) in 1975 said:

Though middle-age is seen as a time for revaluation of self, ideas about ageing are less distinct. The disengagement theory of the 1950–60s not only felt ageing and disengagement to be normal but the best thing for society and the individual. It was this last assumption which has been discarded by modern gerontologists who had seen all too frequently the evidence of withdrawal and isolation and now took the view that the best thing for the individual and society was for the elderly and the aged to remain involved with life and living while they came to terms with the natural process of disengagement in their own time and in their own way.

For many this involvement with life and living stops with retirement. 'Retirement is the filthiest word in the English language' declared Ernest Hemingway. One elderly person (Gladys Elder) deliberately labelled herself OAP and wrote about the experiences of her generation under the title *The Alienated*.[10]

It is important to raise these questions about how society sees ageing because they have implications for social policy. The assumptions that 'the elderly' are a social problem, that they have similar aspirations and that they all need certain services are all

questionable. The Director of Help the Aged, Hugh Faulkner, in a
letter to *The Times* (5.12.1972) said there is a 'frightening attitude
creeping into the actions of some people caring for the elderly. While
most bring true compassion and understanding to their work there
are a vociferous few who regard those over retirement age as just a
massive group of people who have to be coped with in the most
efficient manner.'

NUMBERS

When considering the provision of social services it is important to
try and get as accurate an estimate as possible of how many
recipients there will be. As with any kind of crystal gazing the future
is not always easy to predict. Some elements, however, are relatively
certain. If, for example, there are 4 million young people aged 16–18
about to leave school and go on to higher education or work it is
probable that in 10 years' time something like that number will be
needing services appropriate to people in their late 20s. And so on
until middle and late age. But this assumes no major alteration of
circumstances. War can wipe out almost a complete generation.
Illness or an increase in unhealthy habits such as smoking, drinking
and drug taking can cause premature death or turn a healthy person
into one who is physically disabled. On the other hand medical
advances, such as early diagnosis of illnesses or cures for what
seemed terminal illnesses, can prolong life.

One striking feature has been the increase in the numbers of
elderly people since the beginning of the century. While the total
population has grown it has been at a much slower rate than that
which occurred among the elderly [doc 4]. Table 1 summarises this

Table 1. Population figures 1901–2001* – United Kingdom

	Total population (millions)	% increase	Elderly† (millions)	% increase
1901	38.2	–	2.4	–
1951	50.5	32.0	6.9	188
1981	56.3	11.0	10.0	45
1991‡	57.2	1.5	10.0	0
2001‡	58.3	2.0	9.5	−5

* Figures derived from CSO, *Social Trends* (No. 13), Table 1.2, p. 12 [doc 4].
† Males over 65, females over 60.   ‡ Projected.

growth. From this table it can be seen that forecasts show that the total population will continue to increase until the beginning of the next century but that the numbers of old people, after a slight rise at the end of the century, will then fall back in 2001. However, numbers will subsequently rise (see p. 16).

Figure 1 shows the numbers in each age group now, and from this one can see how and why numbers will fluctuate in the older age

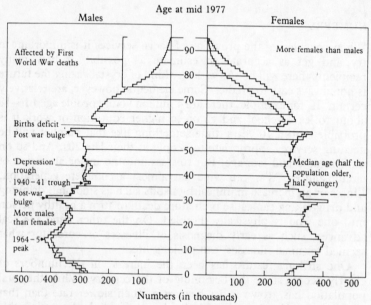

Fig. 1. Population by age and sex, England and Wales. (*Source*: From OPCS, *Population Trends* (No. 15), Spring 1979, p. 37.)

groups as the years pass. The very small numbers of those just below and above 60 in 1977 were due to the low birth-rate during the First World War. A post-war bulge followed which accounts for the larger numbers who were 57–58 in 1977. The Second World War had a similar result with a trough in births in 1940–41 and a post-war bulge. There is neither a steady increase nor a steady decline in numbers in any age group. Students of social policy should look carefully at the evidence on which forecasts are based and ask whether this is firmly based. Demographic forecasting has proved to be fraught with problems.

REGIONAL AND LOCAL VARIATIONS

It has already been stated that generalisations about the elderly are dangerous. It is equally unwise to assume that overall figures, such as the percentage of elderly in the population, will be the same for every part of the country. There are considerable regional variations.

The national average percentage of people above retirement age is 18 per cent. In some areas, such as the South West, it rises to nearly 20 per cent, while in others, such as the East Midlands, it falls to 16 per cent. The reasons for these differences are various. An above-average number of elderly people can be the result of people finding an attractive area to which to retire. Or younger people may have moved out from an inner-city area into the suburbs, leaving behind a disproportionate number of old people. Or there can be a bulge of people reaching retirement age at the same time, as a consequence of a large group of younger people having in the past moved at the same time to new work or to a new town. The area which suddenly became largely one of young families becomes in due time largely one of elderly people, especially if little housing became available there for *their* children when they got married. Within an area, too, there may be pockets where large numbers of old people live, perhaps because of the nature of the housing or the lack of facilities for families.

Those concerned with social policy have to take these variations into account. At a national level allowance has been made for the number of elderly residents when deciding on the level of the rate support grant. Similarly extra help is sometimes given to those professionals who care for the elderly – for example higher capitation fees for doctors with elderly patients.

Those who plan services need to be aware of the local position and take account of how and why it varies from the national picture. The Central Policy Review Staff (CPRS) commenting on this issue said: 'Where allocation of resources at a regional or sub-regional level is involved . . . changes in population in the country as a whole are often less important than local needs and demands which are themselves likely to have been influenced by changes in the distribution of population and in the patterns of internal migration.'[11] Social workers, planners, housing managers, architects, home help organisers and other professionals need not only a current demographic profile of their area but also projections which will enable them to forecast future trends in demand.

THE VERY OLD

It has already been seen that the total number of the elderly will not rise appreciably in the future. What is most significant now is the decline in the number of young elderly and the rise in the number of very old. Using as a basis the figures given before [doc 4] the picture emerges as set out in Table 2.

Table 2. The very old as a percentage of the elderly in the United Kingdom (1901–2001)*

	All elderly people† (millions)	Elderly people 75 and under† (millions)	The very old‡ (millions)	Percentage of all elderly people who are very old
1901	2.4	1.9	0.5	21
1951	6.9	5.1	1.8	26
1981	10.0	6.8	3.2	32
1991§	10.0	6.4	3.6	36
2001§	9.5	5.9	3.6	38

* Figures derived from CSO, *Social Trends* (No. 13), Table 1.2, p. 12 [doc 4].
† Males over 65, females over 60.
‡ All 75 and over.   § Projected.

This demonstrates clearly that the number of young elderly will decline from now until 2001, but that the number of very old people will rise substantially until 1991 and then remain at this level until 2001. Figure 2 illustrates this point. Those over 85 will also increase from 6 per cent of the elderly in 1981 to 8 per cent in 1991 and remain at that level in 2001 [doc 4].

Part of the reason for this increase in the number of very elderly is the bulge in the birth-rate in previous years. But in part it is also caused by a rise in the expectation of life. Expectation of life at birth in 1901 for a male was 48 years and for a female 51.6. In 1951 this had risen to 66.2 and 71.2 respectively. In 1979 it was 70.2 for a male and 76.2 for a female.[12]

The significance of the growing number of old people is that this group makes the highest demands on health and personal social services [doc 5]. Those who are over 75 years make even greater demands; and those over 85 'make particularly heavy demands on the medical and social services'. An official comment on this trend was: 'Even though the total structure of retirement pensioners may not change very greatly, changes in their age structure may lead to an increase in the burden of caring for them.'[13]

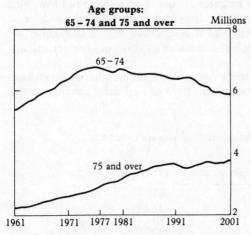

Fig. 2. Population projection for the elderly based on 1977. (From CSO, *Social Trends* (No. 9), p. 33. Chart 1.3

PROPORTIONS OF ELDERLY PEOPLE IN THE POPULATION AND DEPENDENCY RATES

The elderly have formed an increasingly large section of the population since the beginning of the century, but it is forecast that this will become slightly less in 2001 (see Table 3).

Table 3. Elderly people as a percentage of the population of the United Kingdom*

	Total population (millions)	Elderly† (millions)	Elderly as % of total
1901	38.2	2.4	6
1951	50.5	6.9	14
1981	56.3	10.0	18
1991‡	57.2	10.0	17
2001‡	58.3	9.5	16

* Figures derived from CSO, *Social Trends* (No. 13), Table 1.2, p. 12 [doc 4].
† Males over 65, females over 60.   ‡ Projected.

In relation to the social services, which have to be paid for largely by people of working age, the percentage of the population which is dependent is significant. Two groups are commonly regarded as dependants, children under school-leaving age and the elderly over the age of retirement. The latter are not considered to be of working age although some do work. It is also assumed that all those of working age are at work, and if at any time any large number are unemployed (and therefore dependants) this could upset calculations.

Interestingly dependency rates, that is the number of dependants related to those of working age, have altered little throughout this century (see Table 4).

Table 4. Percentage of the population who are dependants – United Kingdom*

	% who are dependants†
1901	41
1951	37
1981	40
1991	39
2001	40

* Figures derived from CSO, *Social Trends* (No. 13), Table 1.2, p. 12 [doc 4].
† Children under 16 (15 for 1901–51), males over 65 and females over 60.

The reason there has been so little change during a period of rapidly increasing numbers of the elderly is that there has been a simultaneous decline in the birth-rate. But looking further ahead it is forecast by Davis [doc 6] that the dependency rates will begin to fall. However, he also points out that another factor which will have to be taken into account is the increase in the expectation of services for dependent groups [doc 6].

THE BALANCE OF THE SEXES

In general there tend to be more women than men among the elderly, especially the very elderly, because women, on average, live longer. Whether this will continue is a matter for debate because no one knows why women live longer. If it is because they have in the past tended to drink less, smoke less and been subject to less stress, then the position could well soon be reversed. There is already evidence that women are drinking and smoking more and becoming more involved in stressful occupations.[14] More women are also becoming drivers with the subsequent dangers of death and accidents. Another factor that can alter the balance is if large numbers of either sex emigrate or are killed. One reason why there are so many more women among the elderly now is the death of so many men in the First World War. If there are no more such events that remove men prematurely, then the sexes may be much more evenly balanced in the future. It is interesting that in all the age groups under 44 in 1981 there were more males than females [doc 4]. A similar pattern is forecast until the end of the century [doc 4].

Of all those over pensionable age at the beginning of the century approximately two-thirds were women. The proportion is the same now. It is in the older age groups that the gap has widened in 1981. One hundred thousand men were 85 or over and 0.5 million women. In 2001 it is forecast that the proportion will be back to 1:3, that is, there will be 0.2 million men over 85 and 0.6 million women [doc 4].

In the foreseeable future women will still heavily outnumber men among the elderly. The significance of this is that women are more likely to be physically disabled and to suffer from ailments such as arthritis. A higher percentage of elderly women than elderly men are permanently bedfast or housebound.[15]

THE ELDERLY WHO LIVE ALONE

Another striking feature of recent years has been the growing number of elderly people living alone.

In 1961 7 per cent of the households were made up of one person over retirement age while in 1981 this figure had risen to 15 per cent.[16] The trend towards smaller households seems likely to continue and the biggest probable rise appears likely among the elderly. 'The number of one person households is projected to be between 4.7 and 5.2 million by 1991 (implying a possible rise from 27 to 30 per cent of all households in 15 years) of which over 3 million will be elderly people.[17]

Turning now to the type of household where the elderly live, 45 per cent of elderly women and 17 per cent of elderly men in private households in 1981 lived alone.[18]

The number of elderly people living alone could be hailed as an advance for social policy in that they are being kept in their own homes and not being forced to live either with relatives or in residential care. There is, indeed, a good deal of evidence from surveys of the elderly that this is what they want. On the other hand, this fact has implications in regard to the provision of services. For example an old person may find it difficult to summon help in an emergency.

CONCLUSION

The elderly have almost quadrupled in number since the beginning of the century, and while in 1901 they represented 6 per cent of the population, by 1977 this figure had grown to 18 per cent. However, future projections suggest that total numbers will remain approximately the same and so will the proportion of the elderly in the population. The percentage of the population who are dependants (elderly and school-children) has remained constant at about 40 per cent and it is forecast that there will be little alteration in the future. The most striking change in the future will be the rise in the number of people over 75 and the decline in the young elderly until the end of the century when numbers will stabilise.

Women in this age group outnumber men by two to one and will continue to do so. Another trend which is likely to continue is the increase in the number of elderly people living alone.

There are still some unanswered questions about the elderly. What, for example, will be the position of the elderly in the ethnic minorities? They are few in number at the present, but in the future planning of social services their needs will have to be taken into account. It is already established that, particularly for first-generation immigrants, these needs may be somewhat different (e.g. health) from those of people who have been born here.[19] These differences may continue into old age. What will happen, for example, to women who do not speak English? Will they remain in their homes cared for by sons and daughters? Will they want sheltered housing or residential care? This may, however, be a transitory problem if an increasing number from the ethnic minorities are born and brought up in this country rather than coming in as immigrants.

It is equally difficult to forecast what medical advances there may be which will enable people to live longer or help them to be less disabled. On the other hand there may be a swing in public opinion against positive medical intervention to help keep the elderly alive.

DEMOGRAPHIC POSTSCRIPT

Long-term population projections relating to Great Britain were produced by OPCS in March 1983.[20] These showed a slow increase in the total population from the census figure of 54.7 millions in 1981 to 58.5 millions in 2051. Of the projected increase of 4 millions about half is accounted for by an increase in people aged 45 to pensionable age and half by those aged 75 and over (numbers of those of pensionable age to 74 remain constant at 6.6 million). The figures mean that elderly people as a percentage of the population will rise from 18 per cent to 21 per cent and that those aged 75 and over as a percentage of all elderly people will rise from 32 per cent to 45 per cent by 2051. This formidable projected increase of the over-75s from 3.2 million in 1981 to 5.4 million in 2051 will represent a considerable challenge in the next century.

The *1981 Census* showed no trend towards more elderly people living in institutions. In 1981 96.5 per cent of people of pensionable age lived in private households.[21] The tendency is for a growing proportion to live alone. In 1982 the proportion of households consisting of one adult aged 60 or more was 16 per cent compared with 12 per cent in 1971.[22] What is particularly significant is the link between growing older and living alone. In 1982 15 per cent of those aged 60–64, 23 per cent aged 65–69, 34 per cent aged 70–74, 40 per cent of those aged 75–79 and 51 per cent of those aged 80 and over, lived alone.[23]

REFERENCES

1. ROBERTS, N., *Our Future Selves*, Allen and Unwin, 1970.
2. HODKINSON, H. M., *An Outline of Geriatrics*, Academic Press, 1975.
3. HUNT, A., *The Elderly at Home*, OPCS, Social Survey Division, HMSO, 1978.
4. ABRAMS, M., *Beyond Three Score and Ten*, Age Concern, 1978.
5. ROBB, B., *Sans Everything*, Nelson, 1967.
6. HOOKER, S., *Caring for Elderly People*, Routledge and Kegan Paul, 1976.
7. KEDDIE, K. M. G., *Action with the Elderly*. A Handbook for Relatives and Friends, Pergamon, 1978.
8. *Ibid.*, p. 64.
9. HODKINSON, *op. cit.*, p. 19.
10. ELDER, G., *The Alienated*, Writers and Readers Publishing Co-operative, 1977.
11. CPRS, *Population and the Social Services*, HMSO, 1977, p. 9.
12. CSO, *Social Trends* (No. 13), HMSO, 1982, p. 91.
13. OPCS, *Demographic Review*, HMSO, 1977, p. 91.
14. DHSS, *Prevention and Health: everybody's business*, HMSO, 1979, pp. 38–9.
15. CSO, *Social Trends* (No. 9), HMSO, 1979, p. 65.
16. CSO, 1982, *op. cit.*, p. 24.

The elderly in modern society

17. CSO, 1979, *op. cit.*, p. 44.
18. CSO, 1982, *op. cit.*, p. 25.
19. DHSS, *op. cit.*, p. 36.
20. OPCS, *Monitor PP2 83/1*, 1983.
21. OPCS, Census, 1981, *Persons of Pensionable Age*, HMSO, 1983, p. 31.
22. OPCS, Monitor, 83/2, *General Household Survey*, 1982, OPCS, 1983.
23. *Ibid.*

Chapter three
GENERAL REVIEW OF THE LITERATURE

INTRODUCTION

It is remarkable that although the elderly population more than doubled between 1901 and 1945 very little information was gathered in these years on either the elderly at home or in residential care. 'A dearth of published information and, apparently of interest too' is how Townsend and Wedderburn described the situation [doc 7].

To obtain a complete picture of what has been written about the elderly one must search a number of different sources. The medical profession, sociologists, psychologists, geographers, social workers and many others have looked at this group from their own different viewpoints. Similarly, research has been undertaken by a variety of bodies: central government, local authorities, voluntary societies and political parties as well as by individuals.

SOCIAL SURVEYS

One of the first large-scale social surveys was undertaken in 1944–46 for the Rowntree Committee on the *Problems of Ageing and the Care of Old People* and published in 1947. As this was a pioneering study the terms of reference to the report are given [doc 8]. Details of this survey and others carried out between 1945 and 1964 are also given [doc 9]. This list of social surveys has been updated by the author.

A high proportion of the surveys carried out in the 1940s and early 1950s was concerned with the medical aspects of ageing, although some, such as that by Walker,[1] and Sheldon,[2] while starting from a medical viewpoint, went on to consider further issues. Others were restricted in geographical scope.

The social surveys of the late 1950s, the 1960s and the 1970s were concerned in the main first with the relationship between need and provision, and secondly with the importance of taking into account informal networks (particularly the family) as well as the statutory provision.

In the 1950s and 1960s a growing number of studies, such as Bracey's *In Retirement* in 1966, began to look in a more open way at questions connected with retirement and suggested that more thought should be given both by society and the individual to where and how the elderly might live.[3] At the same time sociological studies were throwing new light on the place of the elderly in the family. One of the earliest and most important was Townsend's study of *The Family Life of Old People* in 1957.[4] Although there are certain factors peculiar to Bethnal Green, where the research took place, the findings about the close links between the generations surprised a good many people. Willmott and Young's subsequent study of Woodford, *Family and Class in a London Suburb*, in 1960 was an attempt to compare middle-class families with the working-class ones of Bethnal Green.[5] They found that the ties between relatives were much looser, but nonetheless still quite considerable.

All the research relating to social provision showed that this was not as effective as many had supposed. One of the first, published in 1965, was Townsend and Wedderburn's *The Aged in the Welfare State* which was part of a cross-national survey to find out how effective social services were in meeting the needs of the elderly.[6] The authors set out in particular to discover whether certain functions formerly performed by the family had been taken over by the social services. Their findings did not support this view. The cross-national survey itself, by Shanas *et al.*, *Old People in Three Industrial Societies*, came out in 1968.[7] It was important not just for the information it gave on health, incapacity and so on, but in clarifying and substantiating certain concepts related to the family and to isolation among the elderly. They found, for example, that there is flexibility in the patterns of relationships which exist in families between the generations. Even when families are small, they noted, the elderly will adapt and substitute and can often turn to their siblings or the children of siblings for support.

Tunstall's *Old and Alone* in 1966 was another part of the cross-national survey.[8] As well as his conclusion that social policy must do more to help the aged remain independent, his findings and subsequent discussion about living alone, social isolation and loneliness are as relevant now as when they were published.

A much more general survey was carried out by Harris in 1968 for the Government Social Survey and published as *Social Welfare for the Elderly.*[9] The occasion for this study was the anxiety expressed by the National Corporation for the Care of Old People (NCCOP) at the variations in the local authorities' 10-year community care plans. There seemed some doubt as to whether planning was being based on the *needs* of the elderly or on what the local authorities thought they could afford.

In the 1970s both academic and the more popular literature turned to the particular problems of the very elderly. Two major social surveys were published in 1978 which made some comparisons. Hunt in *The Elderly at Home* surveyed 2,622 elderly people living in private households to provide information on their social circumstances as a base for social policy.[10] Abrams in *Beyond Three Score and Ten* surveyed 1,646 elderly people to discover more about their needs, conditions and resources.[11] Both Hunt and Abrams brought out the differences between the under 75s and those over this age.

MEDICAL AND PSYCHOLOGICAL ASPECTS

It is interesting to note that the medical aspect still continues to take a central place in the literature. Some books, such as *The Social Needs of the Over Eighties* by Brockington and Lempert in 1966,[12] *Survival of the Unfittest* by Isaacs, Livingstone and Neville in 1972,[13] and *An Outline of Geriatrics* by Hodkinson in 1975[14] and *The Care of the Elderly* by Williams in 1979[15] are primarily concerned with the medical aspects but are also highly relevant to other professions. Others, such as *Geriatric Medicine* by Anderson and Judge in 1974[16] have chapters which are concerned with other sides of care of the elderly. More recently the BMA published in 1976 a general book called *Care of the Elderly.*[17]

Books such as that by Cartwright, Hockey and Anderson, *Life Before Death*, while written mainly from a medical angle, are important in enhancing our understanding of a specific period in an old person's life.[18] It is also significant that one of the innovatory pieces of action research into housing and other services for the elderly has a strong medical involvement and is led by a doctor. This is the Health Care Evaluation Research Team in Winchester.

A particular medical problem revealed in this growing collection of written material is that of the elderly mentally disordered. Studies on this subject have been made from different standpoints. Robb's *Sans Everything* in 1967, painted a black picture of conditions in psychiatric hospitals.[19] It attracted a lot of publicity although many of the allegations were found not proved by an official investigation.

Meacher's *Taken for a Ride* in 1972 was also a description of institutions for the elderly mentally infirm.[20] After interviews with 329 old people Meacher raised fundamental questions about the nature of 'confusion' and discussed the case for separatist homes and a policy of community care based on integration. The problems which this group pose have also been the subject of reports by groups such as MIND.

Much more attention is being paid to the psychological aspects of ageing with books by Birren in 1964,[21] Comfort in 1965,[22] Bromley in 1966[23] and de Beauvoir in 1972.[24] More recently Comfort popularised his book *A Good Age* [doc 10] in the *Sunday Times* Colour Supplement. This popularisation is an indication of the growing public interest in the subject of the elderly.

INDIVIDUAL SERVICES

There is an increasing amount of specialist literature on particular services. Much of this will be referred to later. Research on some services such as housing is well established. Information and interest in some others have been slower to develop. For example literature on education and leisure in retirement, such as Groombridge pioneered in 1960 is relatively new.[25] So are studies of particular groups such as the elderly with hypothermia which was the subject of Wicks' *Old and Cold* in 1978,[26] and, in a book with that title, those *Found Dead* by Bradshaw, Clifton and Kennedy in 1978.[27]

Similarly, professionals are beginning to consider their role in relation to the elderly. Goldberg in a widely acclaimed study, *Helping the Aged*, in 1970 attempted to measure through an experiment the effect of social work intervention.[28] Brearley in 1975 in *Social Work, Ageing and Society* approached the subject from a more general perspective.[29] He considered both the normality and individual aspects of ageing and how such an understanding could help social workers in their relations with the elderly.

The Open University has also played a role in helping to alert professionals to the growing numbers of elderly people. Their course 'An Ageing Population' was accompanied by a television series and a number of course books in 1978 including Carver and Liddiard's *An Ageing Population*[30] and Pruner's *To the Good Long Life*.[31]

INTERDISCIPLINARY APPROACH

An interdisciplinary approach to questions concerned with the elderly is beginning to develop [doc 11]. The British Council for Ageing was one body formed to encourage this approach. Their report *Research in Gerontology* on the prospects and problems for research brings together useful information.[32] The British Association for the Advancement of Science held a symposium in 1976 on *Old Age– today and tomorrow* and followed this with a report with that title.[33] And Hobman in *The Social Challenge of Ageing* has edited a collection of essays written from different perspectives including education, health and architecture.[34]

LOCAL STUDIES

Recently there has been a spate of reports on individual local areas. A limited number of these have appeared in the past often produced by academics (e.g. Shenfield[35]) but sometimes by local authorities. Many of the recent reports have come from social service departments. East Sussex County Council, for example, has had a prolific output of well-researched papers on the elderly. Some reports are by housing departments while a growing number come from joint planning groups often involving housing and social service departments and health authorities. Some of the local studies such as Watson and Albrow's 1973 study, *The Needs of Old People in Glamorgan*, have been used centrally to draw more general conclusions (e.g. Department of Health and Social Security (DHSS) in 1976, *The Elderly and Personal Social Services*).[36]

PRACTICAL ADVICE

Another noticeable feature of the literature of the last 10 years has been the growing number of books offering practical advice either to the elderly themselves or to their relatives and friends. The Consumers Association published *Arrangements for Old Age* in 1969,[37] and in 1977 *Where to Live After Retirement*.[38] Brandon compiled a handbook *Seventy Plus: easier living for the elderly* in 1972 with chapters on living options, keeping fit, aids and safety in the home and finance.[39]

There has also been a steady stream recently of popular books about retirement. *Thinking about Retirement* by Wallis in 1975 was one.[40] Hooker in 1976 in *Caring for Elderly People* wrote as a physiotherapist about how to understand this group and the practical help that can be given.[41] Keddie in 1978 in *Action with the Elderly* describes his book as 'A Handbook for Relatives and

Friends'.[42] As well as advice on health and a special section on the mentally disordered there is a visitor's charter. Hardie in 1978 in *Understanding Ageing* wrote about facing common family problems from a practical point of view.[43]

THE VIEWS OF POLITICAL AND VOLUNTARY AGENCIES

Some interesting studies, which have probably reached a wider audience than many of the weightier academic works, have been produced by the Fabian Society, the Bow Group and the Conservative Political Centre. Four of the major ones concerned with the elderly are *Old People in Britain*,[44] *Old People: cash and care*,[45] *The Care of the Old*[46] and *New Deal for the Elderly*.[47] These attracted a good deal of publicity and may possibly have more influence on the political parties, and therefore on social policy, than some of the more theoretical approaches.

Similarly, some of the research undertaken by voluntary bodies like Age Concern has great relevance. Their Manifesto Series published in 1974 comprises excellent short accounts by experts of particular problems. Particularly interesting when considering the sort of policies which are likely to find favour with the elderly was a study of the attitudes of 2,700 pensioners.[48] A most useful series, *Profiles of the Elderly*, has now been published which brings together existing evidence on particular topics.[49] Those published so far are about general aspects, such as standards of living and health, accidents and mobility.

Help the Aged and CPA have also produced helpful publications and sometimes sponsored research.

INTERNATIONAL STUDIES

It is beyond the scope of this book to do more than make brief mention of studies of the elderly made abroad. Those who want to pursue comparative studies will find that publications of the United Nations often contain relevant data. For example, those interested in exploring housing and ways of preserving or encouraging family links can read the report of a *European Seminar on Social Aspects of Housing*[50] which contains a discussion about movement to new areas. Another comparative study was *Housing the Aged in Western Countries* by Beyer and Nierstrasz.[51] This showed that many elderly persons were taking up hospital beds and rooms needed by others in nursing homes or residential homes because there was no one to take care of them at home. The authors felt that earlier retirement and the break-up of the extended family had exacerbated the problem.

Some argue that the growing interest shown by other countries does not seem to be matched by a similar degree of interest in this country. Hobman has compared the wide output and interest abroad with that of the few inspired people here.

CURRENT LITERATURE AND RESEARCH AND SOME GAPS

One reason for this book is the lack of a general book about the elderly written from a social point of view. There are some exceptions, but none approaches the subject in the same way. Sumner and Smith's *Planning Local Authority Services for the Elderly* in 1969 was a case study of 41 housing authorities and 24 health and welfare authorities.[52] Bosanquet's *A Future for Old Age* in 1978 is not primarily a research study.[53] It analyses some policy issues and suggests some basic changes.

An excellent handbook of current research is provided by *Old Age: a register of social research* published by the NCCOP.[54] This is updated each year. An interesting analysis by Abrams of the research in progress in 1977 was published in a paper *The Elderly: an overview of current British social research*.[55] This includes an analysis of subject areas, funding, aims, methods and problems. A similar analysis for research in 1978 by Taylor is in the Introduction to the NCCOP 1978 *Register*. A bibliography of research into the elderly in 1978 has been compiled by Norris.[56]

Some aspects of the elderly seem very under-researched and the literature about them noticeably sparse. One of these is the economic aspect, particularly the costing of alternative types of provision. Wager in 1972 produced an innovatory exercise in cost benefits, *Care of the Elderly*,[57] and Davies *et al.* have also written on the subject in *Variations in Services for the Aged*.[58] There has also been some research at the Institute of Economic and Social Research in the University of York concerned with costing alternative patterns of care.

There is also a striking gap in research which sets out to collect information about individuals over a period of years. Abrams identified this as one of the neglected areas.[59] Another matter which has so far been little touched on is what the elderly themselves wish. Elder in *The Alienated* explains very vividly some of the reasons why many members of her generation feel as they do.[60] The media have made some attempt to present the views of the elderly. Television programmes like *What Shall We Do With Granny?* evoked intense controversy. The semi-educational series *The 60, 70, 80 Show*, which started in 1975 on BBC television, also attempted to discuss many issues with the elderly themselves.

The importance of the elderly speaking for themselves was recognised by the DHSS in 1978 when they produced their Discussion Document, *A Happier Old Age*. They specifically asked that the elderly should make their views known.[61]

REFERENCES

1. WALKER, K., *Commentary on Age*, J. Cape, 1952.
2. SHELDON, J. H., *The Social Medicine of Old Age*, Nuffield Foundation, 1948.
3. BRACEY, H. E., *In Retirement*, Routledge and Kegan Paul, 1966.
4. TOWNSEND, P., *The Family Life of Old People*, Routledge and Kegan Paul, 1957, Penguin, 1963.
5. WILLMOTT, P. and YOUNG, M., *Family and Class in a London Suburb*, Routledge and Kegan Paul, 1960.
6. TOWNSEND, P. and WEDDERBURN, D., *The Aged in the Welfare State*, G. Bell and Sons, 1965.
7. SHANAS, E., TOWNSEND, P., WEDDERBURN, D., HENNING, F., MILHØF, P. and STEHOUWER, J., *Old People in Three Industrial Societies*, Routledge and Kegan Paul, 1968.
8. TUNSTALL, J., *Old and Alone*, Routledge and Kegan Paul, 1966.
9. HARRIS, A., *Social Welfare for the Elderly*, Government Social Survey, HMSO, 1968.
10. HUNT, see Ch. 2 note 3.
11. ABRAMS, see Ch. 2 note 4.
12. BROCKINGTON, F. and LEMPERT, S. M., *The Social Needs of the Over Eighties*, Manchester University Press, 1966.
13. ISAACS, B., LIVINGSTONE, M. and NEVILLE, Y., *Survival of the Unfittest*, Routledge and Kegan Paul, 1972.
14. HODKINSON, see Ch. 2 note 2.
15. WILLIAMS, I., *The Care of the Elderly in the Community*, Croom Helm, 1979.
16. ANDERSON, W. FERGUSON (ed.) and JUDGE, T. G., *Geriatric Medicine*, Academic Press, 1974.
17. BRITISH MEDICAL ASSOCIATION, *Care of the Elderly*, BMA, 1976.
18. CARTWRIGHT, A., HOCKEY, L. and ANDERSON, J., *Life Before*

Death, Routledge and Kegan Paul, 1973.

19. ROBB, see Ch. 2 note 5.
20. MEACHER, M., *Taken for a Ride*, Longman, 1972.
21. BIRREN, J. E., *Psychology of Ageing*, Prentice-Hall, 1964.
22. COMFORT, A., *The Process of Ageing*, Weidenfeld and Nicolson, 1965.
23. BROMLEY, D. B., *Psychology of Human Ageing*, Penguin, 1966.
24. DE BEAUVOIR, S., *Old Age*, Penguin, 1972.
25. GROOMBRIDGE, B., *Education and Retirement*, National Institute of Adult Education, 1960.
26. WICKS, M., *Old and Cold*, Heinemann, 1978.
27. BRADSHAW, J., CLIFTON, M. and KENNEDY, J., *Found Dead*, Age Concern, 1978.
28. GOLDBERG, E. M., *Helping the Aged: a field experiment in social work*, Allen and Unwin, 1970.
29. BREARLEY, C. P., *Social Work, Ageing and Society*, Routledge and Kegan Paul, 1975.
30. CARVER, V. and LIDDIARD, P. (ed.), *An Ageing Population – a reader and sourcebook*, Hodder and Stoughton, in association with the Open University Press, 1978.
31. PRUNER, M., *To the Good Long Life*, Macmillan, 1978.
32. BRITISH COUNCIL FOR AGEING, *Research in Gerontology*, Bedford Square Press, 1976.
33. BRITISH ASSOCIATION FOR THE ADVANCEMENT OF SCIENCE, *Old Age – today and tomorrow*, British Association for the Advancement of Science, 1976.
34. HOBMAN, D., *The Social Challenge of Ageing*, Croom Helm, 1978.
35. SHENFIELD, B. E., *Social Policies for Old Age*, Routledge and Kegan Paul, 1957.
36. DHSS, *The Elderly and the Personal Social Services*, HMSO, 1973.
37. CONSUMERS ASSOCIATION, *Arrangements for Old Age*, Consumers Association, 1969.
38. CONSUMERS ASSOCIATION, *Where to Live After Retirement*, Consumers Association, 1977.
39. BRANDON, R., *Seventy Plus: easier living for the elderly*, BBC, 1972.
40. WALLIS, J. H., *Thinking about Retirement*, Pergamon Press, 1975.
41. HOOKER, see Ch. 2 note 6.

42. KEDDIE, see Ch. 2 note 7.
43. HARDIE, M., *Understanding Ageing*, Hodder and Stoughton, 1978.
44. WESTON, T., and ASHWORTH, P., *Old People in Britain*, Bow Group, 1963.
45. BELLAIRS, C., *Old People: cash and care*, Conservative Political Centre, 1968.
46. AGATE, J. and MEACHER, M., *The Care of the Old*, Fabian Research Series 278, Fabian Society, 1969.
47. BOSANQUET, N., *New Deal for the Elderly*, Fabian Tract 435, Fabian Society, 1975.
48. AGE CONCERN, *The Attitudes of the Retired and Elderly*, Age Concern, 1974.
49. AGE CONCERN, *Profiles of the Elderly*, Vols. 1–3, 1977. Vol. 4, 1978, Age Concern.
50. UNITED NATIONS, *European Seminar on Social Aspects of Housing*, United Nations, Geneva, 1960.
51. BEYER, GLENN H. and NIERSTRASZ, F. H. J., *Housing the Aged in Western Countries*, Elsevier, 1967.
52. SUMNER, G. and SMITH, R., *Planning Local Authority Services for the Elderly*, Allen and Unwin, 1969.
53. BOSANQUET, N., *A Future for Old Age*, Temple Smith and New Society, 1978.
54. TODD, H., (ed) *Old Age: a register of social research, 1980–81*, CPA, 1981.
55. ABRAMS, M., *The Elderly: an overview of current British social research*, NCCOP and Age Concern, 1978.
56. NORRIS, M. E., *An Annotated Bibliography of Research into the Elderly*, Tavistock Institute for Operational Research, 1978.
57. WAGER, R., *Care of the Elderly*. An exercise in cost benefit analysis, Institute of Municipal Treasurers and Accountants, 1972.
58. DAVIES, B., BARTON, A. MCMILLAN, I. and WILLIAMSON, V., *Variations in Services for the Aged*, G. Bell and Sons, 1971.
59. ABRAMS, *op. cit.*
60. ELDER, see Ch. 2 note 10.
61. DHSS, *A Happier Old Age*, A Discussion Document, HMSO, 1978.

Part two
NEEDS AND HOW THEY ARE MET

A CRITICAL NARRATIVE OF THE MAIN
DEVELOPMENTS IN SOCIAL SERVICES

It is easy to rationalise when looking back at social provision for any group of people and to see a pattern in what has happened. In practice the directions taken by social policy are often in response to all kinds of events and personalities. A crisis, war, the action of a pressure group or the influence of a dominant person may all change policy, as will the overall political philosophy of a political party.

Policies for the elderly, as for other groups, have evolved as a result of many different factors. Some of these directions will be explored briefly in this chapter to provide a framework for a more detailed account of individual services later.

THE GROWTH IN SERVICES

Greater concern

The needs of the elderly have traditionally in this country been the concern both of central and local government and of voluntary agencies. All of these have paid increasing attention to how appropriate policies and administrative structures may be developed.

Setting up a Royal Commission or a committee to investigate a topic is one conventional way of showing concern. It is interesting that one of the first, which reported in 1895, was the Royal Commission on the Aged Poor. This provided evidence about the poor conditions in which many old people existed. In 1909 both the majority and the minority reports of the Royal Commission on the Poor Laws painted a bleak picture of life for the elderly. Townsend has commented: 'Both reports recommended improvements in institutional conditions and an extension of separate provision for the old, but little was done for many years to carry out these recommendations.'[1] He went on to argue that as far as the infirm aged and chronic sick were concerned far less information on these persons was made available to the public between 1910 and 1946 than was available between 1834 and 1909. No official inquiries were instituted and hardly any books or pamphlets were published which contained more than a few fleeting references to their circumstances or their needs. He believed that the reason for this was the low priority that the welfare of the aged had in British society. It is pertinent that an official publication maintains that provision for the elderly is largely based on legislation passed since 1945.[2]

Since 1945 many important commissions and committees have paid particular attention to the elderly. Three of these were the Guillebaud Report on the cost of the National Health Service (NHS),[3] the Cullingworth Report on council housing[4] and the Seebohm Report on personal and allied social services.[5]

An indicator of present concern is the publication by the DHSS in 1978 of a Discussion Document, *A Happier Old Age*.[6] A White Paper was planned to follow this. Concern at a national level has been matched locally by the blossoming of working parties and groups attempting to work out local patterns of services.

The last 40 years has also seen the birth of major voluntary organisations such as CPA (formerly NCCOP formed in 1947), Age Concern (which started as the National Old People's Welfare Council in 1940 and became Age Concern in 1971) and Help the Aged (which started in 1962). As well as acting as pressure groups these organisations undertake research on behalf of the elderly and are regularly consulted by official bodies.

The development of research

In the review of the literature (Ch. 3) it was noted that increasing attention has been paid to finding out the facts about the elderly. This has taken the form of social surveys, medical enquiries and sociological studies which have often attempted to measure need and provision.

It is worth remembering that increased provision has been accompanied by a more satisfactory data base on which to base policies. But there are still many gaps in our knowledge and as a report from the United Nations put it: 'However, there is no general theory or unified body of knowledge on ageing.'[7]

Much of the research has been very specific and has concentrated on particular groups of old people. For example Townsend wrote about those in residential institutions and homes in *The Last Refuge*,[8]

Bradshaw, Clifton and Kennedy about those *Found Dead*[9] and Wicks in *Old and Cold*[10] about elderly people with hypothermia. Others have chosen to look at recipients of particular services such as home helps (Hunt[11]), telephones (Gregory[12]) and housing (Page and Muir[13]).

Major national surveys sponsored by the government since 1945 have included the Phillips Report on *The Economic and Financial Problems of the Provision for Old Age*,[14] the Boucher Report on *Services Available to the Chronic Sick and Elderly 1954–55*,[15] the Ministry of Pensions and National Insurance (MPNI) Report, *Financial and Other Circumstances of Retirement Pensioners*,[16] Harris, *Social Welfare for the Elderly*,[17] Harris, *Handicapped and Impaired in Great Britain*,[18] DHSS, *A Nutrition Survey of the Elderly*,[19] Hunt, *The Elderly at Home*[20] and a number of surveys undertaken by the Ministry of Housing and Local Government (MHLG) and the Department of the Environment (DOE) of the housing conditions of the elderly.

Widening scope and changes in organisation

At the beginning of the century there was little provision for the elderly apart from the Poor Law, charities and almshouses. Since then the state has played a major role at a national level, particularly in the provision of pensions and health services. At a local level authorities have taken on wide responsibilities for housing and a range of domiciliary services to keep people in their own homes. This is all part of the change from concern in the last century with the environment, through public health and sanitation measures, to concern in this century with individuals and groups.

At a national level Looking back on provision this century there are some notable landmarks. Centrally one of the most important Acts was the 1908 Old Age Pension Act. This was an attempt to make some provision for elderly people outside the Poor Law. It gave the elderly over 70 a small non-contributory pension but applicants had to undergo a means test, and to begin with, provide evidence that they were of good character. Better provision was made in 1925 under the Widows, Orphans and Old Age Contributory Pensions Act. During the Second World War the Unemployment Assistance Board took over the Poor Law responsibility for outdoor relief of the elderly. The Beveridge Report in 1942 recommended [doc 12] that the elderly, and other groups, should be covered by an insurance scheme while an assistance board should provide for those who were not covered. However, after the war pensions were provided on a universal scale (with certain exceptions) out of general taxation, but amounts were not high enough to prevent many having to apply for extra means-tested assistance. Since 1945 a series of Acts have extended pensions to nearly all elderly people. In 1961 graduated pensions were introduced and since 1975 pensions have been earnings related. These measures have enabled the elderly to be financially independent and, in particular, not to be dependent on their children. However, large numbers have had to have their pensions augmented by the DHSS through a supplementary pension (see Ch. 5).

Under the National Health Service Act 1946 a comprehensive health service was set up for everyone regardless of means. The object was to promote the establishment of a comprehensive health service designed to secure improvements in the physical and mental health of the people of England and Wales and the prevention, diagnosis and treatment of illness, and for that purpose, to provide or secure the effective provision of services. This service has been largely free of charge for those in medical need, and even where charges have been made (e.g. prescriptions) pensioners have been exempt. It has enabled the elderly to be spared the kind of indignities remembered by Elder where 'doctors' bills had to be avoided'.[21] There were three main divisions after 1946: the hospital and specialist services administered through regional hospital boards, the general practitioner services administered by local executive councils and the local authority services (such as home nursing and domestic help) administered by the major local authorities. The NHS was reorganised in 1974 – Fig. 4 (p. 70) – with the intention that expertise in health care should be concentrated in the NHS and expertise in social work in social services departments.

At a local level   For local services the Local Government Act 1929 was a milestone because it transferred the powers and duties of the Poor Law Guardians to the county councils and county boroughs. They took over some of the Poor Law institutions and ran them as hospitals. Those that were left were managed by the public assistance committees of the local councils. Conditions in both types of institution, however, remained poor.[22]

The development of local services after 1945 is referred to in Chapter 8, but 1946, 1948, 1962 and 1968 were important dates when the powers of local authorities were extended.

In any discussion about local services for the elderly the effect of local government reorganisation must be taken into account. Many attempts were made from 1945 onwards to change the structure for a number of reasons. Some local authorities were thought to be too small, some boundaries seemed meaningless and the division of responsibility between different types of authority hindered the provision of effective services. Under the Local Government Act 1972 the old all-purpose county boroughs disappeared and the picture as far as the main services for the elderly are concerned became as shown in Fig. 3.

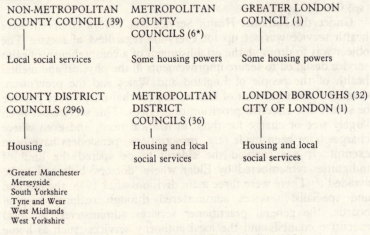

NON-METROPOLITAN COUNTY COUNCIL (39)	METROPOLITAN COUNTY COUNCILS (6*)	GREATER LONDON COUNCIL (1)
Local social services	Some housing powers	Some housing powers
COUNTY DISTRICT COUNCILS (296)	METROPOLITAN DISTRICT COUNCILS (36)	LONDON BOROUGHS (32) CITY OF LONDON (1)
Housing	Housing and local social services	Housing and local social services

*Greater Manchester
Merseyside
South Yorkshire
Tyne and Wear
West Midlands
West Yorkshire

Fig. 3. Structure of local government in England since 1974: responsibility for housing and social services.

At the same time two other changes have occurred that have affected local provision. Following the reorganisation of local government the NHS, as already mentioned, was also reorganised. Some services were taken over by the NHS (such as home nursing) and others, formerly under the NHS (such as medical social work) were transferred to local authorities. Then in 1970 the Local Authority Social Services Act created social service departments in local authorities, bringing together many functions which had previously been scattered between health, welfare and other departments.

Responsibility for services for the elderly is therefore still split between different agencies with the major division being between

NHS (health) and local authorities (local social services). Outside London and the metropolitan areas different authorities are responsible for housing and social services. It has been argued by some that a more effective service could be provided if only one authority was involved. On the other hand it is maintained that division does not matter as long as there is co-ordination of services.

Services for the elderly have expanded greatly, particularly since 1945. Some, such as holidays, telephones and free transport, were scarcely thought of as public services even 20 years ago. But it is possible that the cost of these services combined with the belief of some that the state should play a smaller role may restrict any large-scale future expansion.

By voluntary bodies   Voluntary bodies have pioneered provision for the elderly. Almshouses, charities and trusts to help the elderly date back at least as far as the Middle Ages. Old people's homes, financial help and the provision of meals are all examples of this.

Local authorities sometimes use voluntary bodies instead of making direct provision themselves. Under the National Assistance Act 1948, for instance, a local authority may use accommodation such as a hostel provided by a voluntary body and make payment for it. They may also contribute to the funds of a voluntary body that provides recreation or meals for the elderly.

SOME CHANGES IN THE NATURE OF SERVICES

Greater entitlement as of right

Some of the services for the elderly such as pensions and health are provided as of right. There is no question of pensions or access to a general practitioner (GP) being restricted to a limited number of people. Every old person (with a few exceptions in the case of pensions) has a right to these national services. The same is true in some areas of some local services such as bus passes for free travel.

Eyden in *The Welfare Society* distinguished between three main types of service.[23] Firstly, services which are financed wholly or mainly out of general taxation and are used at will without any test of contribution (e.g. health). Secondly, services framed on a contractual basis with entitlement to benefit being dependent on being within the scope of a particular scheme and satisfying its relevant contribution test (e.g. pensions). Thirdly, services where there is a needs test (e.g. local authority housing).

This provision for everyone in a particular age category (regardless of means) is part of a general change in outlook. In the last century social services were largely looked on as being for second-class citizens on the fringes of society. But even before the First World War, social services were beginning to be regarded not as a form of charity, but rather as one of the rights available to citizens as were services for defence, justice, law and order. During the Second World War the feeling grew that society was not automatically divided into the rich and the poor or givers and receivers. A neat summary of the effect of the war is given in DHSS, *Collaboration in Community Care*: 'The effects of the war were threefold. First, a degree of physical fitness was required in the entire population. Second, the war had an equalising effect on all classes in society which made selective provision of services less acceptable. Third, the cause of social problems, such as unemployment or handicap, was no longer seen to be the individual fault but to lie in the social context.'[24] But among some of the elderly themselves the idea that social services are a form of charity dies hard and is one of the reasons why some seem reluctant to claim benefits to which they are entitled.

Some services are provided on a selective basis – that is certain criteria are laid down and people are invited to apply. Services provided in this way include meals on wheels, chiropody and aids and adaptations to houses. The arguments in favour of this sort of approach are that it ensures that those with specific needs have them met, that scarce resources can be rationed and that services are not 'wasted'. Against this it is held that there may be a low take-up if it is left to individuals to apply, there may be a stigma attached if only a few people receive the service and that such schemes are expensive to administer.

Moves to prevention

Those responsible for many services, for the elderly as well as for other groups, are attempting to move away from the sort of provision which aims to solve particular problems, i.e. is crisis centred, and goes no further.

This is specially noticeable in medicine where people are being persuaded not to drink or smoke and to take greater care on the roads. This approach is in contrast to the provision of a health service which picks up the casualties after the damage has been done. Thus, it can be argued that chiropody and greater attention to the care of the feet may prevent elderly people becoming house-bound. In DHSS, *Prevention and Health: everybody's business* it is stated that, 'Prevention is the key to healthier living and a higher quality of life for all of us',[25] and ways are outlined [doc 13] related to the elderly. The question that has to be asked is what is the object of prevention? Not the avoidance of death, because this is inevitable. One answer is that it may be possible if certain measures are taken early enough to prevent them going into expensive forms of care. It is also held that preventing an accident or entry to institutional care saves money and human suffering. This point will be taken up in Chapter 13 under Priorities.

In social work, too, the tendency has been to try to work with people before a crisis develops, although staff shortages may make this difficult. Leonard in an article in *Social Work Today* (3.6.71) suggests that: 'Primary intervention which concentrates on identifying the pre-conditions of social problems and acting to remedy them, is now seen as a potential further field for social work not only in the form of community work and social policy and planning but as one to which social workers in general can contribute even though they work mainly at other levels of intervention.'

COMMUNITY CARE

A number of factors have combined to shift the emphasis in policy away from institutional care to what is loosely called care in the community. This shift and the reasons for it are not confined to the elderly but apply also to other groups such as children, offenders and the mentally disordered.

There seems to be a lack of satisfactory definition of community care and some confusion as to its meaning. This may be partly because a number of different theories and facts came together at roughly the same time. Firstly, there was the general reaction against institutional care which led to the belief that alternatives ought to be made available for both existing and potential inhabitants of institutions. Secondly, there were practical problems increasingly associated with institutions such as the difficulty of getting residential staff. Thirdly, there was less need to keep some people (including the elderly) in an institution away from society because much behaviour that was disturbed or bizarre could be controlled by drugs and other methods. Fourthly, there was the cost of institutional care. Finally, there was a growing recognition that people had a right, where possible, to live among ordinary people in society and not to be in a separate institution. The institution was seen as a barrier to normal living.

In short, for both positive and negative reasons the fashionable swing towards attempting to look after people within society (or the community as it was usually put) snowballed. There can be scarcely a group of people now who do not have some form of 'community' service whether it is community (children's) homes, community health councils or (offenders') community service.

In the past it seems that community care has meant very much what people have wanted it to mean. There are two extremes of meaning. There is the narrow definition of community care as the provision of domiciliary rather than institutional services and there is the ill-defined cosy picture of a group of local people 'caring' for their neighbours.

The official view for a long time was nearer to the first description and has correlated the concept with the provision of services by local authorities. The Ministry of Health (MOH) 1962 *Hospital Plan*, for example, was intended to be complementary to the local services 'for care in the community'. Similarly, when local authorities were asked to produce plans along these lines the title of the official publication was *The Development of Community Care*[26] and so was the revision.[27] The introduction to the 1963 edition states: 'At the reorganisation of 1948, local government, while losing responsibility for any part of the hospital service, retained the environmental services, and took on much wider responsibilities for the prevention of ill-health and for care in the community.' But it went on to include a short section headed 'Voluntary Effort' which was an indication that something other than statutory help could be included in the definition.

A wider definition of community emerges from the Seebohm Report, although even here the official definition was: 'Community care has come to mean treatment and care outside hospitals or residential homes.'[28] It is this concept of community which is so difficult to define and perhaps contributes to the extreme view of a caring group of people given above. As Clegg points out: 'There is no agreed definition of "community" among academic sociologists, social workers or the makers of social policy.'[29] She indicates that the sociological concept relates to 'a small population in a defined geographical area whose social relationships are distinguished by the fact that they share a common culture which has emerged over a long period of time'.

The chapter on The Community in the Seebohm Report starts with the definition of community both in the physical sense of location but also 'the common identity of a group of people'.[30] However, it then goes on to introduce yet another factor. 'The notion of a community implies the existence of a network of reciprocal social relationships which among other things ensure mutual aid and give those who experience it a sense of well-being.'[31] Although official thinking has moved beyond the narrow concept of domiciliary provision there is still need for what Freeman has called in *New Society* (10.4.69) 'a working definition of Community Care' which needs to be spelled out with precision.

It will be suggested in Chapter 12 that any redefinition of community care needs to take into account in a realistic way the role both of the family and of the elderly themselves.

REFERENCES

1. TOWNSEND, P., *The Last Refuge*, Routledge and Kegan Paul, 1964, p. 16.
2. COI, *Care of the Elderly in Britain*, HMSO, 1977, p. 1.
3. MOH, *Report of the Committee of Enquiry into the Cost of the National Health Service*, Cmnd 9663 (the Guillebaud Committee), HMSO, 1956.
4. MHLG, *Council Housing Purposes, Procedures and Priorities*, Report of the Housing Management Sub-Committee of the Central Housing Advisory Committee (the Cullingworth Committee), HMSO, 1969.
5. HOME OFFICE, DES, MHLG and MOH, *The Report of the Committee on Local Authority and Allied Personal Social Services* (the Seebohm Committee), HMSO, 1968.
6. DHSS, *A Happier Old Age*, see Ch. 3 note 61.
7. UNITED NATIONS, *The Ageing: trends and policies*, UN, New York, 1975, p. 7.
8. TOWNSEND, *op. cit.*
9. BRADSHAW, CLIFTON and KENNEDY, see Ch. 3 note 27.
10. WICKS, see Ch. 3 note 26.
11. HUNT, A., assisted by FOX, J., *The Home Help Service in England and Wales*, Government Social Survey, HMSO, 1970.
12. GREGORY, P., *Telephones for the Elderly*, G. Bell and Sons, 1973.
13. PAGE, D. and MUIR, T., *New Housing for the Elderly*, Bedford Square Press, 1971.
14. CHANCELLOR OF THE EXCHEQUER, *Report of the Committee on the Economic and Financial Problems of the Provision for Old Age*, Cmnd 9333, HMSO, 1954.

15. MOH, *Survey of Services Available to the Chronic Sick and Elderly, 1954–55*. Summary report prepared by Boucher, C. A., HMSO, 1957.

16. MPNI, *Financial and Other Circumstances of Retirement Pensioners*, HMSO, 1966.

17. HARRIS, see Ch. 3 note 9.

18. HARRIS, A., *Handicapped and Impaired in Great Britain*, OPCS, Social Survey Division, HMSO, 1971.

19. DHSS, *A Nutrition Survey of the Elderly*, Report by the Panel on Nutrition of the Elderly, HMSO, 1972.

20. HUNT, see Ch. 2 note 3.

21. ELDER, see Ch. 2 note 10, p. 62.

22. TOWNSEND, *op. cit.*, pp. 16–19.

23. EYDEN, J., *The Welfare Society*, Bedford Square Press, 1971, pp. 15–16.

24. DHSS, *Collaboration in Community Care*, A Discussion Document, Central Health Services Council and Personal Social Services Council, HMSO, 1978, p. 4.

25. DHSS, *Prevention and Health*, see Ch. 2 note 14, p. 96.

26. MOH, *Health and Welfare. The Development of Community Care*, Cmnd 1973, HMSO, 1963.

27. MOH, *Health and Welfare. The Development of Community Care*, Cmnd 3022, HMSO, 1966.

28. HOME OFFICE *et al.*, *op. cit.*, p. 107.

29. CLEGG, J., *Dictionary of Social Services*, Bedford Square Press, 1971, p. 16.

30. HOME OFFICE *et al.*, *op. cit.*, p. 147.

31. *Ibid.*, p. 147.

Chapter five
THE FINANCIAL AND EMPLOYMENT POSITION

THE FINANCIAL POSITION

Introduction

Financial security in old age is a fundamental need because few elderly people are able to continue to earn their living. An adequate income may be secured from a number of sources including personal savings, a state pension and a pension from a job. In the past elderly people who could no longer work and had no savings were thrown on the resources of the Poor Law or of their families.

Landmarks in legislation

The development of statutory provision of pensions from 1908 has been outlined in Chapter 4. Some points are elaborated below.

A major initiative was the Committee of Inquiry set up by the government in 1941 and chaired by Sir William Beveridge, to look at the whole system of social security. Its terms of reference were 'to undertake, with special reference to the inter-relation of the schemes, a survey of the existing national schemes of social insurance and allied services, including workmen's compensation and to make recommendations'.[1] The Committee's proposals for pensions must be seen against the background of an overall strategy for a system of insurance covering everyone whatever their income, and for benefits, including pensions, to be paid to everyone who contributed based on a national minimum [doc 14]. Contributions were to be compulsory and benefits universal and not means tested. The responsibility of the state was seen as the provision of a minimum, while voluntary action by people to supplement this was to be encouraged. The monetary benefit was to be seen as only part of 'a comprehensive policy of social progress' which included provision of better services in health, education and housing.

The Beveridge Report was published in 1942 and accepted with one important exception. This was the rejection of the 'national minimum' standard of benefits, which would have meant frequent changes to keep up with the cost of living. Benefits were to be fixed and reviewed at intervals. National insurance became compulsory for everyone of working age except married women. Pensions were to be paid on retirement (65 for men and 60 for women). To encourage people to work beyond this age an addition to the basic rate was given for each year of deferment.

In 1948 the National Assistance Act set up the National Assistance Board (NAB) with a duty to assist persons in need, i.e. 'who are without resources to meet their requirements or whose resources (including benefits receivable under the National Insurance Act 1946) must be supplemented in order to meet their requirements'. For those who were not insured, or who needed additional help, this Act laid down the machinery. It was the last break with the Poor Law [doc 15].

One of the provisions of the National Insurance Act 1957 was to enable retirement and widowed pensioners under the age of 70 (65 for women) to revoke their declaration of retirement if they wished and to earn additions to their retirement pensions to be paid when they ceased working.

A major change of principle was embodied in the National Insurance Act 1966. In order that people might be able to receive a pension more closely related to the level of what they had been earning, as distinct from a basic minimum, a Graduated Pensions Scheme was brought in. Higher pensions were to be payable in return for higher contributions related to higher earnings. Employees might, however, be contracted out if their employers provided a comparable or better occupational scheme. Another change was the granting of a standard addition for supplementary pensioners and some other long-term cases. This was intended to reduce the number of discretionary additions to the weekly rate of benefit and to limit the need to ask detailed questions about special expenses.

In 1966 the NAB was merged with the MPNI to become the Ministry of Social Security, and a semi-autonomous board, the Supplementary Benefits Commission (SBC) (which replaced the NAB) was set up under this Ministry.

The National Insurance Act 1970 provided three new social security cash benefits, one of which was for old people aged 80 or over who were too old to come into the National Insurance Scheme when it began in 1948. About 110,000 old people benefited. The National Insurance Act 1971 authorised a further payment above the normal retirement pension for the over 80s. And the following year a tax-free Christmas bonus for pensioners, and some others, was provided under the Pensioners and Family Income Supplement Payments Act 1972. This bonus has been paid in most subsequent years.

The Social Security Act 1973 provided for all employed people to be covered by a second, and earnings-related, pension on top of the basic state provision. It was thought that most people would come under an occupational scheme but, for those who did not, there was to be a reserve state scheme. The outline of the basic scheme is given in document 16. This Act also gave statutory backing to an annual review of pensions. In 1975 under the Social Security Act 1975 pensions were statutorily linked to the rise in prices or earnings, whichever was greater.

Following the Social Security Act 1975 a new earnings-related pension scheme was introduced in 1978 and contributions to the former Graduated Pension Scheme ceased. One of the main features was that pension rights should be protected during absence from work to look after children, the old or the sick. This will be particularly beneficial to women. There is provision for members of occupational pension schemes to be 'contracted out' of the additional pension of the state scheme by their employers [doc 17].

Some poverty and other studies

A noticeable feature of much research into poverty is how prominent the elderly are. Some of these studies will now be referred to in chronological order.

The studies   As early as 1895 a Royal Commission had investigated 'the Aged Poor' and recommended some alterations to the Poor Law system. Then a notable researcher, Seebohm Rowntree, carried out a survey of poverty in York in 1899 and again in 1936 and 1948. He concluded that the main causes of poverty had been low wages in 1899, unemployment in 1936 and old age in 1948. In 1947 Rowntree chaired a committee on the problems of ageing and the care of old people [doc 8]. One of their main conclusions was that acute poverty had been substantially abolished among the aged and that state

pensions were 'now probably adequate'.[2] They felt that there was
still a considerable measure of austerity, but the flexible administration of the Assistance Board had been successful in adjusting benefits
to need in a humane but not unreasonably extravagant manner. The
year 1953 saw the setting up of an official committee chaired by Sir
Thomas Phillips 'to review the economic and financial problems
involved in providing for old age, having regard to the prospective
increase in the numbers of the aged, and to make recommendations'.[3]
They considered the economic problems to be those resulting from
the need to accumulate or free resources out of which adequate
provision could be made for the old, and the financial problems to be
those arising from the need to transfer to the old the purchasing
power that would give them the appropriate command over those
resources.[4]

In 1962 Cole and Utting in a study, *The Economic Circumstances of
Old People*, noted that all the problems they looked at – loneliness,
ill health and poverty – appeared to be suffered in *extreme* form by
only a relatively small minority.[5] Two periods were examined by
Abel-Smith and Townsend and reported on in *The Poor and the
Poorest*. Comparing 1953–54 and 1960 they found that 7.8 per cent
of people in the United Kingdom (4 million persons) were living
below 'national assistance' level in 1953–54. About half of them were
living in households whose heads were retired. In 1960 they found
that 14.2 per cent of people in the United Kingdom (7.5 million
persons) were living below 'national assistance' level. About 35 per
cent were living in households primarily dependent on pensions.
One of the reasons for the apparent increase from 7.8 to 14.2 per
cent living at this low level appeared to be the relative increase in the
number of old people in the population. Another reason was the
slight relative increase in the number of chronically sick middle-aged
men and the relative increase in the number of large families.
Abel-Smith and Townsend concluded: 'On the whole the data we
have presented contradicts the commonly held view that a trend
towards greater equality has accompanied the trend towards greater
affluence.'[6]

Townsend and Wedderburn in their survey *The Aged in the
Welfare State* in 1962[7] of over 4,000 people, found that in general the
elderly had income levels a half or more below the levels of younger
persons in the population. Few old people had substantial assets and
over one-third were solely dependent on state benefits. About
two-fifths of the men and of the couples and one-tenth of the women
received a pension from their employers, but these were relatively

small. The very old were worse off as a result of inflation and because they were less likely to work.

There was mounting evidence that some old people were living on a smaller income than the scale provided by the NAB. The MPNI, in co-operation with the NAB, carried out an enquiry in 1965 to find out their numbers and the reasons why they did not apply for assistance. The report, *Financial and Other Circumstances of Retirement Pensioners*, was published in 1966.[8]

The enquiry consisted of a survey of nearly 11,000 pensioners and the findings were similar to those of other researchers. Incomes of pensioners were low. Nearly one-half of the men had occupational pensions. The corresponding proportions were one-quarter for single women other than widows, and one-ninth for widows.

Turning to the main purpose of the enquiry it was estimated that rather more than 700,000 pensioner households (about 850,000 pensioners) could have received assistance if they had applied for it.[9] The main reasons why pensioners did not apply for assistance were: lack of knowledge, the dislike of 'charity', a feeling that they were managing all right on what they had and (a small proportion) a dislike of going to the NAB.[10]

The Townsend and Wedderburn survey and that of the MPNI both found that the older the person the smaller the income, that few old people had substantial assets or savings and that single and widowed women were the worst off. In Townsend's 1968–69 national sample, elderly people comprised one-third of those in poverty. One of his findings, reported in *Poverty in the United Kingdom* was that: 'People tend to separate into two groups, one anticipating a comfortable and even early retirement, the other dreading the prospect and depending almost entirely for their livelihood on the resources made available by the State through its social security system.'[11]

The 1976 OPCS survey for DHSS gives further data about the financial position of the elderly.[12] Many of the findings, such as the dependence of the elderly on state benefits and the decline of income with age, were similar to previous surveys. It is interesting, however, that financial difficulties did not figure prominently in the list of things disliked by the elderly, although suggestions about ways in which elderly people could be helped *did* include a number having financial implications [doc 18].

Some definitions The strict definition of poverty as below subsistence level is not the one normally used today. Some researchers have used as a guide supplementary benefit level, which is higher than would be needed for sheer physical survival. Others have claimed that a better yardstick would be a certain percentage above supplementary benefit levels. Thus Abel-Smith and Townsend added 40 per cent, taking into account discretionary payments and statutory disregards.

These differing definitions make strict comparison between the poverty studies difficult. It is generally accepted that any definition must take account of more than just financial matters. Abel-Smith and Townsend considered that income or expenditure should be regarded as only one of a number of indicators of poverty, including differences in home environment, material possessions and educational and occupational resources.[13] Townsend has more recently suggested a definition based on 'relatiye deprivation' – that is 'the absence or inadequacy of those diets, amenities, standards, services and activities which are common or customary in society'.[14]

Studies must also take account of the poverty cycle of people being in poverty as children but out of it when they earn, in again when they have a family but out when the family has grown up, and finally in again when they become pensioners.

The present position

Income and expenditure A retirement pension is payable to people of pensionable age provided that they have paid sufficient national insurance contributions and have retired from regular full-time work. Anyone over 80 who satisfies certain residence conditions is entitled to a non-contributory pension. In 1981 9.1 million elderly people received a pension. A supplementary pension may also be claimed if an elderly person's income does not reach a minimum amount. Additions to the basic supplementary pension may be given and wide-ranging discretionary powers are available to the SBC. These include additions to weekly benefits (exceptional circumstances additions (ECA)) and of single lump-sum payments (exceptional needs payments (ENP)). Examples of ECAs are for heating, special diets and laundry. Examples of ENPs are for furniture, household equipment, repairs and redecoration of accommodation, removal expenses, fares (e.g. to visit relatives in hospital) and funeral expenses.

The main source of income for most elderly people is national insurance and supplementary pensions. The elderly are also more likely than other households to be dependent on social security benefits. This is more pronounced for single women than men, who are more likely to have a pension from an employer and/or an investment income. Some pensioners also have earnings from paid employment, but the proportion who do has declined.

Elderly people have much lower average household incomes (£42.68 per week in 1976) than other households (£82.30 per week in 1976).[15] But a comparison of data from the 1970 and 1976 Family Expenditure Surveys (FES) indicates that their position has improved.[16] In 1970, 56 per cent of elderly households were in the lowest 20 per cent of the distribution of equivalent normal net income. By 1976 this had fallen to 43 per cent.

Pensioners also have a slightly different pattern of expenditure to other households. They spend much more on fuel and light and more on food and housing. They spend less on clothing, footwear and transport.[17]

Personal savings   One way in which people can provide for their old age is through personal savings. The 1965 MPNI survey showed that few old people had much in the way of savings[18] and the position in 1976[19] was very similar. In part this may be due to low levels of wages and unemployment in the past, but in part it may also be due to the effect of inflation which erodes the value of savings. In 1977 most claimants for supplementary pensions had no capital at all and very few had more than £1,249.00, the amount that was at that time totally disregarded in the calculation of weekly benefit.

Index-linked savings bonds recently available to pensioners are a hedge against inflation, but the proportion of pensioners holding them is not high.

Occupational pensions   Many public services and commercial organisations now run occupational pension schemes with pension based on final salary. About half the workforce, 11¾ million people, were covered by such schemes in 1979,[20] but not all the present pensioners, and in particular few women, are covered by this sort of scheme. Nor is the amount very much. In 1979 it averaged £10.00 per week for widows and dependants and £20 for ex-employees.

Other forms of financial help

There are other ways in which financial help is given, apart from pensions, and some of these are listed below.

The elderly in modern society

Help with health charges Pensioners, and others, on supplementary benefit are entitled to help with certain NHS charges. They are eligible for free prescriptions and for remission of charges for glasses, dentures, dental treatment, wigs and fabric supports.

Help with heating costs Housing surveys show that the elderly tend to live in older, poorer accommodation than other households. This means that they will need to spend a higher proportion of their income on fuel than other groups. They are also likely to be at home more than most households and therefore need heat for longer periods. These facts, as well as the great increase in the cost of fuel, have given rise to a widespread concern about the many elderly who are living in homes which are cold (see Ch. 6).

Supplementary pensioners are eligible for help with extra heating costs, but this benefits only those who qualify in this way. In the winters of 1977, 1978 and 1979 discounts were given on electricity bills, but for the elderly this benefit again was restricted to supplementary pensioners.

Aid can also be given to people wanting to insulate their lofts. Under the Homes Insulation Act 1978 local authorities have the power to make grants for this purpose and to give priority to the elderly.

Help with housing costs Financial help is also available from local authorities in the form of rate rebates, rent rebates and rent allowances. Pensioners and others on low incomes are entitled to rate rebates unless they receive a supplementary pension which covers the rates. Elderly people are eligible for rent rebates if they are local authority tenants and rent allowances if they are tenants of housing associations or private landlords. In 1977 85 per cent of local authority tenants aged 60 and over received help with housing costs (rent and/or rate rebate or supplementary benefit), and for those renting privately unfurnished accommodation or from a housing association 66 per cent received help. Half of elderly owner-occupiers without a mortgage received help.[21]

A major problem faced by elderly owner-occupiers is the large repair bill. A small amount is allowed to supplementary pensioners to cover the cost of insurance and minor repairs and a small lump sum can also be given. But this sum is inadequate for major repairs. Among the powers local authorities have to help is that of lending money to owner-occupiers who are unable to obtain a mortgage to cover repairs. These loans are usually maturity ones where the principal is recovered from the value of the property when it is sold. There are other ways in which help can be given.[22]

Income tax   There are certain special tax reliefs available for people of pensionable age. A number of special deductions may be made before income tax is charged. There is also a higher threshold for the elderly before the surcharge is made on investment income.

Attendance allowance   A tax-free attendance allowance is payable for people who need frequent attention or continual supervision by day and at night. A lower amount is payable if the help is needed only for the day *or* the night. Many of those who receive this are elderly.

Other financial concessions   Travel at a reduced rate, or free between certain hours, is allowed by some local authorities. Some also give concessions for other services such as for pensioners attending further education courses or public entertainments. There has been a growth in these types of service, but there is much variation between local authorities. British Rail allow pensioners to travel at half fare if they buy a special railcard. Television licences at a reduced rate are available for pensioners in old people's homes and sheltered housing.

Some issues

Level of pensions   The main need of the elderly is for an adequate income when they are no longer able to earn their own living. What is required is a scheme through which people can contribute a sufficient amount to a fund while they are at work to provide for an adequate standard of living when they retire, and the new pensions scheme which began in 1978 is designed to help achieve this.

There have been substantial increases in pensions in relation to the real incomes of the rest of the population in the last three or four years. As Bosanquet comments: 'Such increases must be considered a major achievement at a time of economic recession.'[23] But others such as Townsend are more critical and many writers and pressure groups argue strongly for an increase in the basic pension.

As the overall future increase in the number of pensioners will be much less than that of the last 25 years, pressure on the pensions fund will be less great. This is reflected in the planned public expenditure on social security benefits where the increase for national insurance and supplementary pensions is not as great as for some other benefits.[24]

Age for retirement   Most people are now retired compulsorily at the minimum state pension age. A few continue for longer (e.g. clergy, those in domestic service, the self-employed) but they are the exception. Some people, especially those in heavy manual jobs, may wish for early retirement while others would prefer to stay on for longer. A flexible age of retirement may be more in keeping with the varying physical and mental capacities of the elderly.

There is also the question of the disparity between the ages at which men and women are eligible for a state pension. The gradual equalisation of pension ages has been suggested among others by the Equal Opportunities Commission. This was one of the matters raised in DHSS, *A Happier Old Age*, which asked for comments 'on the desirability of an equalisation of men's and women's pension ages at whatever age can be afforded between 60 and 65, and on the possibility that pensions at less than the new scheme's full level should be made available to those who choose to retire earlier'.[25] Any change in the age for retirement has repercussions both on employment and on occupational pensions.

Dependence on supplementary pensions   It has been seen that the original Beveridge plan was for the national insurance retirement pension to be sufficiently high for pensioners not, in general, to have to rely on means-tested assistance. This has not happened and so large numbers of elderly people have had to apply for the latter. The safety net of supplementary benefit has become an important part of pensioners' resources.

At the end of 1981 there were nearly 3.7 million people receiving supplementary benefit of whom 1.7 million were pensioners (about 46% of the total). This means that over a fifth of all retired people were dependent on a supplementary pension.

Growing number of discretionary payments   The growing number of discretionary payments, most of which go to pensioners, is a source of concern to the SBC. The percentage receiving discretionary additions in respect of exceptional circumstances (mainly extra heating) was 72.4 in 1977. When two-thirds of supplementary pensioners are paid a heating addition the word 'exceptional' payment hardly seems appropriate. The growing number of ECAs and ENPs have been criticised for a number of reasons including the difficulty for claimants in understanding their entitlement, complications in assessment and unfairness between claimants. Not only this, but the SBC point out that they are restricted by legislation to giving help with heating costs only to those entitled to benefit. This means that help cannot be given either to those people who are living just above the supplementary benefit level or those who do not claim. The Commission felt in 1977 that the way forward was to replace the schemes of supplementary benefit heating additions and *ad hoc* winter fuel discount schemes with a comprehensive fuel rebate or bonus scheme.

Take-up of benefits One of the regular findings of surveys has been that elderly people do not all claim the benefits to which they are entitled. The SBC issued a Discussion Paper, *Take-up of Supplementary Benefits*, in 1978 based on 1975 estimates.[26] They concluded that nearly 1 million people – over 60 per cent of whom were pensioners – seemed not to be receiving the supplementary benefit to which they were entitled. In 1979 it was estimated that 65 per cent of pensioners received the supplementary pension to which they were entitled, compared with 78 per cent of non-pensioners. Of the estimated unclaimed benefit in 1976 of £250 million, 32 per cent was where the head of the family was over pensionable age. Commenting on take-up the SBC pointed out that while a national publicity drive to improve take-up might be desirable it would also create a good deal of work and increase costs, because a large number of abortive claims would have to be assessed. In 1979 the weekly entitlement of pensioners failing to claim was £3.10 per week. However, the value of this small weekly entitlement, stretching over years, may not be inconsiderable. The SBC suggested some ways in which this problem could be overcome, including better contact with existing pensioners.

Housing costs The SBC have considered that problems arise, mainly for retirement pensioners, when it is difficult to judge whether they would be better off on supplementary benefit, including an addition for rent, or alternatively with rent rebates and allowances. Because of the different means tests and allowances householders have to make complicated comparisons and even the experts may find it difficult to reach a firm conclusion. The SBC said that they 'regard this state of affairs as intolerable and . . . are keenly interested in the possibility of creating a single scheme of housing benefit which would cover all low-income householders whether or not they were eligible for supplementary benefit'. David Donnison, when Chairman of the SBC, suggested that this is one of the 'boundary problems' between services concerned with income maintenance and housing. The problem of owner-occupiers has already been mentioned.

Abuse There is great public concern about wrongful claims to social security and in 1971 the Fisher Committee was set up to report on this form of abuse and to recommend any changes in procedure that seemed necessary. In 1973 they produced their *Report of The Committee on Abuse of Social Security Benefits*.[27] In one area (non-disclosure of earnings) the Committee found that there was abuse 'to a substantial extent' though no evidence is given about the extent of this among pensioners. The Committee considered how the DHSS attempted to make sure that pensioners were aware of the earnings rule and correctly reported any earnings which might affect the amount of benefit payable. The Committee felt that there was little public sympathy for those who both worked and drew benefit, but they added: 'More sympathy is felt for pensioners, for disabled men and for women without male support who do part-time or casual work and earn a little over the "disregard" limits. Though this is "abuse" it could take a lower place in the attentions of the Departments.'[28]

EMPLOYMENT

Introduction

Retirement from work, as the Acton Society Trust has pointed out, can be viewed from a number of standpoints – economic, medical, administrative and social. Economically, it implies both the loss of trained and experienced workers and also considerable expenditure by the state on pensions. Medically, there is the effect of ageing on productivity and of retirement on the individual's health. Administratively, there is the problem of deciding what type of retirement policy should be adopted. Socially, it can be examined for its impact on the happiness of the individual.

Decline in proportions of economically active elderly people

An important change took place in the economic activity rate (i.e. the percentage of the age group gainfully employed) of the elderly between 1951 and 1971. There was a steady decline in the number of men continuing in work. Whereas 48 per cent of men aged 65–69 were gainfully employed in 1951 only 31 per cent were in 1971. For those aged 70 and over the employment rate dropped from 20 to 11 per cent. There was a similar decrease among single women. In contrast to this, however, a higher percentage of married women and widows were employed in 1971. In 1951 among those aged 60–64 the percentage employed was 7 (married women) and 19 (widows), while the figures for 1971 were 25 and 34 per cent respectively. There was also an increase for the over 65s. Recently there has been a decline in economic activity for all pensioners. In 1982 for people over 65, 10 per cent of men and 5 per cent of both non-married and married women were economically active.[29] The figures in 1973 were 19, 6 and 8 per cent respectively.

Why elderly people stop working　As might be expected, the percentage of people working decreases sharply with age. Most elderly people have to leave their jobs on reaching the official retiring age, unless they are self-employed. Some leave earlier. Surveys, such as MPNI, *Reasons Given for Retiring or Continuing at Work*,[30] and subsequent research have confirmed that many who retire early do so for health reasons. Although there are no detailed figures for the age of people who were made redundant before the Redundancy Payments Act 1965 there is some evidence that, prior to that Act, age played a rather less significant part in redundancy selection than it has subsequently.

The elderly who want to continue to work　Work provides income, status, interest and companionship and the need for these does not necessarily become less important on retirement. People may wish to continue to work for all of these reasons. Showler, and others, have argued that while many older people prefer to retire rather than continue in work others would suffer a substantial fall in living standards and prefer to work.

Even those who have been compulsorily retired from their jobs may seek another one, and for those who have to retire in their 50s (e.g. from the police or armed forces) a long spell in another occupation may be possible. The most likely outcome is part-time work. In 1976 10 per cent of men over 65 and 4 per cent of women over 65 in England worked part-time (6% of men that age and 1% of women worked full-time).[31]

Some who wish to continue working may opt for a different type of job – perhaps a less stressful or less physically demanding one. The 1971 census shows that where occupations were classified retired women were mainly employed in service, sport and recreation. This category included such jobs as office cleaning and domestic work. The figure for men was 16 per cent.

Some have suggested that jobs suitable for older people should be kept open for them and that special training programmes should be provided. This, however, assumes that the elderly are alike in all respects and can be provided for as a group, whereas all the evidence shows that each is an individual with particular skills and a different level of performance from others. But what can be done and is done is the provision of workplaces specially for the elderly. Under the Health Services and Public Health Act 1968 local authorities have the power to provide such places either themselves or through a voluntary body. Most are in fact run by voluntary bodies and many receive grants from local authorities or charities. A few are self-supporting.

Some have argued that work after retirement should be encouraged. The Rowntree Committee, for example, pointed out that from the economic standpoint it was important for people of pensionable age to remain at work so long as they could make a worthwhile contribution to the creation of wealth.[32] However, these views have to be seen against the background of full employment in the 1950s. In the late 1970s problems of unemployment make it less likely that people will argue along these lines. Indeed in some cases there has been official encouragement for workers to retire early to allow younger people to fill their jobs. Voluntary work should also be considered in this context. A detailed discussion follows in Chapter 11, but it is appropriate to mention one special scheme here. This is the Link Scheme which began in 1976 with the backing of Age Concern and other organisations. Through it the elderly are given the opportunity to carry on using their skills and crafts for the benefit of other elderly people. They inform a central point when they either need something done or are willing themselves to do a job for others. Services are matched up to callers, a time agreed for the job and payment given in the form of stamps which in turn provides the volunteer with the means of getting some necessary job done. This has proved to be an ingenious job-exchange scheme and at the beginning of 1979 there were schemes in 30 centres. These schemes have been devised to tackle two of the problems of retirement – poverty and inactivity. The exchange system that has resulted means that jobs get done without money changing hands and people are able to give as well as to receive help. When the jobs that the pensioners have wanted done have involved heavy work it has been possible to obtain help from younger members of other need groups, such as Gingerbread (single parents).

Some problems

Attitudes In Chapter 2 reference was made to society's perceptions of ageing and it was remarked that the elderly are often regarded as second-class citizens unable to make much contribution to the world around them. A blanket approach like this is unhelpful and inaccurate. Research in two particular spheres, the physiological and psychological aspects of ageing, demonstrate this in relation to employment.

Research into the physiological aspects of ageing is clearly important for the light that can be shed on physical and mental performance. The general conclusion seems to be that while performance in certain ways, e.g. physical strength, does decline with age, yet chronological age is by no means an accurate indicator of capacity to perform a task. Psychological evidence is just as important because the way in which both prospective employee and employer view the older worker will affect their attitudes. There is evidence that stereotypes are common about ageing and that these influence the behaviour of people in the employment market. These beliefs can affect recruitment, transfer, training and redundancy policies.

Age bars Evidence drawn from advertised job vacancies has shown that the incidence of age-qualified vacancies is fairly widespread. A number of reasons for this practice has been suggested: the presence of career structures and internal labour markets (people may be recruited and trained to fit in with the structure of a particular organisation); the likely age at which the peak of professional output is reached; the standard of health and fitness required; restrictive practices; length of training required; wage-for-age scales; a filter mechanism (to reduce the number of applicants); and problems over pension funds.

In 1978 legislation in the United States outlawed discrimination on grounds of age among workers up to the age of 70, but no similar legislation has so far been passed in this country.

The need for preparation for retirement More attention is now being paid to the need for preparation for retirement. Some firms organise courses for their employees and some adult education institutes do the same for a wider constituency. The Pre-Retirement Association offers seminars, courses and individual counselling and publishes a monthly magazine, *Choice*. Studies of elderly people, however, show clearly that many are ill prepared to cope with what may be one-third of their lives. In one of the classic studies of the elderly, *Work, Age and Leisure*, Le Gros Clark argued that for most men the end of their working life no longer coincides with physiological old age. He believed that advances in technology would mean fewer jobs and that other methods for prolonging working life outside industry such as sheltered workshops were little more than pilot schemes. He ended with a plea for active pursuits in retirement to be considered in the wider context of increasing leisure for people of all ages.

Conclusions It is clear that older workers are not a group who can be neatly categorised according to skill, ability or physical strength. It would be helpful if employers could choose people for a particular job regardless of their age and train them accordingly. But for those older people who are disabled, some of whom will be elderly, special policies may be appropriate.

There are, however, real practical difficulties for employers. For example an employer undertaking to train someone for a job expects that person to work in it for a sufficient time to pay off the cost of the training. Again the employer will have to weigh up the cost of additional safety measures such as extra lighting that may be required against the value of the end product. On the other hand he may find that older workers provide stability and do not move on so quickly from one job to another as younger people sometimes do.

What also has to be remembered is that employment policies cannot be considered in isolation. Pension transfer schemes, the effect of the earnings allowance and the effect of the state pension age all have a bearing both on what the individual elderly person chooses to do and on the retirement policies of employers.

REFERENCES

1. BEVERIDGE, SIR WILLIAM, *Social Insurance and Allied Services*, Cmnd 6404, HMSO, 1942, p. 5.
2. ROWNTREE, B. SEEBOHM, *Old People*. Report of a survey committee on the problems of ageing and the care of old people,

The Nuffield Foundation, Oxford University Press, 1947, p. 99.
3. CHANCELLOR OF THE EXCHEQUER, *Provision for Old Age*, see Ch. 4 note 14.
4. *Ibid.*, p. 77.
5. COLE, D. and UTTING, J., *The Economic Circumstances of Old People*, Codicote Press, 1962.
6. ABEL-SMITH, B. and TOWNSEND, P., *The Poor and the Poorest*, G. Bell and Sons, 1965, p. 66.
7. TOWNSEND and WEDDERBURN, see Ch. 3 note 6.
8. MPNI, *Retirement Pensioners*, see Ch. 4 note 16.
9. *Ibid.*, pp. 83–4.
10. *Ibid.*, pp. 84–5.
11. TOWNSEND, P., *Poverty in the United Kingdom*, Penguin, 1979, p. 820.
12. HUNT, see Ch. 2 note 3.
13. ABEL-SMITH and TOWNSEND, *op. cit.*, p. 63.
14. TOWNSEND, *op. cit.*, p. 915.
15. DHSS, *A Happier Old Age*, see Ch. 3 note 61, p. 22.
16. CSO, *Social Trends* (No. 9), see Ch. 2 note 15, p. 102.
17. *Ibid.*, p. 126.
18. MPNI, *Retirement Pensioners*, see Ch. 4 note 16.
19. HUNT, see Ch. 2 note 3.
20. THE GOVERNMENT ACTUARY, *Occupational Pension Schemes, 1979, Sixth Survey by the Government Actuary*, HMSO 1981.
21. CSO, *Social Trends* (No. 9), see Ch. 2 note 15, p. 156.
22. TINKER, A. and WHITE, J., 'How can elderly owner occupiers be helped to improve and repair their homes?' *Housing Review*, 28 (No. 3), May/June, 1979, pp. 74–5.
23. BOSANQUET, see Ch. 3 note 53, p. 54.
24. CSO, *Social Trends* (No. 13), see Ch. 2 note 12, p. 69.
25. DHSS, *A Happier Old Age*, see Ch. 3 note 61, p. 19.
26. DHSS, SBC, *Take-up of Supplementary Benefits*, HMSO, 1978.
27. DHSS, *Report of the Committee on Abuse of Social Security Benefits* (The Fisher Committee), Cmnd 5228, HMSO, 1973.
28. *Ibid.*, p. 227, para. 492.
29. OPCS, *Monitor 83/2, Preliminary Results for 1982 GHS*, OPCS, 1983.
30. MPNI, *Reasons Given for Retiring or Continuing at Work*, HMSO, 1954.
31. CSO, *Social Trends* (No. 9), see Ch. 2 note 15, p. 64.
32. ROWNTREE, *op. cit.*, p. 84.

Chapter six
HEALTH

INTRODUCTION

Health is a matter of prime importance for the elderly because it is staying reasonably well that enables them to remain independent. As has been seen in Chapter 2, a common view of ageing is a quick decline of physical and mental powers. Professional workers can be particularly prone to this view, since it is the ill and the frail whom they normally meet.

THE HEALTH OF THE ELDERLY

General

There is clear evidence of a greater incidence of both acute and chronic sickness among the elderly than in other age groups.[1] The average number of days of acute illness for people aged 65 and over in 1981 was 35 for men and 47 for women. The average for all ages was 19 for men and 24 for women. For chronic illness 54 per cent of men and 63 per cent of women over 65 reported a long-standing illness in 1981. The average for all ages was 28 per cent for men and 30 per cent for women.

Elderly patients differ in three major ways from the young: in the type and number of diseases, in their reactions to disease and in special features to do with their background.[2] They often have a multiplicity of diseases, partly accounted for by the accumulation of non-lethal diseases such as osteo-arthritis and deafness. Many researchers have pointed to the dangers to them of toxic effects from the many drugs they have to take. On the other hand, diseases such as infective hepatitis are less common among the aged and so is severe bronchitis – probably because 'susceptible individuals are eliminated at earlier ages'.[3] There are also differences in the way the elderly react to disease (e.g. pain mechanisms and temperature response). General background, too, has an effect, for poverty, lack of status and disability can all lead to depression. Coronary heart diseases and many cancers, while strongly age related, also have important environmental causes.

The views of the elderly

The elderly themselves seem to fear illness and loneliness more than any other condition, although most older people think their health is 'good'.[4] Anderson has noted that in most surveys there is a 'difference of opinion between the doctors and the old people examined with regard to their state of health'. Commenting on this and drawing from a large number of studies Johnson argues that self-referred illness is only the tip of the iceberg and is likely to have reached a fairly advanced state before consultation with a doctor is considered necessary.[5] Because there is a stereotype of old age which promotes expectations of ill health and decrepitude it is little wonder that old people refuse as long as possible to be labelled as sick.

The very old and the least mobile

In general there is an increase in ill health among the over 75s. In the 1981 *General Household Survey* (GHS) 60 per cent of males and 70 per cent of females aged 75 or over reported that they suffered from a chronic health problem, compared with 51 per cent of males and 58 per cent of females aged between 65 and 74. In 1976 elderly people who were neither bedfast nor housebound were asked whether they had any illness or disability which handicapped them or interfered with their activities. The results showed that only one-quarter of males and one-third of females over 85 had no disability, compared with 44 per cent of all elderly people over 65.[6]

The main causes of loss of mobility were arthritic and rheumatic conditions, followed by cardiac and pulmonary conditions. Evidence about the least mobile is given in a study by the Social Survey Division of the Office of Population Censuses and Surveys (OPCS)[7] which provided estimates of the incidence of impairment and handicap among persons living in private households in Great Britain. Impairment was defined in the study as 'lacking part or all of a limb, or having a defective limb, organ or mechanism of the body'. Handicap was the 'disadvantage of restriction of activity caused by the loss or reduction of functional ability'. Table 5 shows the increasing rate of impairment with age.

Table 5. Handicapped and impaired:* October 1968–February 1969 – Great Britain

| | Age group | | | |
	30–49	50–64	65–74	75 and over
Number impaired per 1,000 population				
Men	30	86	211	316
Women	26	85	227	409
All persons	28	85	221	378

* All living in private households.

Source: Harris, A., *Handicapped and Impaired in Great Britain*, Table 2, p. 5.

Less mobile are the bedfast and housebound. In 1976 Hunt found that 1.9 per cent of the over 80s were bedfast permanently (compared with 0.4% of those aged 75–79 and none between 65 and 75).[8] There was a steady increase in those permanently housebound from 1.1 per cent of the 65–69 year olds to 17.7 per cent of those aged 85 and over. Nearly half the bedfast and housebound had not been out of their houses for more than a year.[9]

SOME RELATED HEALTH ISSUES

Some health problems faced by the elderly have attracted a good deal of cross-disciplinary research and have a particular relevance to social administration. Three of these are nutrition, incontinence and hypothermia.

Nutrition

The health of individuals is clearly affected by what they eat. The early poverty studies (e.g. those by Rowntree) showed that many old people did not enjoy a diet which enabled them to remain healthy. More recent evidence suggests that this is now no longer the case.

Surveys in 1952 and 1962 indicated that the popular idea that many old people who live alone exist almost entirely on bread, butter, jam, biscuits and cups of sweetened tea was not substantiated. In 1972 *A Nutrition Survey of the Elderly* found that elderly people followed a dietary pattern that was similar to that of the general population except that they ate smaller quantities.[10] There was no evidence to suggest that those elderly people in the survey who ate a less good diet did so for economic reasons. There was little overt malnutrition and where it did occur the cause was usually an underlying medical condition rather than a poor diet. Nevertheless, some old people were malnourished. The researchers felt that elderly people at risk should be identified through regular visits by community nurses. Similar findings were reported in 1979.[11]

Incontinence

It is estimated that more than 2 million people of all ages in this country, many of them elderly, suffer from incontinence. Often they do not get assistance because society treats it as a taboo subject. But it is serious because it can prevent an old person from living an independent life. For instance it is sometimes laid down that no one who is incontinent can be accepted in sheltered housing. It can also lead to great stress on relatives and may be the determining factor in whether or not a family will continue to care for an old person.

It is therefore important to find out whether the cause is physical or is the result of psychological factors. There is some evidence that on occasion urinary incontinence can be the result of rejection by society. So a social as well as a physical assessment may be necessary. Practical considerations like steps to negotiate or the absence of a conveniently placed lavatory may suggest the need for adaptations to the home. Local authorities can supply aids such as disposable pads and protective bedding and may give advice. Some have special laundry services and arrangements for collecting disposable items. The DHSS can pay a special needs allowance to cover extra laundry costs.

Hypothermia

Unlike incontinence hypothermia *is* a subject which is discussed in public. Hypothermia means low body temperature. It is usually defined as the condition present when the body temperature falls below 35 °C, or 95 °F, but there is no sharp cut-off point at this temperature. There are two main causes: diseases and conditions in the body (such as a failure in the temperature-regulating system) and environmental factors such as cold winters and lack of heating.

Hypothermia is a dangerous condition with a high mortality rate.

The importance of hypothermia as a medical condition seems to have been noted only comparatively recently. In the 1950s articles appeared in medical journals reporting hypothermia in babies and these were followed by accounts relating to the elderly. The British Medical Association (BMA) reviewed existing knowledge and the Royal College of Physicians undertook a screening survey. The Medical Research Council and the Centre for Environmental Studies then combined to undertake a joint research programme. The aim was to measure the body temperatures and the social and environmental conditions of a sample of old people and 1,020 were interviewed. The results can be found in Wicks, *Old and Cold* [doc 19].

There appeared to be no simple way of identifying those in the coldest homes in terms of sex, marital status, household composition or age.[12] Many of those 'at risk' and most in need of help were unlikely to report that they felt cold and required warmer conditions. The Hunt survey found that a high porportion of elderly people had no means of heating their bedroom, and that a majority of halls, passages and lavatories, and many kitchens were unheated. Households with heads aged 85 and over were in many respects worse off. Many of those who were not warm enough blamed it on inadequate heating facilities, often arising from financial stringency.[13] What can be done? Fox in *Warmth and the Elderly* recommends publicity (especially about the extent of the problem), research, changes in benefit to give more help with heating, a concerted attack on environmental problems and greater attention paid to the housing and economic difficulties of the elderly.[14] Gray *et al.* in *A Policy for Warmth* (Fabian Society, 1977) claim that there is a lack of overall policy for warmth. They identify a number of possible solutions including greater attention to insulation, income support, changing attitudes of fuel boards towards debt and disconnection, and training for all who have contact with the elderly (especially home helps) about ways of helping them.

Wicks concluded that while specific policies such as using electric blankets, providing heating additions, insulating housing, etc. would help, a more general approach was required.[15] He emphasised in particular the need for smaller units of accommodation and housing specially built for the elderly, and for a significant increase in the level of pensions.

A joint DOE/DHSS circular, *Heating for Elderly People in Winter*, which came out in 1972 advised local authorities to focus attention on 'those in the less active higher age groups (e.g. 75 or over) living alone – including elderly couples living alone – and particularly those who are housebound or severely handicapped'; but it warned that all old people may be at risk. Various courses of action were proposed, and the role of social services authorities was seen as drawing together information and initiating and co-ordinating action. The DOE in *An Exploratory Project on Heating for the Elderly* made recommendations about small first-aid works including draught-stripping and other minor improvements.

GROUPS WITH SPECIAL NEEDS

There are some groups of elderly people about whom there is particular concern. Three of them are the dying, the bereaved and the mentally disordered.

The dying

Over one-third of those who die do so in their own homes, and many of those who die elsewhere may have spent many months seriously ill at home before they went to hospital. Over half a million people die in Great Britain each year and a high proportion are in the upper age ranges.

The care of the dying is a major social problem, not only for those faced with death but for those who attempt to provide support and help. Until recently there was little in medical or social work education about care for the dying nor was there much public concern. Now the subject is more openly discussed. See for example Hinton's book *Dying*.[16] Hodkinson points out that the attitudes towards death of staff, patients and the community at large have a considerable bearing on terminal care. 'Thus doctors and nurses are at risk of being so geared to the philosophy of cure that death is regarded as a humiliating failure.'[17]

In *Life Before Death* the last 12 months in the lives of 785 adults is described by Cartwright, Hockey and Anderson.[18] This study shows that relatives often struggle on with inadequate help from professionals and community services. The message is for more and better co-ordinated services.

One of the pioneers in this country in care of the dying is Dr Cicely Saunders. Her approach outlined in *Management of Terminal Disease* is based on the control of pain, allaying the fear of a painful death and a positive and caring approach to patients who are encouraged to feel that their lives are still worth living.

One study analysed the circumstances of 203 people who had been found dead or dying in their homes in York:[19] 143 of them were over retirement age. In *Found Dead* the authors suggest that the number of old people found dead is rising, but the length of time between death and discovery is decreasing. Most had been living alone but they were not isolated and most had extensive contact with relatives and neighbours. The authors state that this finding supports the results of other studies that the majority of families do maintain contacts with their elderly relatives.[20] Regular medical screening has been suggested to identify the risk of sudden collapse, but the researchers thought it unlikely that many old people would be willing to accept formal arrangements or surveillance to prevent their being found dead. The report adds that even residential care and sheltered housing do not eliminate the possibility of old people dying alone. They concluded that there is no dramatic case for the development of services to prevent such deaths [doc 20].

The bereaved

To bereave is defined as 'to rob of'. The elderly are more likely than other age groups to be robbed of the life of someone close to them. Those who lose a partner or who see their contemporaries dying may feel grief, shock, anger and bitterness. In 1977 13 per cent of men aged 65–74 and 40 per cent of women aged 65–74 were widowed or divorced. As would be expected, those aged over 75 are more likely to be widowed or divorced (34% of men and 67% of women).

The importance of understanding mourning and the need for skilled professional help is underlined by Parkes in his book *Bereavement*, and by Pincus in *Death and the Family*. At a BASW meeting in 1976 a call was made for a much higher priority to be given to bereavement counselling in the training of social workers, the clergy, teachers and the medical profession. This view is echoed in the Age Concern Manifesto Group publication, *Death and Bereavement*.[21]

The mentally disordered

One of the most difficult problems for families and professionals alike is the mentally disordered elderly person. This term 'mentally disordered' is usually taken to cover both the mentally ill and the mentally handicapped.

The mentally ill have been defined as 'those whose minds have previously functioned normally but who suffer a breakdown, the symptoms of which are often odd behaviour that ordinary people find difficult to tolerate'.[22] The DHSS have distinguished three main groups among the aged with mental illness symptoms to whom the term 'psychogeriatric' is often loosely applied. These are patients who entered hospitals for the mentally ill before modern methods of treatment were available and have grown old in them, elderly patients with functional mental illness and elderly persons with dementia.

It is difficult to estimate the number of elderly people who are mentally ill, but one-quarter of the beds in mental illness hospitals are occupied by patients over 75.[23] Anderson quotes evidence from research studies that indicated an incidence in 1971 of mental illness in 22 per cent of men and 39 per cent of women in the 65 and over age group.[24] He also states that numerous studies have revealed a high incidence of depression (from 10 to 30% in older people in the community) and the close association between depression and physical disease. There is also evidence that confusion often has physical causes such as dehydration, cardiac failure and urinary retention. It is also believed that some 3–7 per cent of the elderly have dementia.

The mentally handicapped have been defined as 'those whose intelligence in relation to their age is so far below average that they are incapable of assuming the kind of responsibilities accepted as normal'.[25] Their numbers are difficult to estimate.

It is expected that the number of elderly people suffering from mental disorder will grow.[26] They are likely to present problems both for relatives and for the social services if other types of provision are inadequate. In the past the care of both these groups has been by the family and in institutions isolated from society. In the 1950s, however, a number of factors combined to emphasise the trend away from hospitals. There was dissatisfaction in many quarters about the effects of institutional care. There were also major developments in drug treatment allowing the symptoms of mentally ill patients to be controlled so that their behaviour became less disturbing. So the underlying movement was to community care.

In 1971, *Better Services for the Mentally Handicapped* (DHSS, Cmnd 4683) explained why the present services needed to be extended and improved. It showed that there had been a large growth in numbers of elderly people in hospitals, but also that considerable numbers had been discharged. 'Many of these probably required residential rather than hospital care.'

In 1972 the DHSS in a circular, *Services for Mental Illness Related to Old Age*, stressed the importance of assessment, defined the groups involved and examined their needs in turn. It advised that those needing hospital treatment were best treated in the psychiatric departments of district general hospitals. For the rest the emphasis was on rehabilitation with the use of day hospitals and, where necessary, residential care. The importance of co-ordination and joint planning with local authorities was stressed. The eventual closure of hospitals for the mentally ill was envisaged.

In 1975 a White Paper, *Better Services for the Mentally Ill* (DHSS, Cmnd 6233), was published and the question was posed: 'How far have expectations been fulfilled?' It was recognised that adequate support facilities in the community had not generally become available owing to the limits on resources and increasing and competing demands for new developments. In a section on the elderly it was stated that: 'Mental illness in old people is often too easily regarded as untreatable, but experience has shown that early intervention can be particularly effective.'

One problem has been the running down of institutional provision before adequate domiciliary care has become available. In 1978 fears of the effect of a run-down seem to have been realised for it was stated in *A Happier Old Age* that places in some large mental hospitals were being reduced ahead of the availability of alternative provision in local hospitals.[27]

Another problem has been the prevailing conditions in the institutions provided for the mentally disordered. There has been much concern both about the physical conditions, such as bleak dormitories and lack of furniture and about other matters such as staff attitudes. After Barbara Robb's *Sans Everything* in 1967[28] independent committees of enquiry investigated the allegations. In 1968 in *Findings and Recommendations Following Enquiries into Allegations Concerning the Care of Elderly Patients in Certain Hospitals* (NHS, Cmnd 3687) some, though not all, of the allegations were proved. Although it is clear from the Health (formerly Hospital) Advisory Service annual reports from 1969 onwards that conditions had improved there were still comments in the 1976 report about lack of provision for the elderly, particularly those mentally ill. Specific recommendations about the elderly mentally handicapped are given in a report, *Helping Mentally Handicapped People in Hospital* [doc 21].

TRENDS AND PRIORITIES IN HEALTH CARE

Health promotion

'Current policy reflecting both modern medical practice and the wish of most elderly people to be in their own home is to promote an active approach to treatment and rehabilitation.'[29] This statement taken from *A Happier Old Age* is an indication of a positive approach towards the health of the elderly.

To enable the elderly to remain healthy attention has to be given to prevention, detection and rehabilitation. Prevention has already been mentioned (Ch. 4) as an objective of many services. Detection to pick up early signs of illness is achieved by a variety of methods, including screening clinics. It is important because not all old people report their medical problems.[30] This can lead not only to serious illnesses being unnoticed in their early stages but also to failure to treat minor conditions which later can have a cumulative effect. Recent research into the health of the elderly underlines the importance of rehabilitation, which is generally defined as the achievement of the optimum level of independence for the individual. Most experts who write about rehabilitation agree that a successful outcome owes more to mental factors than to the degree or nature of the physical disability.[31] Good motivation may lead to recovery in the face of quite severe physical difficulties.

Expenditure

There is overwhelming evidence that the elderly use the NHS more than younger people. For example while only about 2.5 per cent of old people are in hospital at any one time they occupy more than half of all the beds.[32] And whereas an average of £160 per head was spent on health services in 1980–81, the amount for those aged 65–74 was £310 and for those age 75 and over it was £765 [doc 5]. The Royal Commission on the NHS gave evidence that expenditure per head on health services is almost six times as much for people aged 75 and over as for people aged 16 to 64.[33] But, as was seen in Chapter 2, it is the older group that is increasing most rapidly.

There is evidence that some health services for the elderly are worse than for other age groups. Criticism which the Hospital (and later the Health) Advisory Service made of hospitals for the elderly were similar to those made about hospitals for the mentally disordered. There is evidence that both in quality and quantity staffing standards may be lower than in some other fields. In 1977 only

22.8 per cent of geriatricians received distinction awards, compared with an average 35.2 per cent for other specialists. And the DHSS pointed out in 1977 that nationally the need for physicians trained in geriatrics greatly exceeded the supply.

When considering future expenditure it is clear that the increase in numbers of the very elderly means that extra resources will be needed just to maintain, let alone improve, present standards.

THE DEVELOPMENT OF SERVICES

General

The origin and organisation of the NHS were described in Chapter 4. Specific points relating to the development of services are now touched on briefly.

An early matter of concern was the cost of the service which in 1946 had been estimated at £110 million, but by 1951–52 had grown to £384 million. The Guillebaud Committee in *Report of the Committee of Enquiry into the Cost of the National Health Service*[34] concluded that in practice there is no objective and attainable standard of 'adequacy' in the health field, that there was no evidence of extravagant spending, and that in some cases (e.g. hospitals' capital expenditure) more money needed to be spent. For the elderly they drew heavily on a paper on costs prepared for them by Abel-Smith and Titmuss which concluded that 'by-and-large, the older age group are currently receiving a lower standard of service than the main body of consumers and that there are also substantial areas of unmet need among the elderly'.[35] The Committee examined the pattern of care between the different parts of the NHS and laid down guidelines.

The Guillebaud Committee referred to a survey on chronic sick which was then being carried out and which was published in 1957. The report was called *Survey of Services Available to the Chronic Sick and Elderly 1954–1955*.[36] The wide-ranging conclusions of this survey covered both medical and other provision. In regard to the former the report indicated that the number of hospital beds for the chronic sick was sufficient in total but needed to be properly used and better distributed. Their recommendations about other provisions arose out of their conviction that 'the key to the problems stemming from an ageing population lies with the preventive and domiciliary services'.[37]

The *Hospital Plan, 1962* (MOH, Cmnd 1604) laid down standards (for geriatric patients 1.4 beds per 1,000 total population) and it was visualised that the main hospital services would be brought together in district general hospitals (of 600–800 beds) designed to serve a population of 100,000–150,000. Although the plan was subsequently modified in 1966 many new hospitals were built and conditions for patients and staff greatly improved. More of these general hospitals had geriatric units providing treatment and rehabilitation so that the elderly would not need long-term hospital care. More day hospitals were established.

In 1962 local authorities were asked to take part in a long-term planning exercise similar to that for the hospitals.[38, 39] Wide variations were disclosed in what they planned to provide for health and welfare services [doc 22].

The administration of the NHS had since its inception been the subject of much comment and criticism and it was reorganised in 1974. Then followed what Abel-Smith has called 'the lean years following reorganisation: 1974–8', with a shortage of resources and criticisms of the new tiered system of administration. Geographical equity was one matter of concern: the Resource Allocation Working Party made suggestions for financial allocations to be based on criteria which included age and mortality.[40] The question of priorities formed the subject of two Consultative Documents – *Priorities for Health and Personal Social Services in England* in 1976[41] and *The Way Forward* in 1977.[42] Both Consultative Documents visualised an expansion in community services, and advice by the DHSS to local authorities and health authorities in 1979 acknowledged the growing pressure on services.

The Royal Commission on the NHS, which reported in 1979, had a great deal to say about the demands of the elderly on health and local authorities for the rest of this century. They agreed with current national priorities, including the emphasis on the elderly and community care for them [doc 23], but found that there were considerable practical difficulties to be overcome in shifting the resources from one patient or client group to another.[43]

In 1982 the NHS was reorganised following the Health Services Act 1980. The main effect was to reduce the tiers of management from five to three (see Fig. 4).

Primary health care

Elderly people account for about 20 per cent of all general practice consultations and are likely to need more home visits than average.

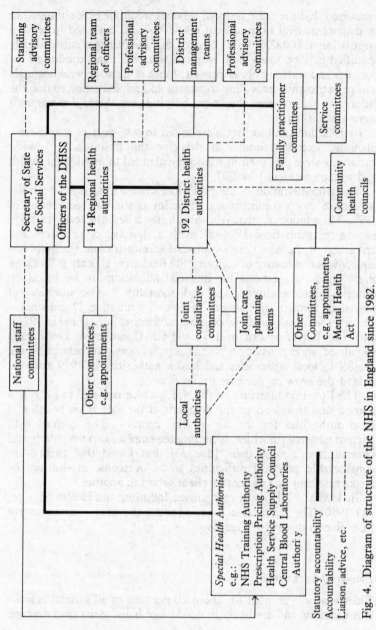

Fig. 4. Diagram of structure of the NHS in England since 1982.

Two-thirds of consultations take place at home for those over 75.[44] This may partly be due to difficulty in getting to a surgery because of lack of transport. A number of developments have taken place since the early days of the NHS which have affected the elderly. There has been the shift away from single-doctor practices to group practices and health centres. These make it possible to experiment with different methods of providing primary care, and they can also house a wide range of services, such as consultant out-patient clinics, diagnostic and paramedical services. For the elderly their advantage is that they are more likely to have purpose-built premises which are more comfortable and have better facilities, and it is more likely that a range of both medical and non-medical staff are employed. The elderly person may therefore be able to see a nurse for dressings or injections and not join the queue to see the doctor. Home nurses also do much of value in visiting the elderly at home and making follow-up visits on a regular basis. However, there are disadvantages. The grouping of doctors in one building inevitably means that it is less likely that elderly people will have their own GP just 'round the corner'. A group or health centre practice is also likely to run an appointments system, although there may be an open surgery as well. A rigid appointments system may cause problems for elderly people who are less likely to be on the telephone than the rest of the population and who may then just 'turn up' at the surgery. Elderly people may also feel that they get a more personal service from a doctor practising alone whom they will see on every occasion except when he is ill or on holiday. Some single-handed doctors are, however, in poor, lock-up premises in inner-city areas and may not in fact be as accessible as a group practice. The Royal Commission on the NHS also mentioned difficulties in rural areas.

Another development has been the growth in the number of staff other than doctors who are involved in the primary health care team. In 1980 over 80 per cent of district nurses and health visitors worked with GPs and their patients. An early study of schemes in 1969 by DHSS published in *Nursing Attachments to General Practice* identified some of the factors which make a scheme successful or possibly a failure. The report also showed that one effect for health visitors had been to make their case-load more varied and to give them more time with the elderly.

It is not known how many social workers are members of primary health care teams, but progress has been slower, possibly partly due to a different approach to patients between the two professions and some mutual distrust. Some schemes have been monitored, notably one in Kentish Town, London, and described by Goldberg and Neill in *Social Work in General Practice*. The importance of receptionists and secretaries is also being increasingly recognised for they can act as 'gatekeepers' – that is, be a help or a barrier between the elderly patient and the doctor.

Community and other services

Community services include nursing, health visiting, occupational therapy and pharmaceutical, ophthalmic, chiropody and dental services.

District nurses, many of whom work in group practices or health centres, are state registered nurses who provide care for people in their own homes. In some areas this extends to a night nursing service. The district nurse is the leader of the district nursing team and she may have state enrolled nurses and nursing auxiliaries working with her. Over 1.5 million elderly people were treated in 1981.

Health visitors are nurses with additional training, who are concerned with the promotion of health and the prevention of ill health. They work in an advisory supportive role rather than in a nursing capacity. Some work directly in the community while others are attached to general practices or health centres. In 1981 of cases dealt with by health visitors about 12 per cent involved elderly people compared with 10 per cent in 1971.[45] In 1977 about half a million old people were in touch with a health visitor.

The Royal Commission on the NHS thought that there was considerable scope for expanding the role and responsibilities of health visitors and district nurses. They said: 'We consider that there are increasingly important roles for community nurses, not just in the treatment room but in health surveillance for vulnerable groups and in screening procedures, health education and preventive programmes, and as a point of first contact, particularly for the young and elderly.'[46]

Another invaluable service is occupational therapy. This is usually arranged through a hospital, but some local authorities have occupational therapy services associated with the provision of aids and appliances. Occupational therapists now play an important role in rehabilitation and can help elderly people to cope with everyday activities such as cooking, cleaning and eating, as well as providing advice on, and arranging for, aids and adaptations.

For *pharmaceutical services* two matters are of particular concern –

access to the service and the role of the pharmacist. Both these were considered by the Royal Commission on the NHS.[47] They found that while few people experienced difficulty in getting a prescription dispensed there were some problems in rural areas. The concentration of GPs in group practices had led, in some places, to a process of leap-frogging with pharmacists trying to move nearer practice premises. The role of the pharmacist has traditionally been to dispense medicine on the prescription of doctors. The Royal Commission on the NHS found that this role had expanded and that the pharmacist was now regarded as a main source of advice in relation to minor ailments. The Royal Commission considered this an important and useful service and recommended that pharmacists should respond helpfully, though taking care not to act as quasi-doctors.

Many elderly people have eye problems and these increase with age.[48] They may be dealt with under the NHS by hospitals or by the general *ophthalmic service*, which provides sight-testing and the supply, replacement and repair of spectacles. A particular need, however, of many elderly is for a domiciliary consultation.

Many surveys have confirmed that one of the greatest unmet needs of the elderly is *chiropody*. Quite apart from medical conditions which need treatment, cutting toenails can present major difficulties. Hunt found that 20 per cent of her sample could not cut their own toenails.[49] The importance of this service has also been emphasised by researchers. Townsend and Wedderburn said: 'Foot conditions affect almost all activities – getting about inside and outside the house, climbing and descending stairs and even standing to prepare and cook a hot meal.'[50] They felt that the preventive role of chiropody may come to be regarded just as seriously as preventive dental care.

Most (90%) patients receiving the service under the NHS in 1981 were aged 65 or over.[51] But there is evidence that the demand for NHS chiropody outstrips the supply. And one survey found that for the over 65s during the past two years 13 per cent had used a private service, 15 per cent the NHS and 71 per cent had no treatment.[52]

Dental services are also important to the elderly. In 1978 74 per cent of elderly people aged 65–74 and 87 per cent aged 75 and over had no natural teeth.[53] There is evidence, too, of poor dental health among the elderly. The Royal Commission on the NHS noted that 'handicapped patients of all ages, and many elderly patients in particular, need special dental care'.[54]

Payment for these services is a matter of controversy. In 1979 the elderly received free prescriptions, but NHS dental and optical care was free only for those in low incomes or in hospital. In *A Happier Old Age* the DHSS said: 'It has been argued that dental and optical charges should be waived for elderly people but the cost of doing so would need to be set against other ways of providing help for elderly people.'[55]

Hospital services

Very few old people (2.5%) are in hospital at any one time, but they occupy more than half the beds and stay longer than younger people. Those aged 75 and over occupy one-third of all hospital beds and the effect on hospitals of the increasing numbers of very old people in the next 20–25 years will be marked.

Elderly people now go either to geriatric hospitals (some of which were formerly workhouses, though some are modern), to psychiatric hospitals or to geriatric or specialty wards (such as orthopaedics) in acute hospitals. One of the objectives of policy has been to bring the three types of hospital together. This has been for a number of reasons; not least to even up standards and to bring the first two types of hospital into the mainstream of modern medicine. The development of geriatrics, which is the study and treatment of diseases common to old age, as a medical specialty also has a bearing on the service provided. The Royal Commission on the NHS felt that the development of geriatrics had in many places enhanced the quality of care of elderly people, but that it had also 'influenced some physicians to take less interest in the old and to look to geriatricians excessively for the care of the elderly'.[56]

Another development has been connected with maintaining the elderly in their own homes while at the same time providing them with hospital treatment. This can often relieve the pressures on a family who are looking after a frail elderly person. It is achieved through short-term care in hospitals, for example admitting an old person for a specified period on a regular basis, or through day hospitals where treatment is given in the daytime on certain days to patients who continue to live at home. The first purpose-built day hospitals were erected in 1958. The number of regular geriatric day patients has grown from 65 per 1,000 population in 1967 to 183 in 1977. Day hospitals can be economical because they only require a single staff shift, provide fewer meals and no sleeping accommodation.

There is general agreement that conditions for the elderly in hospitals have improved greatly. New buildings, more patients being nursed in wards of acute hospitals and growing medical interest in old age have all contributed to this improvement. Nevertheless, there are still some problems and these are mainly to do with buildings, staff and lack of suitable accommodation for some patients who should be discharged. The problem of old buildings is still acute despite the considerable progress that has been made and many geriatric beds are still in old workhouses, former fever hospitals or sanatoria. The trend is now towards community hospitals varying from 50 to 150 beds. It had been envisaged that those elderly, and other patients who did not need the facilities of the district general hospital, would be treated in these community hospitals, but very few have so far been established. The Royal Commission on the NHS found support for small hospitals manned by GPs, but expressed concern that they might simply turn into long-stay units for the elderly.[57]

Staff problems are related to shortages, lack of trained personnel and attitudes. Despite an increase in the number of consultants in geriatric medicine there are still insufficient and in some areas there may be few applicants for such posts. Lack of nurses in geriatric medicine is another unsatisfactory feature as is the high number of untrained staff. In 1975 a report by the British Geriatric Society and a Royal College of Nursing Working Party on *Improving Geriatric Care in Hospital* stressed the importance of preserving human dignity and of encouraging independence and mobility in elderly patients.

A further dilemma is 'bed-blocking' which comes about when a patient cannot be discharged from hospital because no suitable accommodation is available. The Royal Commission on the NHS recommended that there should be some experimentation in the provision of nursing homes mainly staffed and run by nurses.[58] Some patients will need residential care while others will find sheltered housing or a small, easy-to-manage home acceptable. To enable this sort of provision to be available close links are necessary between the various services.

COLLABORATION BETWEEN SERVICES

Teamwork and co-ordination within the NHS

Since the creation of the NHS it has been realised that any division of services would bring the danger of gaps and overlaps. One of the reasons for the many attempts to bring the three parts of the structure closer together was to make effective co-ordination more possible. Since the reorganisation of the NHS in 1974 the three parts of the NHS have been brought together under regional health authorities. Planning services for the elderly should, therefore, in theory, be easier particularly now that there is a single source of finance. There are planning and other reasons why close links between the parts of the new NHS structure are vital for the elderly, and the same is true at an inter-professional level when the service is delivered. A few examples demonstrate the need for co-operation. When an elderly patient is referred to a hospital the latter must be made aware of all the relevant medical and social circumstances which only the GP will know. When the patient is discharged the primary health care team need to be alerted in good time and advised what, if any, treatment is needed. The authors of *Life Before Death* found that three-fifths of GPs were critical about lack of consultation by hospitals over discharge.[59]

Those working in community nursing and other services also need to be kept in the picture and the growing practice of attaching nurses, health visitors and others to the primary health care team should help to ensure better co-ordination. The Royal Commission on the NHS concluded that the development of the primary health care team was encouraging, but there was a continuing need to foster closer working relationships and teamwork between the professions.[60]

Links between health and other services

After the reorganisation of the NHS in 1974 the health of the elderly became the concern of the NHS and welfare that of local authority social service departments. The latter took the responsibility for the medical social workers employed in hospitals and certain other services (see Ch. 8). Preventive and after-care services vital to the health of the elderly are therefore now provided by local authorities. The main services involved are social services and housing. The latter will be discussed in the next chapter, but the links between health and social services will be considered here. See also DHSS, *Collaboration in Community Care*.[61]

The new local and health authorities were required to set up joint consultative committees, made up of members from both authorities, to advise on arrangements for collaboration and the planning and operation of services of common concern. Authorities were recommended to set up joint care planning teams, one of whose tasks was to plan and co-ordinate for groups such as the elderly. These planning care teams consist of geriatricians, GPs, nurses, health visitors, dentists and representatives of housing and social service departments and administrators. A new feature since 1976 has been joint financing, which is based on a special allocation of money which health authorities can use in sharing the cost with local authorities of schemes which are of benefit to both, such as provision for people who do not need hospital care to be looked after in the community. The objective is to encourage a shift of resources from hospital services to community care, to foster and develop joint planning and to encourage the resolution of issues where the responsibilities of the health and social services overlap. In the first year £8 million was allocated, while in 1978–79 it had risen to £32 million. Examples of such projects are a home from hospital scheme, day centres, a meals on wheels kitchen and provision of a lift in a home for the elderly.

Some further examples will show the importance of links between health and social services. When elderly people are discharged from hospital they probably need the support of some of the domiciliary services. If the number of home helps and the other domiciliary services are insufficient, or if they are not alerted, an old person may either have to remain in hospital unnecessarily or may return home to inadequate care. Equally, there can be occasions when an elderly person is incapable of remaining either at home or in Part III accommodation, but the hospital will not or cannot accept them.

REFERENCES

1. *GHS, 1981*, HMSO, 1982, pp. 142 and 145.
2. HODKINSON, see Ch. 2 note 2.
3. *Ibid.*, p. 6.
4. HUNT, see Ch. 2 note 3.
5. JOHNSON, M., 'Self-perception of need among the elderly', *Sociological Review*, 20.4.72.
6. HUNT, see Ch. 2 note 3, p. 71.
7. HARRIS, see Ch. 4 note 18.
8. HUNT, see Ch. 2 note 3, p. 68.
9. *Ibid.*, p. 71.
10. DHSS, *A Nutrition Survey*, see Ch. 4 note 19.
11. DHSS, *Nutrition and Health in Old Age*, HMSO, 1979.
12. WICKS, see Ch. 3 note 26, p. 96.

13. HUNT, see Ch. 2 note 3, p. 51.
14. FOX, R., *Warmth and the Elderly*, Age Concern, 1974.
15. WICKS, see Ch. 3 note 26, p. 172.
16. HINTON, J., *Dying*, Penguin, 1972.
17. HODKINSON, see Ch. 2 note 2, p. 61.
18. CARTWRIGHT, HOCKEY and ANDERSON, see Ch. 3 note 18.
19. BRADSHAW, CLIFTON and KENNEDY, see Ch. 3 note 27.
20. *Ibid.*, p. 13.
21. WILLIAMS, J., *Death and Bereavement*, Age Concern, 1974, p. 6.
22. CLEGG, see Ch. 4 note 29.
23. DHSS, *A Happier Old Age*, see Ch. 3 note 61, p. 36.
24. ANDERSON, SIR FERGUSON, 'Helping old people to continue living at home', *Royal Society of Health Journal*, Jan. 1978, p. 3.
25. CLEGG, see Ch. 4 note 29.
26. DHSS, *A Happier Old Age*, see Ch. 3 note 61, p. 39.
27. *Ibid.*, p. 38.
28. ROBB, see Ch. 2 note 5.
29. DHSS, *A Happier Old Age*, see Ch. 3 note 61, p. 37.
30. WILLIAMS, see Ch. 3 note 15.
31. HODKINSON, see Ch. 2 note 2.
32. DHSS, *A Happier Old Age*, see Ch. 3 note 61, p. 36.
33. ROYAL COMMISSION ON THE NHS, *Report* (The Merrison Committee), Cmnd 7615, HMSO, 1979, p. 61.
34. MOH, Guillebaud Committee, see Ch. 4 note 3.
35. *Ibid.*, p. 40.
36. MOH, *Survey of Services Available to the Chronic Sick*, see Ch. 4 note 15.
37. *Ibid.*, p. 37.
38. MOH, *Health and Welfare*, see Ch. 4 note 26.
39. MOH, *Health and Welfare*, see Ch. 4 note 27.
40. DHSS, *Sharing Resources for Health in England*, Report of the Resource Allocation Working Party, HMSO, 1976.
41. DHSS, *Priorities for Health and Personal Social Services in England*, A Consultative Document, HMSO, 1976.
42. DHSS, *Priorities in the Health and Social Services. The Way Forward*, HMSO, 1977.
43. ROYAL COMMISSION ON THE NHS, *op. cit.*, p. 358.
44. DHSS, *A Happier Old Age*, see Ch. 3 note 61, p. 32.
45. CSO, *Social Trends* (No. 13), see Ch. 2 note 12, p. 105.
46. ROYAL COMMISSION ON THE NHS, *op. cit.*, p. 79.
47. *Ibid.*, pp. 93–6.
48. HUNT, *The Elderly at Home*, see Ch. 2 note 3, p. 71.

49. *Ibid.*, p. 73.
50. TOWNSEND and WEDDERBURN, *The Aged in the Welfare State*, see Ch. 3 note 6, p. 55.
51. CSO, *Social Trends* (No. 13), see Ch. 2 note 12, p. 105.
52. RITCHIE, J., JACOBY, A. and BONE, M., *Access to Primary Health Care*, HMSO, 1981, p. 111.
53. *Ibid.*, p. 104.
54. *Ibid.*, p. 118.
55. DHSS, *A Happier Old Age*, see Ch. 3 note 61, pp. 33–4.
56. ROYAL COMMISSION ON THE NHS, *op. cit.*, p. 216.
57. *Ibid.*, p. 135.
58. *Ibid.*, pp. 135–6.
59. CARTWRIGHT *et al.*, see Ch. 3 note 18.
60. ROYAL COMMISSION ON THE NHS, *op. cit.*, p. 359.
61. DHSS, *Collaboration in Community Care*, see Ch. 4 note 24.

Chapter seven

HOUSING

INTRODUCTION

Any discussion about housing for the elderly should have as its starting point the fact that most of them live in homes of their own and not in any form of residential care. There has been little change since 1948. Approximately 89 per cent live in ordinary accommodation either owned by themselves or rented, 5 per cent live in their own home in sheltered housing and 6 per cent live in some form of institutional care – mainly old people's homes or hospitals.[1]

Adequate housing is of importance to the elderly in many ways. Such features as the absence of stairs and the presence of an indoor lavatory may enable even a very frail person to continue living independently. Warmth, too, is particularly necessary for less active people. Familiar surroundings and nearness to shops, post office, pub and church also contribute to their ability to live alone. What is shown more clearly than anything else by surveys is the desire of the elderly to be able to live in the way they want in their own home. At the same time community physicians have been pointing to the benefits of the physical and mental activity involved in housework, shopping and generally caring for themselves. Those who have been concerned with the financial aspects of old age, such as the Phillips Committee in 1954, have stressed the need for suitable housing on the grounds of both social happiness and finance.[2]

Many old people, however, live in less than desirable housing and some groups have particular problems. There is evidence, too,[3, 4] that some people remain in residential care only because alternative accommodation is lacking.

THE DEVELOPMENT OF POLICIES

There has been remarkable consistency in policies for housing the elderly irrespective of which political party has been in power. Advice from central government, given mainly in circulars, has emphasised the need to provide small units of accommodation, to allow elderly people to maintain independent lives in their own homes and to make movement from larger to smaller dwellings easier. Other points made have been the importance of siting dwellings near amenities and, since 1944, the value of grouping accommodation, usually referred to as sheltered housing, with communal facilities and a warden [doc 24]. Another piece of advice regularly given is the need for effective co-operation between all the authorities and departments concerned.

In 1956 the Ministry decided to find out whether old people were receiving a reasonable share of the accommodation provided and whether this was of the kind best suited to their physical needs and financial circumstances (Circular 32/56, *The Housing of Old People*). The following year advice was given (Circular 18/57, *Housing of Old People*) which stressed the need for adequate provision of small dwellings and a sympathetic and an efficient system for moving tenants from larger to smaller homes. Observations were made about the success of local authority and housing association schemes for accommodating the less active elderly in bedsitters or flatlets in converted large houses where some shared facilities can be provided. Handbooks were then issued (in 1958 *Flatlets for Old People* and in 1960 *More Flatlets for Old People*) illustrating sheltered housing schemes and the hope was expressed that councils would consider carrying out such schemes. In 1961 general advice was given in a joint MHLG/MOH circular, *Services for Old People* (Circular 10/61) [doc 25].

The Ministry then became involved in an interesting experiment in which they built (for Stevenage Development Corporation) a prototype sheltered housing scheme and then monitored reactions to it. The results were published in three Design Bulletins (No. 1, *Some Aspects of Designing for Old People* in 1962, No. 2, *Grouped Flatlets for Old People* in 1962 and No. 11, *Old People's Flatlets in Stevenage* in 1966).

The following year Circular 36/67, *Housing Standards, Costs and Subsidies*, established what have become known as the Parker Morris Standards (these were minimum standards of design and construction). Then in 1969 the principal circular (*Housing Standards and Costs: accommodation specially designed for old people*)[5] came out [doc 26]. In that circular two types of accommodation were declared eligible for subsidy. Category 1 is self-contained dwellings for old people who are more active. The standard is Parker Morris with some additional features. Limited communal facilities may be provided and so may a warden. Category 2 accommodation, for less active elderly people, is smaller than Parker Morris standards and comprises grouped flatlets with full communal facilities and a warden.

As a preliminary to a new circular the DOE issued *Housing for Old People: a Consultative Paper* in 1976.[6] This particularly stressed the importance of widening the choice of accommodation available for the elderly.

General housing policies have also had an effect on provision, for example the 1963 White Paper, *Housing* (Cmnd 2050), laid great stress on new building and in particular of small units for the elderly. A White Paper, *The Housing Programme 1965 to 1970* (Cmnd 2838), in 1965 set out the first stage in formulating a national housing plan but stated that more needed to be known about the needs of the elderly. Meanwhile a committee was set up by the MHLG to review the practice by authorities of allocating tenancies. Their report, *Council Housing Purposes, Procedures and Priorities* (the Cullingworth Committee), appeared in 1969.[7] Concern about the need for more and better homes led to another White Paper (in 1973), *Widening the Choice: the next steps in housing* (Cmnd 5280), which expressed disquiet about the many people who had no choice at all. When considering the way in which provision could be made the government proposed a range of measures to expand owner-occupation and the role of housing associations, but the view was expressed that local authorities had a special responsibility for groups who had 'general needs or suffer from special disadvantages'. Included among these were the elderly. A further White Paper, *Better Homes: the next priorities* (Cmnd 5339), in 1973 proposed a range of measures to tackle the worst housing conditions and in particular outlined changes in the improvement grants system. The setting up of housing action areas and general improvement areas, recommended in the White Paper, took place after the Housing Act 1974 which also expanded the role of the Housing Corporation. The importance of these changes was the attempt to help urban areas with poor property (where incidentally many elderly people lived) and to expand the role of housing associations (which were fast becoming major providers of accommodation for the elderly). The Rent Act 1974 gave security of tenure to tenants in furnished accommodation many of whom were elderly.

The growth in small households, including the elderly, was one of the reasons for *Housing Needs and Action* (DOE Circular 24/75) in

1975 which stressed the need for more small accommodation and showed how better use could be made of existing dwellings. The latter theme was expanded in 1977 in *Better use of Vacant and Under-Occupied Housing* (Circular 76/77) which sought to bring into full use empty and under-occupied dwellings, whether or not they belonged to the local authority, and to ensure that the accommodation people occupied accurately reflected their housing requirements. In the same year the new system for deciding on capital allocations to local authorities by central government was put forward by the DOE in *Housing Strategies and Investment Programmes* (Circular 63/77). In the annual strategy statement which local authorities were requested to complete they were asked to include any measures 'to meet the housing requirements of groups with special needs, for example, the aged and disabled'.

In 1977 a Consultative Document, *Housing Policy*, was published.[8] Previous policies for the elderly were endorsed, but the proposed abolition of local authority residential qualifications was stressed as was the need for co-operation between authorities [doc 27].

THE PRESENT POSITION

A good deal of information about housing conditions now exists which updates the 1971 census. The 1976 DOE *National Dwelling and Housing Survey* (NDHS)[9] of England, the Hunt study[10] and the annual GHS are all useful sources of information. They show that housing conditions have improved for the elderly as for the rest of the population.

Tenure

A lower proportion of the elderly than all households are owner-occupiers but more elderly households are outright owners and fewer have mortgages. Overall it would appear that whereas 54 per cent of all households are owner-occupiers 46 per cent of elderly households are buying or own their own home. More of the elderly are local authority or housing association tenants and a higher percentage rent private unfurnished accommodation. These findings are shown in Table 6.

For all households the major change since 1948 has been the rise in owner-occupation and the decline of the private rented sector. This seems to reflect people's wishes. Figures from the *NDHS* show that satisfaction with housing is highest among owner-occupiers and

Table 6. Age of household by tenure in Great Britain, 1981 (%)

	Owned outright	Owned with mortgage or loan	Rented from council	Rented from housing association	Privately rented* unfurnished	Privately rented* furnished
Head of household aged 65 or over	44	2	39	3	12	½
All households	23	31	34	2	6	2

Taken from OPCS, *General Household Survey, 1981*, p. 59, Table 3.14.
* A negligible number of elderly households and 3% of all households were in tied accommodation.

lowest among those renting privately (particularly in unfurnished accommodation).[11] A new feature has been the growth in housing association tenancies. Housing associations are non-profit-making organisations providing housing and some date back to the beginning of the century. Their expansion dates from 1964 when the Housing Corporation was set up to make loans to cost-rent and co-ownership housing associations.

Under the Housing Act 1974 the Housing Corporation was given wider powers which included the supervision and registration of housing associations. Local authorities usually nominate about half the tenants to the housing association. In a national survey by the Housing Corporation and DOE of new housing association tenants (*Housing Association Tenants*) in 1978 one-third were elderly people. Some major housing associations such as Anchor and Hanover provide only sheltered housing.

One of the most important roles of a housing association is that of complementing what the local authority does. The Housing Corporation in a 1975 circular, *The Selection of Tenants by Housing Associations for Subsidised Schemes*, was at pains to point out that housing associations should not simply duplicate what local authorities do. A useful role was seen as offering accommodation to a wider range of people than the local authority was able to house (particularly those from the private rented sector) and to concentrate on meeting the needs of particular groups of people for whom inadequate provision was made.

Even more recent are leasehold schemes for the elderly which are being developed experimentally for sheltered housing. Buildings are being erected with the aid of housing association grants which cover 30 per cent of the cost. The elderly person buys a lease at 70 per cent of the value and the lease reverts to the association at the end of the leaseholder's occupation. While the elderly person becomes the leaseholder of the flat the association retains responsibility for the management of the scheme (including, if wanted, a warden service and communal facilities) and for maintenance and repairs.

Amenities

Research in 1965,[12] 1968[13] and the 1971 census showed that many elderly people are inadequately housed. The DOE *NDHS* confirms the expected pattern that younger households tend to share amenities while elderly households are more likely to be without them. For example 59 per cent of the 441,000 households lacking a bath/shower were of pensionable age. Similarly, 56 per cent of the 447,000 households without a hot-water supply were elderly. However, to put the latter figure in perspective the Hunt survey found that 93 per cent of elderly households had a hot-water supply.[14] More worrying was the finding that 12 per cent of households with elderly people had only an outside lavatory.

The older the household the fewer the amenities and the more likely that the elderly person will be in old accommodation. A likely reason is that their incomes are generally lower than those of people in full-time employment.

Types of accommodation

Houses, bungalows and flats The majority of elderly people live in houses or bungalows – 63 per cent in the former and 12 per cent in the latter. Leaving aside those living in flats in converted houses and those in sheltered housing, 8 per cent lived in purpose-built flats and 1 per cent in maisonettes in 1976.[15] It is not known on what floor level these were. The *NDHS* revealed, however, that 15.5 per cent of all households living on the second floor, 16.5 per cent of those on the third floor, 23.5 per cent of those on the fourth to ninth floors and 25 per cent of those on the tenth or higher floors were aged 60 or over.[16]

What many old people, though by no means all, seem to want, is somewhere small and easy to manage. In one survey of preferences among elderly people wishing to move from their present accommodation half would have liked a bungalow. In recent years a higher proportion of public sector stock has been small accommodation following a swing away from the concentration on building three-bedroom family houses that took place between the wars. From 1945 to 1960 small accommodation was 10 per cent of the total, from 1966 to 1971 it was 27 per cent. Since 1970 almost a third of all new building by local authorities has consisted of one-bedroom accommodation, most of which was probably for occupation by old people. But it is by no means certain that these buildings will have the special design features advocated in Circular 82/69.[17]

A survey for the DOE by the Oxford Polytechnic showed that in England and Wales in 1978 approximately 419,000 specially designed units had been provided by local authorities, which was equivalent to 59 per 1,000 population aged 65 and over.[18] Of these approximately 199,000 were provided with a warden service (28 per 1,000 population aged 65 and over) while approximately 221,000 had no warden service (31 per 1,000 population aged 65 and over). They also found that 47,000 units had been built by housing associations, the majority having a warden service. Wide differences between regions and between individual authorities were disclosed, but they point out that their research did not seek explanations of why this should be so.

Housebuilding, however, in both the public and private sectors has dropped steadily in the last few years while the number of small households has increased. It is likely, therefore, that there will be increasing pressure on what small accommodation there is.

Sheltered housing The 5 per cent of elderly people who live in sheltered housing have many advantages. They have their own flat (although not all – particularly in early schemes – are self-contained) or a bungalow with a warden on hand for emergencies. For those who enjoy living in groups with people of their own age this type of living arrangement seems very satisfactory. It has been hailed by some housing managers as the great success story in housing. The fact that schemes are beginning to develop in the private sector is some indication of the demand.

Most of the early literature concerned design features, but in the last few years a more critical approach to the social implications has been apparent. This can be seen both in academic research such as that of Boldy, Abel and Carter,[19] and Page and Muir,[20] and research sponsored by the DOE.[21, 22] Sheltered housing, although excellent for some people, is not quite the panacea that some envisaged, and research published by Byteway and James[23] and by the Leeds

University team[24] as well as others have raised a number of question-marks over the future of sheltered housing.

Three crucial questions relate to the purpose of sheltered housing, the design and layout of schemes and the problem of frail elderly tenants. It is clear from Circular 82/69 that sheltered housing was conceived as a form of accommodation where the elderly could maintain independent lives. The less active were expected to form the main body of the tenants although there was believed to be value in mixing ages and states of dependency. Sheltered housing has been seen as having a preventive role (to prevent people going into Part III accommodation), a social role (primarily for those who are isolated and have no or few relatives) and a housing role in offering an attractive alternative for elderly people who are under-occupying or who need to be rehoused for some other reason. In reality, as Bytheway and James have shown, clear criteria for selection do not appear to be applied[25] and Butler has claimed at the 1979 Institute of Social Welfare Conference that many local authorities no longer attempt to keep a balance between ages and levels of dependency.

On design and layout there has been a good deal of comment that the distinction between categories 1 and 2 is artificial. Some have questioned the need for communal facilities, and research indeed seems to indicate that their use depends to some extent on the warden. Most recent schemes consist of about 30 dwellings, but research has not found that the size of the schemes is an important factor in their success or otherwise.[26]

The question of what should happen to tenants as they become older and more frail is a difficult one. Because they are tenants they cannot be forced to move even though they should really be in Part III accommodation or a hospital. There may also be some difficulty in getting them into this form of care or alternatively securing them adequate domiciliary help. Wardens are becoming more outspoken about the demands on their time, and at least three working parties have reported on whether extra care, such as nursing facilities, should be provided. The Working Party set up by the Abbeyfield Society concluded that extra care must be provided and they are now doing so. But the other two working parties came down against extra care. Anchor Housing Association did not rule out short-term extra help, but considered that when tenants needed continuous nursing they should be moved to some other form of care. In the joint report produced for Age Concern and the NCCOP it was acknowledged that in some schemes wardens did give more care than their role required, but that the solution must be sought in clear liaison with outside groups. However, some local authorities are now providing what has become known as 'very sheltered housing' (i.e. housing plus extra care) on an experimental basis.

The role of the warden has been the subject of much research and comment. The original idea was that the warden should be a good neighbour and, despite evidence that some wardens perform more duties than others, the general conclusion is that the warden should be the enabler and should not perform duties, such as home nursing, that are the responsibility of others.

Granny annexes Another form of special housing is granny annexes. These are self-contained homes next to a family home. The idea is that the elderly person will be able to live independently yet be able to give and receive help from their family next door. In an evaluation by Tinker of local authority schemes some problems of flexibility were found when either the family had to move or the grandparent died.[27] Should the family be asked to move out, or should an unrelated person be moved in? Most local authorities took the latter course and, although relations generally proved good, there were rarely close links between the two households. Private schemes seem to be becoming increasingly popular as families see the advantages of having a grandparent next door. Some owner-occupiers use the granny flat for a nanny, au pair or teenager when they do not need it for a grandparent, or else they just let it.

Hostels Hostels are another type of provision. Shared rather than self-contained accommodation is provided. One variety is provided by the 300 or so Abbeyfield societies where 8–10 elderly people live in bedsitters in one house. A housekeeper provides the main meals.

Comparisons between different types of accommodation

Comparisons between different types of housing for the elderly are in their infancy, but the study done by Wager for the Institute of Municipal Treasurers and Accountants in 1972[28] provided important evidence. The research was limited to Essex where comparison was made of the relative standards of living of those old people in their own homes and those in residential care. It was found that costs for those living in sheltered housing or lower value normal housing allowed, on average, a margin of £3 to £4 per week that could be spent on domiciliary services before reaching the cost of residential care. In more expensive housing the margin was smaller or negative.

The report concluded that for those in need of substantial help a better return would be obtained by selective domiciliary care rather than by an expansion of residential facilities.

In 1973 Plank made a large comparative study for the Greater London Council (GLC) of residents in old people's homes and sheltered housing, and of those on the waiting list for old people's homes and for sheltered housing.[29] Over 2,000 old people were interviewed in this comparison of residential and domiciliary provisions for old people in need of some support. The researchers compared the social advantages and disadvantages and the financial costs of caring for the elderly in these four situations. The conclusion was that the most expensive form of care was residential, followed by sheltered housing and then domiciliary care. But Plank has reservations about his findings [doc 28] and other cost-effective studies have run into problems.

With whom the elderly live

One clear trend is for a growing number of elderly people to live alone. Taking households by type those consisting of one person over retirement age formed 7 per cent of all households in 1961 and 15 per cent in 1976.[30] Numbers are expected to rise further. The forecasts, on current trends, give an increase of 32 per cent for 1971–81 for the elderly compared with 9 per cent for all households.

Over one-third of pensioners in private households in Great Britain in 1981 lived alone and one-half with their spouse. The remainder lived with others. In the case of married couples this was nearly always with their child or children, but for the unmarried it was most likely to be with a sibling. A few lived in households with children.

SOME ISSUES

Assessing and meeting needs

One dilemma facing local authorities and housing associations is how to assess what sort of housing is needed and by whom, and then how these needs may be met. It is also a question that private developers may consider when they decide what to build and where.

The Cullingworth Committee put forward certain criteria to be used by local authorities as a basis for assessing housing need. This included looking at the needs of the whole community and not just of those on the housing list and regardless of whether the solution to any problems lies in their own hands or elsewhere. To avoid confusing 'need' with 'aspiration' the DOE Housing Services Advisory Group in *The Assessment of Housing Requirements* restricted the meaning to include only those households who lacked and required separate accommodation for their well-being and lived in accommodation which was not up to socially acceptable standards of fitness, the five basic amenities and space.[31]

One way of finding out about needs is being aware of, and participating in, general research which shows national, regional or even local trends. For example, national forecasts show that it is likely that there will be some reallocation between tenures and that local authorities will have increased demand (mainly because of the decline of the private rented sector). But there are many problems in this type of forecasting because of the complexities of the housing market. Trying to forecast potential households is particularly fraught with hazards, and so is forecasting the type of provision.

Another way that the local authority may become aware of the needs of their community is by pursuing their own researches and carrying out local studies. But the evidence of a survey by Sumner and Smith of services provided for the elderly by local authorities was that only a few surveyed their own needs, and when it came to selecting tenants again only a few went outside their housing list. The study concluded that 'local authorities did not see the point of seeking out unexpressed needs when there were already more expressed needs than they had resources to provide for'.[32]

Once needs are assessed the best method of meeting them has to be decided. This may not necessarily be by local authority provision. It has become more widely accepted that local authorities should take a wider view and in 1978 the DOE Housing Services Advisory Group spelt out what this means in *Organising a Comprehensive Housing Service*. They also pointed out that the introduction of Housing Strategies and Investment Programmes (HIPs) further highlights the need for integrated housing policies.

Local authorities use a number of different methods for allocating accommodation. Some work on a points basis, some work strictly on a date order of first come first served while others have separate categories for different people and different types of accommodation. In 1978 the DOE Housing Services Advisory Group in *Allocation of Council Housing* suggested various criteria such as the need to treat applicants equitably and to be easily understood by both applicants and staff. Specific recommendations were made about elderly people.

It may be necessary to treat special groups in a special way for housing, but that does not necessarily mean that they will need special types of housing. Some may need a special design, or special location or to be grouped in a special way, but not all. The larger the variety of provision the wider the choice. Nor should the assumption be made that those who are already housed are necessarily in the most appropriate form of accommodation. Plank found that wardens assessed that over a quarter of their tenants did not require sheltered housing. At the same time social workers assessed that nearly a third of those on waiting lists for Part III accommodation required sheltered housing rather than a residential place.[33] The accommodation may be the wrong size, in an inconvenient place or lack amenities.

It may indeed be possible to solve some of these housing problems simply through a more flexible and sensitive use of existing stock and without much new building. Even a small amount of building of one- and two-bedroom homes may lead to a general shifting round of people to a more appropriate size of accommodation. But this raises the question of under-occupation, where accommodation is located and whether elderly people should be encouraged to move.

Under-occupation

Many elderly occupy only a part of their home after their family die or move away. This can be a problem to them when it comes to decorating, cleaning and heating. The *GHS* (1977) shows that 67 per cent of individuals and 80 per cent of couples aged 60 or over have accommodation with one or more bedrooms in excess of their requirements. But this is on the basis that a couple need only one bedroom. Age Concern suggest that a more realistic standard is one bedroom for each elderly member of a household. Under-occupation is more prevalent and extensive in the private sector and above all among owner-occupiers. For such people home repairs can be a financial problem.

There may be a shortage of accommodation for families in those same areas where the elderly are under-occupying. Yet many local authorities do nothing to encourage the elderly to move. Sumner and Smith's case study of 41 local authorities showed that more than half did not use compulsion, persuasion or inducement of any kind.[34] The reasons are not hard to seek. There is a general reluctance to persuade elderly people to move from a home in which they have lived for many years.

Location and design

When physical mobility decreases, and the likelihood of owning a car diminishes, the location of the home near facilities becomes of vital importance.

There are a number of problems to be solved in designing small units of accommodation which are suitable for all ages, but there is no reason why some of the features specially recommended for the elderly, such as high electric sockets, should not always be provided.

Moving

General   About 7 per cent of the population move each year and of these about 10 per cent are elderly. Hunt found that 20 per cent of elderly people had lived for less than 10 years in their present neighbourhood. Not all old people find it easy to move to a local authority dwelling because they lack a residential qualification. Local authorities were advised in the 1977 Housing Green Paper that no one should be precluded from applying, or being considered for a council tenancy on any ground whatsoever.[35] Some local authorities have used their powers to provide grants to help with the removal costs of their tenants.

While many move willingly this is not always the case. For example in a study of sheltered housing tenants reported at the Institute of Social Welfare Conference, 1979, Butler and Oldman found that nearly one-third would have preferred to have remained in their own homes. The possibility of remaining where they are, perhaps with adaptations, insulation or extra domiciliary help should always be examined before a decision to move is taken.

To another tenure   There are several reasons why people may wish to switch tenure as they become elderly. They may, for example, have to give up tied accommodation when their employment ends. They may be worried about the upkeep of their own home and garden and willingly accept a council or housing association tenancy. They may need some special form of accommodation only provided in the public sector. It is also interesting that in 1975 a survey of tenure preference in two years' time showed that about 10 per cent more of the 55s and over would have liked to have been owner-occupiers,[36] but insufficient resources may prove insurmountable. Some of the new forms of tenure such as equity sharing (the purchase of a leasehold interest in part of the value of a house), co-ownership and housing co-operatives may prove attractive to the elderly. One new form of equity sharing – 'leasehold schemes for the elderly' – has already been mentioned earlier in Chapter 3.

To a retirement area   While the majority of older people remain in the same neighbourhood others may choose to move to the seaside, country or other retirement area. In some cases this movement has been encouraged by the local authority. For example the GLC has built bungalows outside London for older people to retire to.

Retirement migration may have some effect on the recipient area and therefore on the elderly who move there. This is shown in studies of the effect on small towns in Norfolk and Suffolk and on the seaside resorts of Morecambe and Llandudno. Karn in *Retiring to the Seaside* found that while the majority of the sample were happy in their new environment, and would have made the same decision again, there were problems for the health and social services which were well below the national average and were under enormous pressure [doc 29]. Karn and Law and Warnes in their retirement studies have established that elderly migrants are less likely to have younger relatives who can help them. These elderly movers are predominantly owner-occupiers, are childless or have few children and retire at or before pensionable age.

To be near relatives   One of the groups identified by both the Cullingworth Committee [doc 30] and in the Housing Green Paper as wanting to move was elderly people wanting to join relatives or their family.[37] In most cases this was to enable them to give mutual help. In Hunt's survey the major reason given for moving (by 40 per cent of movers) was to be near relatives. In a study of every housing authority in England and Wales and a number of housing associations, Tinker in *Housing the Elderly near Relatives* found that although many elderly people already lived near their families, there was a demand from those who did not to move closer.[38] Two groups of elderly people who faced particular problems over moving were owner-occupiers who wanted to move into council accommodation in their own area and people from any tenure who wanted to rent in another local authority area.

Some groups in need

Four groups of elderly people who may be particularly vulnerable in the housing market are the disabled, owner-occupiers, the homeless and tenants in tied accommodation.

The disabled The elderly figure prominently among the disabled, but their housing problems may differ widely. Evidence about the housing conditions of the disabled is given in Buckle's *Work and Housing of Impaired Persons in Great Britain*.[39] In general she found that accommodation was neither better nor worse than for the rest of the population. However, 10 per cent of people were unable to use part of the accommodation because of disability. The DOE Housing Services Advisory Group's *The Assessment of Housing Requirements* advised that for many disabled people, the adaptation of the dwellings in which they live usually provide the quickest, cheapest and best solution.[40] Much more help has been available for adaptations of housing both in the public and private sector, especially since the Housing Act 1974. Apart from the whole range of house renovation grants (improvement, intermediate and repairs) power to help with adaptations had been available through both housing departments and social service departments. In a circular published in 1978, *Adaptations of Housing for People who are Physically Handicapped*, housing authorities were asked to accept responsibility for structural modifications and social services, under the Chronically Sick and Disabled Persons Act 1970, for non-structural features and aids.

The Advisory Group also argued that, for those who rely on the public sector, 'mobility housing' is suitable.[41] This is normal housing with low-cost adaptations such as level thresholds and ramped access. They consider that for the very disabled 'wheelchair housing', which has extra space and other provisions, might be needed, but at most for 1 per 1,000 population.[42]

Owner-occupiers Elderly owner-occupiers may face particular problems. Among those identified by the Cullingworth Committee were physical inability to cope with maintenance, cleaning, stairs or garden, too large accommodation, financial problems of upkeep, the need to move to a more convenient area and inability to cope with improvements.[43]

Some specific problems faced by this group in addition to those mentioned above are lack of knowledge about the grant system, difficulty in finding builders to carry out the work and dislike of the upheaval of having workmen in the house. There is, however, more assistance available than is sometimes realised, though this may vary from area to area.

What elderly owner-occupiers who wish to move may want is a smaller home. The National Economic Development Office in

Housing for All (1977) has noted that private developers have failed to provide dwellings for smaller households on any appreciable scale. Nor has there been very much in the way of private sheltered housing.

The homeless Surprise is often expressed that some elderly people are homeless. But in one of the most detailed studies carried out the elderly figured prominently. A survey for the NAB *Homeless Single Persons* (1966), found that of those sleeping rough (nearly 1,000) 18 per cent of the men were 60 and over. Of the 25,490 users of lodging-houses and hostels 35 per cent of these men and 39 per cent of these women were 60 or over. In addition 12 per cent of men and 3 per cent of women who used reception centres were 60 or over. In a follow-up survey in 1972, 32 per cent of men using lodging-houses and hostels were over 60 and 36 per cent of women.

Under the Housing (Homeless Persons) Act 1977 specific duties are laid on housing departments, and categories of homeless people who, for the purpose of the Act, have to be regarded as having priority needs for accommodation are distinguished. In the first half of 1982 there were elderly people in 8 per cent of the households for whom English local authorities accepted responsibility under the Housing (Homeless Persons) Act 1977. The code of guidance asks local authorities to treat as vulnerable those above or approaching retirement age who are frail, in poor health or vulnerable for any other reason.

Tenants in tied accommodation Those who live in accommodation provided by their employers generally lose their right to their home when they stop working. Their employer may try to help them find alternative accommodation, but he will need their home for his next employee. Some elderly people will have managed to save for a retirement home, but others will have to apply to a local authority or housing association for a tenancy. The Hunt survey found that those who lived rent free came out as worse than average, e.g. for heating and hot-water supply.

The need for advice

Over many of the issues just discussed, such as whether to move or not and how to get repairs done, advice is pertinent. Advice may also be needed by elderly people who rent. There is some evidence, such as that produced by Age Concern, Greater London, that the elderly do not use housing advice centres to any great extent.[44] It is important to ensure that the staff in housing departments, housing advice centres and housing associations are fully briefed on the needs of the elderly and the means available to help them.

Links with other services

To offer choice and to avoid duplication and omissions, housing and social service departments and health authorities need to collaborate to plan whatever services are appropriate for their areas. Account should also be taken of the contribution of housing associations. In the overall planning of particular forms of housing and especially over the criteria for acceptance to sheltered housing and Part III accommodation co-operation is essential. Staff in each agency must be clear about this policy. The Royal Commission on the NHS pointed to examples where there had not been collaboration[45] and similar points were noted in the Scottish Development Department's *Housing and Social Work: a joint approach* (1975).

There are a number of other issues in housing which have been discussed previously. For problems of heating see Chapter 6, and for questions of financial help through rent rebates, etc. see Chapter 5.

REFERENCES

1. DHSS, *A Happier Old Age*, see Ch. 3 note 61, p. 9.
2. CHANCELLOR OF THE EXCHEQUER, *Provision for Old Age*, see Ch. 4 note 14, p. 71.
3. TOWNSEND, *The Last Refuge*, see Ch. 4 note 1.
4. PLANK, D., *Caring for the Elderly: A report of a study of various means of caring for dependent elderly people in eight London boroughs*, Greater London Council Research Memorandum, GLC, 1977.
5. MHLG, *Housing Standards and Costs: accommodation specially designed for old people*, MHLG Circular 82/69, WO Circular 84/69, HMSO, 1969.
6. DOE, *Housing for Old People: a Consultative Paper*, DOE, 1976.
7. MHLG, Cullingworth Committee, see Ch. 4 note 4.
8. DOE, *Housing Policy – A Consultative Document*, HMSO, 1977.
9. DOE, *National Dwelling and Housing Survey*, HMSO, 1978.
10. HUNT, see Ch. 2 note 3.
11. DOE, *National Dwelling and Housing Survey*, p. 36.

12. TUNSTALL, see Ch. 3 note 8.

13. MHLG, Cullingworth Committee, see Ch. 4 note 4.

14. HUNT, see Ch. 2 note 3, p. 7.

15. *Ibid.*, p. 41.

16. DOE, *National Dwelling and Housing Survey*, p. 45.

17. MHLG, *Housing Standards*.

18. DOE and WO, *Report on a Survey of Accommodation for Old People provided by Local Authorities and Housing Associations in England and Wales*, DOE, 1980.

19. BOLDY, D., ABEL, P. and CARTER, K., *The Elderly in Grouped Dwellings – A Profile*, University of Exeter, 1973.

20. PAGE and MUIR, see Ch. 4 note 13.

21. ATTENBURROW, J., *Grouped Housing for the Elderly*, Department of the Environment, Building Research Establishment, 1976.

22. DOE, *Housing for the Elderly – the size of grouped schemes*, HMSO, 1975.

23. BYTHEWAY, W. and JAMES, L., *The Allocation of Sheltered Housing*, University College of Swansea, Medical Sociology Research Centre, 1978.

24. BUTLER, A., OLDMAN, C. and WRIGHT, R., *Sheltered Housing for the Elderly: a critical review*, University of Leeds, Department of Social Policy and Administration, Research Monograph, 1979.

25. BYTHEWAY and JAMES, *op. cit.*, p. 104.

26. DOE, *Housing for the Elderly*, p. 3.

27. TINKER, A., *Housing the Elderly: how successful are granny annexes?*, DOE, Housing Development Directorate, Occasional Paper 1/76, 1976 (HMSO, 1980).

28. WAGER, see Ch. 3 note 57.

29. PLANK, *op. cit.*

30. CSO, *Social Trends* (No. 13), see Ch. 2 note 12, p. 24.

31. DOE, Housing Services Advisory Group, *The Assessment of Housing Requirements*, DOE, 1977.

32. SUMNER and SMITH, see Ch. 3 note 52, p. 163.

33. PLANK, *op. cit.*

34. SUMNER and SMITH, see Ch. 3 note 52.

35. DOE, *Housing Policy*.

36. CSO, *Social Trends* (No. 9), see Ch. 2 note 15, p. 149.

37. DOE, *Housing Policy*.

38. TINKER, A., *Housing the Elderly near Relatives: moving and other options*, DOE, Housing Development Directorate, Occasional Paper 1/80, HMSO, 1980.

39. BUCKLE, J., *Work and Housing of Impaired Persons in Great Britain*, OPCS, Social Survey Division, HMSO, 1971.
40. DOE, *Assessment of Housing Requirements*.
41. GOLDSMITH, S., *Mobility Housing*, DOE, Housing Development Directorate, Occasional Paper 2/74, 1974 (HMSO, 1980).
42. GOLDSMITH, S., *Wheelchair Housing*, DOE, Housing Development Directorate, Occasional Paper 2/75, 1975 (HMSO, 1980).
43. MHLG, Cullingworth Committee, see Ch. 4 note 4, p. 101.
44. AGE CONCERN (Greater London), *Housing Advice for the Elderly*, Age Concern, 1975.
45. ROYAL COMMISSION ON THE NHS, see Ch. 6 note 33, p. 260.

Chapter eight
PERSONAL AND OTHER SOCIAL SERVICES

THE DEVELOPMENT OF LOCAL SOCIAL SERVICES

Before 1971

In comparison with services concerned with income maintenance, health and housing, local personal social services are of more recent origin. Much of the provision before 1946 was by voluntary bodies. One of the first post-war Acts to give local authorities powers to intervene in this field was the National Health Service Act 1946 which among other things allowed local authorities to employ home helps [doc 31]. It also gave very general powers for the care and aftercare of persons suffering from illness and for preventive measures relating to health. So services such as chiropody and laundry became possible.

Under the National Assistance Act 1948 local authorities were enabled to make arrangements for 'promoting the welfare' of people who were deaf, dumb, blind or substantially handicapped [doc 32]. The provision of workshops, hostels and recreational facilities were specifically mentioned. Elderly people who came into any of these categories benefited from this legislation. Power was also given to local authorities to make contributions to the funds of voluntary bodies providing meals or recreation for old people [doc 32].

Under the 1948 Act a duty was laid on local authorities to make accommodation available for all persons who by reason of age, infirmity or any other circumstances are in need of care and attention not otherwise available to them [doc 33]. Because residential accommodation is provided under Part III of this Act it is usually just referred to as Part III. Some local authorities had been providing residential care on an experimental basis, but they now inherited from public assistance committees large workhouses. Local authorities were also given power to provide residential care in homes run by voluntary bodies.

Under the National Assistance Act 1948 (Amendment) Act 1962 local authorities were themselves enabled to provide meals and recreation for old people in their homes or elsewhere, as well as day centres, clubs and recreational workshops. They might, however, continue to employ voluntary bodies as agents, if they so wished.

It has been noted (Ch. 4) that the development of local services was seen as being complementary to the hospital service. In 1962 local authorities were asked by the Ministry of Health to draw up plans for local health and welfare services for the next 10 years. The advice given (in Circular 2/62, *Development of Local Authority Health and Welfare Services*) was that:

Services for the elderly should be designed to help them to remain in their own homes as long as possible. For this purpose adequate supporting services must be available, including home nurses, domestic help, chiropody and temporary residential care. These supporting services will also often be needed for those who live in special housing where there is a resident warden. Residential homes are required for those who, for some reason, short of a need for hospital care, cannot manage on their own, even in special housing with a resident warden.

Specific standards were not laid down.

Sumner and Smith's survey of 24 health and welfare authorities and 41 housing authorities in England, Wales and Scotland, *Planning Local Authority Services for the Elderly*, concluded that there had been a very considerable growth of local authority services for the elderly between 1945 and 1965.[1] But planning of these services was at an embryonic stage largely because of lack of basic information, lack of the means to obtain information, doubts about the best way to provide for the elderly and lack of confidence in central government. Wider-ranging recommendations were made about a possible approach to planning.[2]

The general power for local authorities to provide welfare services for the elderly was not given until 1968 in the Health Services and Public Health Act 1968 [doc 34]. These powers did not come into force until 1971. They include powers to provide home helps, visiting, social work and warden services, arrangements to inform elderly people about services and to carry out adaptations. Local authorities may use voluntary bodies as agents and may make charges. Another section of the 1968 Act which came into effect in 1971 made mandatory the provision of domestic help on an adequate scale. Power was also given to provide laundry services.

The Local Authority Social Services Act and after

Concern about the lack of a co-ordinated approach to the family by the local authority, which meant that welfare departments were responsible for the elderly and mentally disordered, children's departments for children and health, for home helps and other domiciliary provision, was one of the reasons for the appointment of a committee in 1965 'to review the organisation and responsibilities of the local authority personal social services in England and Wales, and to consider what changes are desirable to secure an effective family service'. Its report *Local Authority and Allied Personal Social Services* (the Seebohm Report) was published in 1968.[3] Its main recommendation concerning administration was the establishment of a single social service department in each authority and this took place in 1971 following the Local Authority Social Services Act 1970.

The overall philosophy of the Report was that the new departments should be less concerned simply to meet individual needs in crises and more concerned about ensuring a co-ordinated and comprehensive approach to people's problems [doc 35], detecting need and encouraging people to seek help. In this way they would be better able to attract and use resources and to plan systematically for the future.[4] Another reason for the setting up of a single department was the belief of the Seebohm Committee that the piecemeal and haphazard development of services was unlikely to use scarce resources to the best advantage. The need to support families caring for old people was also a consideration [doc 35].

Following the Act the main services for the elderly for which social service departments became responsible were: provision of domestic help, residential accommodation, general welfare, meals and recreation, registration of old people's homes and social work support.

Another change which came about as a result of the Seebohm Report was the increase in the number of generic social workers.

Developments since 1972 have included further attempts at long-term planning. In 1972 (Circular 35/72) 10-year plans were requested by the DHSS for health and social care and in 1977 3-year plans were introduced. Financial constraints have subsequently made planning more difficult.

THE DISABLED

Evidence has already been presented about disability increasing with age (Ch. 6). Because the largest number of physically disabled in any age group are among the elderly (65% of the sample in Harris' *Handicapped and Impaired in Great Britain* were over 65),[5] it is appropriate to consider any special provision that has been made for this group. Generalisations about the disabled are as dangerous as those about the elderly. Elderly people with impaired hearing or vision may need different services to those in wheelchairs. There is also a distinction between physical impairment which can be clinically assessed (e.g. loss of a limb) and the degree of handicap or disadvantage which the person suffers as a result of this disability (see Sainsbury, *Measuring Disability*).[6] Handicap has some relationship to a number of environmental variables and so is not capable of exact measurement. Most services, therefore, are based on the degree of disablement, e.g. mobility allowance on impaired locomotor mobility. Housing has already been touched on (Ch. 7) and will not be discussed further.

The main way in which provision can be made is under the Chronically Sick and Disabled Persons Act 1970, although local authorities had responsibilities under the National Assistance Act 1948 to promote the welfare of handicapped people. The 1970 Act extended these powers and placed a duty on local authorities to find out the numbers of disabled people in their area, to publicise the services available and, where there was need, provide services described in the Act. These included practical assistance in the home (including aids such as walking frames), television and radio, help with travel, holidays, meals, telephones and adaptations to the home. The latter is now the main responsibility of housing departments (see Ch. 7). Three-quarters of all households for which aids, adaptations or telephones have been provided contain an elderly disabled person. A DHSS circular (12/70) stated that local authorities were to assess need in the light of their resources. Charges may be made for services. Occupational therapists are skilled at assessing these needs and are valuable members of social service teams.

The main thrust of official advice has been for the provision of domiciliary and other services to enable the disabled to remain in their own homes, but there is considerable evidence that provision is patchy. Links with voluntary bodies are proving invaluable. The Crossroads Care Attendant Scheme which was pioneered in Rugby is one such link. Care attendants provide the sort of regular help that would be expected of relatives and act as a support to families caring for a severely handicapped person.

Financial provisions for certain categories of the disabled include a mobility allowance for people unable to walk, a non-contributory invalidity pension and an attendance allowance (a non-contributory benefit paid to someone who is severely disabled and needs frequent attention or continual supervision).

DOMICILIARY SERVICES

General

The purpose of domiciliary services is to provide help to people in their own homes so that they can remain there. Townsend and Wedderburn saw their role in this way: 'The domiciliary services therefore perform two main positive functions. They furnish expert professional help which the family cannot supply, and they furnish unskilled or semi-skilled help for persons who do not have families and whose families living in the household or nearby are not always able or available to help.'[7]

This role of providing services for the elderly who have no relatives and of supplementing what the family does came out again in the study by Shanas *et al.*[8] *The Times* leader (28.6.68) commented on this study: 'For many old people they [domiciliary services] complement the care provided by the family – in supplying meals, for instance, while an only child is out at work all day; or skilled attention such as nursing or chiropody.'

Standards for these services are laid down by the DHSS (Ch. 12). Because of the difficulties of increasing residential care the DHSS suggested in 1977 that the need for meals, home helps and chiropody services would be greater than previously envisaged.[9] Guidelines and provision in 1976 are shown in Table 7.

In a comparison of changes in provision of social services for the elderly, Bebbington[10] has compared the situation in 1965 based on *The Aged in the Welfare State*[11] with that in 1976 based on *The Elderly at Home*.[12] He concludes that there has been an enormous expansion in domiciliary services (e.g. twice as many people received a home help and meals on wheels) especially for the very elderly. More old people lived alone, there seemed increasing incapacity and there was some evidence (e.g. home helps) that a large number were receiving the service, though at the expense of people receiving it less frequently.

Hunt's findings on visits received from social services and similar bodies during the last six months of 1976 were that, as was the

Table 7. Local authority personal social services for the elderly in England (average level of provision and expenditure per head 1975–76)

Service	Population base	Level of provision (per 1,000 appropriate population)		Cost per occupied place, available place, meal or staff (£)	Expenditure per head of population (£)
		Departmental guidelines	1975–76 Out-turn		
		Available places	*Available places*	*Occupied place*	
Residential	65 years and over	25.0	18.1	1,210	20.8
Day care	65 years and over	3–4	2.6	560	1.5
		Staff (WTE)*	*Staff (WTE)**	*Staff (WTE)**	
Home helps	65 years and over	12.0	6.5	2,210	14.3
Social workers	Total†	Not laid down	0.44	4,590	2.0
		Meals/wk	*Meals/wk*	*Meal*	
Meals	65 years and over	200	119	0.34	2.1
Aids, adaptations, etc.	Total†	Not laid down	Not applicable	Not applicable	0.26

* WTE = Whole Time Equivalent.
† Total = all age groups.

Figures taken from DHSS, *Priorities in the Health and Social Services: the way forward*, HMSO, 1977, p. 24.

case with personal tasks, those who appeared to be in greatest need were more likely to have received help, but not all appeared to have received all the help they needed.[13]

Home helps

There is evidence from numerous studies that the home help services are the most popular and effective elements of community care.

Home helps undertake a range of tasks including cleaning, laundering, shopping and cooking, and sometimes give help with dressing and washing. They also often informally provide companionship and advice. Almost 90 per cent of the users of home helps are elderly people.

The service expanded rapidly and by 1949 all the English and Welsh local authorities provided home helps. Guidelines laid down by the DHSS in 1977 specified that there should be 12 home helps per 1,000 population over the age of 65, but in 1975/76 the national average was only 6.5 (Table 7). In 1966, 329,000 cases were attended in England and Wales and by 1977 it had risen to 619,000. Research suggests that there is a substantial amount of unmet need. Townsend and Wedderburn in 1965 considered that at least another 10 per cent of their sample needed a home help in addition to those already receiving one.[14] A doubling of the service was required suggested Harris in her 1965/66 survey.[15] A survey, *The Home Help Service in England and Wales*, carried out in 1967 for the Government Social Survey said that: 'There are probably at least as many households in need of home help among the elderly population as are currently receiving it. (This is on the basis of the current standards and makes no allowance for extending the service to people who are ineligible by these standards.)'[16] Taking into account other groups the conclusion was that, in order to satisfy the unmet needs of present recipients and to provide help for those eligible but not receiving it, the size of the service would need to be increased to between two and three times that at present. In 1976 Hunt found that 8.9 (1981-9) per cent of her sample had a home help during the past six months and commented: 'Although those groups who appear on the face of it to be in greatest need of home help are most likely to receive it, in all these groups a majority do not do so.'[17]

One difficulty is how to assess the extent of need, but local authorities are under a duty to make provision 'on such a scale as is adequate for the needs of their area'. Other problems include restrictions on the number of visits elderly people receive per week –

spreading the service thinly – and charges which may deter some elderly people in need. Also, despite the excellent support home helps give in the majority of cases there are many tasks such as redecorating, gardening and household repairs, which are outside their scope. *The Home Help Service in England and Wales* commented on the tasks which home helps were not equipped to do and for which outside help was essential.[18]

Meals

Meals, usually lunch, are provided for old people either at day centres or clubs or are delivered to their homes. Sometimes a meal is cooked by a neighbour who may receive payment from the local authority. Among the purposes of the provision of meals are the nutritional one and that of enabling someone to keep an eye on recipients to make sure all is well. The meals service is a good example of co-operation between local authorities and voluntary bodies. Much of the distribution is done by the latter, particularly the Women's Royal Voluntary Service. As we have seen earlier, voluntary provision came first and local authorities were given powers to contribute to their costs under the National Assistance Act 1948. One of the suggestions put forward in a research report by the Social Survey in 1959 on *Meals on Wheels Services* was that local authorities should be responsible for administering 'meals on wheels' services. In 1962 this Act was amended to allow local authorities to provide meals themselves, as well as widening their powers to help voluntary bodies with the cost of vehicles, equipment, premises and staff.

Guidelines by the DHSS in 1977 for meals were 200 for every 1,000 old people over the age of 65. In 1975/76 119 were provided (Table 7). But there has been a slight increase in the proportion of people receiving more meals. Whereas in 1970 in England and Wales 60 per cent of a sample in one week received only one or two meals per week and 17 per cent five or more meals, in 1978 50 per cent received one to two and 22 per cent five or more.[19] Many more very old people now receive the service. Hunt found that while 2.6 per cent of all old people received meals on wheels, for those aged 85 and over it was 11.5 per cent. In 1981 the figures were 3 and 12 per cent.

Research is being carried out on the social and economic aspects of the meals-on-wheels service and some local authorities have looked at how need can be assessed and at the current organisation of the service. Some authorities raise doubts about the nutritional value of the meals, about the value of the surveillance when visits only take place infrequently, and also more fundamental questions about whether provision of meals can sometimes increase dependency.

Day centres and clubs

Day care is care provided on a daily basis not in the elderly person's home. Attendance may be daily or less frequently. Sometimes this is provided in a day hospital (see Ch. 6), sometimes in a residential home and sometimes in a day centre.

Voluntary organisations are the biggest providers of clubs for the elderly and a wide range of recreational facilities is offered. There is usually a regular membership. For elderly people who do not want to attend any of the day facilities some authorities and voluntary organisations have opened premises where people can drop in without having to join. They are called by various names – rest centres, drop-ins, pop-in parlours. In 1977 there were 22,100 day-centre places, including those at residential homes. DHSS guidelines in 1977 were three to four places for every 1,000 elderly persons aged 65 years and over. Provision in 1975/76 was between two and three. In 1981 5 per cent of elderly people attended a day centre.

The purpose of day centres and clubs is to provide a means of social contact and recreation, and in some of the former other services such as meals, laundry facilities and chiropody are available. Services provided may be for different sorts of need, including physical (meals, chiropody, etc.), emotional (companionship, advice, etc.), recreational (drama, choir, etc.) and further education. Day care may also be helpful in relieving relatives of their care of an elderly person for a few hours each day.

In *Day Care*, a survey of the facilities provided, Morley concluded that there is a 'profusion of activity, perhaps not always being handled to the best advantage of the elderly'.[20] (For example, the need for lunch clubs may not be quite the same if there is a good meals-on-wheels service. She felt that 'real choice' should be available – not one thing in one part of the area and another in another – which may make provision appear better than it is.) She also identified a number of problems such as transport and location and type of buildings. The value of day care is underlined in more recent research and some problems are identified.[21] Help the Aged is one organisation that has campaigned vigorously for more day centres, notably in *The Case for Day Centres: an urgent report* (1975).

Good neighbour and similar schemes

Although the official Good Neighbour Campaign sprang into life in 1976 good neighbour, street warden and similar schemes had been in existence for many years. Some are run entirely by voluntary bodies, but some social service departments contribute money or staff to help. The campaign's aim, in the words of their secretary, was not to supplant but to strengthen the good work being done by health and social services and the voluntary organisations through the promotion of mutual concern and mutual care. Many schemes are designed to help the elderly, but in others they are themselves the helpers.

The reasons for visiting elderly people in their homes may vary. They range from just talking to shopping and cooking. It is interesting that a DHSS circular (5/70) *Organisation of Meals on Wheels* in 1970 emphasised the desirability of good neighbour services because of the value of the home-cooked meal. Meals on wheels were 'inevitably a second-best service' but were needed for a number of reasons, including the reliability of the service. In some cases good neighbours undertake household tasks such as repairs or gardening.

Telephones and alarm systems

Old people, particularly those living alone and those who find difficulty in getting out of their homes, may need to summon help in an emergency. They may also want to communicate with professionals such as their doctor or with relatives, friends and shopkeepers.

The most versatile means of two-way communication is the telephone. Many local authorities now supply these to elderly people under the Chronically Sick and Disabled Persons Act 1970. Before the Act telephones had been provided in Hull for some time for the elderly and poor disabled and the scheme there was evaluated by Gregory in *Telephones for the Elderly*. In a comparison of people who had had a telephone installed and a control group without one, he concluded:

In terms of expected, reported and objectively demonstrated use, there seems therefore a strong case for the provision of telephones to the elderly on a wider basis. The core of the case rests with the impact on life-and-death emergency situations, although there is evidence that a service even if provided primarily for this purpose would also benefit the social life of the housebound and poor elderly (they would feel less lonely) and would ease the problems involved for such people in obtaining food and other services.[22]

A growing number of local authorities are providing alarm systems. Some are speech systems allowing the elderly person to say what the problem is, while others provide different types of sign (usually saying 'Help') which can be put in a window or, if a permanent installation, which lights up. Not everyone is happy about the signs because they might sometimes draw the attention of some unscrupulous person to one who is very vulnerable. Other types of alarm are buzzers and bells which will alert a neighbour, passer-by or (in a few cases) a central point.

Holidays

An increasing number of elderly people, who might not otherwise have had a holiday, have been able to enjoy one through schemes organised by local authorities. Before 1962 they had no power to do this and any schemes there were were mostly organised by voluntary associations. Some authorities meet the cost of a holiday taken independently, but most offer holidays for groups of old people Some run their own homes but more use ordinary holiday accommodation, usually out-of-season in the spring or autumn. In some schemes the organisation and accommodation are provided by voluntary bodies while the authority (social services department) selects the individuals and pays all or part of the cost.

A study by Stone, *Local Authority Holidays for the Elderly and Physically Handicapped*, in 1973 described some schemes and explored ways in which they might develop.[23]

BOARDING OUT

A small number of local authority social service departments search out suitable private households where an elderly person can live as a boarder. This form of care is used extensively for children but rarely for the elderly. Where there have been schemes they are often labelled by the Press 'rent a granny' or 'foster a granny'.

In a handful of towns voluntary organisations ran schemes like this in the late 1940s, but there is little public provision. A survey by Rattee in 1977 of all social service departments in England and Wales revealed that less than 10 per cent had a scheme operating. Rattee concluded that boarding out in the short term allows a family to have a break or holiday and longer-term schemes may free a hospital bed, or provide home care for someone who refuses residential care. Schemes are now being monitored further in a DHSS-sponsored research project at the University of Leeds.

SOCIAL WORK SUPPORT

Before the creation of social service departments most statutory work with the elderly was done by welfare officers from the welfare department of the local authority, few of whom were professionally qualified. The Seebohm Committee recommended a radical altera-tion to the pattern of specialisation whereby social workers, many of whom were unqualified, dealt only with one client group.[24] They suggested that a generic training should be followed by the under-taking of a wide range of functions. The Younghusband Committee in *The Report of the Working Party on Social Workers* had previously (in 1959) also come down in favour of a generic approach. However, it was considered that some specialisation would be necessary above the basic field level.

A study for the DHSS, *Social Service Teams: the practitioner's view* by Stevenson and Parsloe in 1978, found that four types of specialisation have developed: informal specialisation within social work teams, formal specialisation at practitioner level, organisational specialism at team level (e.g. sub-teams concerned with particular groups of clients) and formal 'advisory' specialisms outside the teams.[25] They also found social workers to be preoccupied with the needs of families and children to the exclusion of other groups such as the elderly and physically disabled. The BASW found that many agencies seem to give the elderly a low priority and often workers with little experience or training are expected to undertake all, or a large proportion of, the work with this group.

The nature and aims of social work are a matter of controversy. The Younghusband Committee saw them as to help 'individuals or families with various problems, and to overcome or lessen these so that they may achieve a better personal, family or social adjustment'. The worker's function might include assessing the problems, and offering appropriate help of a practical or supportive nature (e.g. practical assistance, giving information or bringing about environ-mental changes). Stevenson and Parsloe described case-work as 'broadly concerned with helping the individual or family with a range of problems rather than narrowly directed to discussing the client's emotional functioning and interpersonal relationships'.[26]

A more detailed statement by the BASW laying down guidelines for work with the elderly also gave a summary of the role of the qualified social worker [doc 36]. This role was based on social work values of acceptance, self-determination and confidentiality.

The assessment of social work support has only been attempted by a few researchers. One which took place between 1965 and 1970 by Goldberg and others found that trained social workers did not bring about any further change in physical circumstances but did create a general improvement in morale.[27] Brearley in *Social Work, Ageing and Society* has stressed the danger of limited crisis intervention and the value of 'restoring a normal, ongoing process of growing old, with the satisfactions that this will imply'.[28]

There are no DHSS guidelines for the provision of social workers, but the level of provision per 1,000 population in 1975/76 was 0.44 (Table 7). The Hunt survey found that 3.9 per cent of elderly people had been visited by a council welfare officer during the past six months. But as 'welfare officer' was not defined it may include social services, housing and other local authority personnel.

RESIDENTIAL CARE

Residential homes for the elderly are provided by both local authorities and voluntary bodies. In 1981 there were about 6,000 homes in England and Wales with about 170,300 residents aged 65 and over. Of these, 110,400 were in homes provided by local authorities, 14,100 in accommodation provided for local authorities by voluntary and private homes and 45,800 in voluntary and private homes. Provision is below DHSS guidelines (Table 7). Some old people also live in private guest-houses, some of which it is alleged are in effect residential homes, but not registered as such. Conditions in these vary greatly. A homes advice service is offered by CPA to all voluntary and private old people's homes about matters relating to their management and improvement.

Residential care is only for old people who, even with domiciliary support, cannot manage to live in the community, but who still do not need hospital care. The respective roles of residential home and hospital were laid down by the MOH 15.9.65 Memorandum for Local Authorities and Hospital Authorities, *Care of the Elderly in Hospitals and Residential Homes*. Evidence has already been presented that some elderly people were in residential care only because of the lack of alternative housing, e.g. Townsend in *The Last Refuge* [doc 37]. More recently a DHSS study, *Residential Care for the Elderly in London*, came to a similar conclusion. A survey of 93 local authority, 18 voluntary and 13 private homes found many cases of residents whom the staff thought would have been more suitably placed in other accommodation, such as sheltered housing.[29] They also found that one-third of the homes had some residents who should have been in hospital.

The argument for a move away from residential care is, as Stapleton has argued, two-fold: 'Firstly such care does not necessarily meet the client's needs, and is a less preferable solution to their problems than living in their own homes. Secondly, there is the sheer expense of this form of provision which concentrates resources on a very small group of the elderly population.'[30]

There is no doubt that institutional care is not cheap. In the year ending March 1978 the average cost of maintaining a resident in a home for the elderly was £6–15 per day (residents pay according to their means). In the same period it cost £15–35 per day for an old person in a geriatric hospital. On the other hand the cost of keeping a person in the community with full domiciliary support may also be expensive (see Ch. 7). And recent evidence points to the increasing age and frailty of residents in old people's homes. In the year ending March 1976 nearly 35 per cent of new admissions to local authority homes were over 85 years of age.

Some of the problems connected with residential homes relate to buildings. Perhaps more difficult to deal with are problems stemming from staff attitudes. The Personal Social Services Council in *Living and Working in Residential Homes*[31] and in *Residential Care Reviewed*[32] made suggestions about the objectives of residential care and about administration and the role of the staff. Brocklehurst has written about the rights of old people in institutions,[33] and Meacher in *Taken for a Ride* criticised residential provision for the mentally confused elderly.[34] Other problems include lack of privacy, lack of self-determination, lack of choice over many everyday matters and arrangements for health care. There has also been criticism about compulsory admissions. Most elderly people move to institutional care voluntarily or with persuasion. But in certain circumstances – such as where an old person is physically incapacitated or is living in insanitary conditions and is unable to devote to himself, and is not receiving from other people, due care and attention – the local authority may apply for a court order for their removal to a hospital or other suitable place.

New thinking about residential care concentrates attention on the quality of care, and ways have been discussed to make life more satisfying and individual for both residents and staff. In DHSS, *A Lifestyle for the Elderly* (1976), for example, the way in which staff and buildings can meet the real needs of residents is discussed. The point of the title of the report is that elderly people are not just consumers of a service which may or may not affect their lives but of a life style which affects every aspect of living. In DHSS, *Residential Care for the Elderly in London*, suggestions are made for improving the management of homes and encouraging the independence of residents.[35] Other ways of improving conditions such as inspection, consumer representation, sponsors and a national residents' organisation are put forward by Lynes and Woolacott.[36]

In some homes residents stay only for a short time, perhaps while relatives have a break, or for rehabilitation between hospital and their own home. In Salford a scheme has been devised for an elderly person, who is reasonably ambulant and not confused, but on the list for residential care, to go into a home for a month. While there they are built up physically or helped to improve their walking or whatever is needed. They then go home but are not precluded from returning to the home for another spell if needed.

MOBILITY AND TRANSPORT

The mobility of elderly people which affects their access to facilities they need to use decreases with increasing age. Not only do many of them become physically less able to move about but fewer own cars than other age groups. Age Concern found that walking is the basic method of travel used by the elderly, and for longer distances the majority relied almost exclusively on buses. In Age Concern's *Profiles of the Elderly: their mobility and transport* suggestions are made for policies to improve their mobility.[37] These include improving public transport, developing new forms of transport such as dial-a-ride buses and paying greater attention to the location both of the homes the elderly occupy and the places they regularly visit.

Concessionary fares (Ch. 5) are helpful, but less so for the elderly who are disabled and for those who live in areas with an infrequent bus service. Norman in *Transport and the Elderly* writes of 'the chaos of travel concessions' because of the complexity and unevenness of schemes. She summarises suggested action, some of which would require changes in the law, such as relaxing regulations relating to hired cars and supplementary rural transport, and some which would simply require action by ministries, local authorities, bus companies, pressure groups and individuals.[38]

SOME ISSUES

Some of the points of concern about local social services are discussed elsewhere such as variations between authorities (Ch. 12) and voluntary involvement (Ch. 10). Some which are more specific are discussed below.

The organisation of social service departments

A formidable problem of size was posed when local authority departments were not only amalgamated but took on fresh responsibilities at the time when the new social service departments were created. Most departments have attempted to get over the problem of size by creating area teams which are locally based.

The detailed study by Stevenson and Parsloe of 31 teams in 8 parts of the United Kingdom formed the basis of *Social Service Teams: the practitioner's view*.[39] The researchers found a lack of clarity about objectives and roles (and of social work in particular), a lack of imagination about roles and structures and criticism of senior management who were rarely seen in a supportive role. They also noted that restraints and cutbacks had come at an unfortunate time.

Staff

Lack of trained staff is a major problem in social service departments. Only 40 per cent of social workers are trained and the Central Council for Education and Training in Social Work aims at 50 per cent by the end of the 1980s. The report of a DHSS committee, *Manpower and Training for the Social Services* (1976) (the Birch Report) emphasised that: '. . . a substantial and continuing programme of development in training should be a major national priority, to which Government, employing authorities, voluntary organisations and the educational sector should all contribute'. Not all who are trained have a great knowledge of the elderly and there is some criticism of an over-concentration on childhood and adolescence. Views were sought in *A Happier Old Age* on 'the place of fully trained social workers, knowledgeable about the ageing process, and the effect of physical and mental disorders in old age, in providing the counselling necessary to enable some people to reach decisions acceptable to themselves'.[40]

Another difficulty arises when jobs, such as those of social work, have no generally accepted job analysis. It then becomes even more difficult to allocate work between the qualified professional, the unqualified social worker and the volunteer.

Residential staff, of whom about 4 per cent are trained, face particular problems and the Williams Report, *Caring for People: staffing residential homes* (1967), commented on the lack of career structure, the variation in the accommodation provided and the need for skills of which they felt the public was ignorant. The demands on residential staff are likely to increase as a higher proportion of residents become very frail and also possibly confused. Also the use of homes for varying purposes, including day and short-stay care, is another factor to take into account.

Linking residential and domiciliary care

There is a need to examine whether the division between community and residential care has to be so absolute. A psychiatrist at Severalls Hospital, Colchester, in *Sans Everything* described the system which they operated where community care, outpatient care, day care and admission to hospital were all part of one system and the elderly could slip fairly easily from one to another.[41] Brearley described in *Social Work Today* (14.12.72) the way in which residential institutions could be used for rehabilitation. He said that relatively few people enter a home on other than a long-term basis and with other than the expectation of dying there. He felt that some at least could leave after a period of care, and that the resulting increase in turnover would relieve congestion and allow more people to be helped. But problems of paying the rent and keeping the home going while an elderly person was in residential care would have to be overcome.

Innovatory schemes

In *A Happier Old Age* stress was laid on exploring innovatory methods, especially in providing practical help to meet personal needs.[42]

A growing number of authorities are experimenting with ways of keeping old people in their own homes by providing intensive domiciliary services (e.g. extra home help service as in a scheme in Coventry), alarm systems and peripatetic wardens (sometimes linked to an alarm system). Some authorities are providing extra help for relatives such as night sitting or a service which is a cross between nursing and home help. The Crossroads Care Attendance Scheme which started in Rugby provides help for relatives out of normal working hours.

One innovative scheme is based at the University of Kent under Professor Bleddyn Davies and is funded and supported by Kent County Council. In this 100 elderly people who would otherwise be on a waiting list or admitted to an old people's home are being given a package of different sorts of help to keep them at home. The social worker has a budget and can buy in whatever help seems appropriate. This includes help from home helps, relatives, voluntary bodies, etc.

Charges for services

Charges may be made by local authorities for certain services. For the elderly these include home helps, meals, day centres and residential care. Little is known about the effect of these charges, which vary between areas, or how far they act as a dissuasive.

Links with other agencies

It is likely that more of all the supportive services are needed. More home helps, better laundry services, more adequate meals services, perhaps more paid 'good neighbours' and so on. But what is vitally important is that all the services should be planned together. Links between social service departments and health were discussed in Chapter 6 and housing in Chapter 7. The other main agency with whom social workers come in contact is the Supplementary Benefits Section of the DHSS.

The researchers looking at social service teams found that in the opinion of many social workers, relationships between the two departments had improved markedly in the immediate past.[43] Nevertheless there were still difficulties in relationships arising from such things as uncertainty about the right 'level' for contact, changes in the staff involved, lack of understanding of the ways in which each worked, and, related to all these, the problem of identification of named people. The SBC have commented in their annual reports on their 'frontier problems' with neighbouring agencies and written of the difficulties in defining each agency's sphere and influence and responsibilities. In particular they felt that their relationships had been:

beset in the past by a feeling not uncommon amongst social workers that financial needs were to be met primarily, if not exclusively, by the

Commission, and the Social Services Departments should be concerned only with social needs. This is a simplification which leads to the conclusion that there is no financial problem which is not for the Commission to solve and ignores the legislative limits to our functions (*Annual Report*, 1976).

REFERENCES

1. SUMNER and SMITH, see Ch. 3 note 52.
2. *Ibid.*, pp. 372–4.
3. HOME OFFICE *et al.*, Seebohm Committee, see Ch. 4 note 5.
4. *Ibid.*, p. 12.
5. HARRIS, see Ch. 4 note 18.
6. SAINSBURY, S., *Measuring Disability*, G. Bell and Sons, 1973.
7. TOWNSEND and WEDDERBURN, see Ch. 3 note 6, p. 135.
8. SHANAS *et al.*, see Ch. 3 note 7.
9. DHSS, *Priorities in the Health and Social Services*, see Ch. 6 note 42.
10. BEBBINGTON, A., 'Changes in the provision of social services to the elderly in the community over fourteen years', *Social Policy and Administration*, 13 (No. 2), 1979, pp. 111–23.
11. TOWNSEND and WEDDERBURN, see Ch. 3 note 6.
12. HUNT, see Ch. 2 note 3.
13. *Ibid.*
14. TOWNSEND and WEDDERBURN, see Ch. 3 note 6.
15. HARRIS, see Ch. 3 note 9.
16. HUNT, see Ch. 4 note 11, p. 24.
17. HUNT, see Ch. 2 note 3, p. 89.
18. HUNT, see Ch. 4 note 11, pp. 347 and 350.
19. CSO, *Social Trends* (No. 11), 1981, HMSO, p. 48.
20. MORLEY, D., *Day Care and Leisure Provision for the Elderly*, Age Concern, 1974, p. 22.
21. BOWL, R. *et al.*, 'Not just a day out', *Community Care*, 14.6.79, pp. 26–7.
22. GREGORY, see Ch. 4 note 12, pp. 108–9.
23. STONE, S., *Local Authority Holidays for the Elderly and Physically Handicapped*, HMSO, 1973.
24. HOME OFFICE *et al.*, Seebohm Committee, see Ch. 4 note 5.
25. STEVENSON, O. and PARSLOE, P. (eds), *Social Service Teams: the practitioner's view.* HMSO, 1978.
26. *Ibid.*, p. 133.
27. GOLDBERG, see Ch. 3 note 28.
28. BREARLEY, see Ch. 3 note 29, p. 110.

29. DHSS, Social Work Service, London Region, *Residential Care for the Elderly in London*, DHSS, 1979, p. 67.

30. STAPLETON, B., 'Avoiding residential care for the old', *Community Care*, 10.5.79, pp. 14–16.

31. PERSONAL SOCIAL SERVICES COUNCIL, *Living and Working in Residential Homes*, Personal Social Services Council, 1975.

32. PERSONAL SOCIAL SERVICES COUNCIL, *Residential Care Reviewed*, Personal Social Services Council, 1977.

33. BROCKLEHURST, J. C., *Old People in Institutions – their rights*, Age Concern, 1974.

34. MEACHER, see Ch. 3 note 20.

35. DHSS, *op. cit.*

36. LYNES, T. and WOOLACOTT, 'Old people's homes – the resident as consumer', *Social Work Today*, 21.12.76, pp. 17–18.

37. AGE CONCERN, *Profiles of the Elderly*, see Ch. 3 note 49.

38. NORMAN, A., *Transport and the Elderly*, NCCOP, 1977, pp. 109–11.

39. STEVENSON and PARSLOE, *op. cit.*

40. DHSS, *A Happier Old Age*, see Ch. 3 note 61, p. 33.

41. ROBB, see Ch. 2 note 5.

42. DHSS, *A Happier Old Age*, see Ch. 3 note 61, p. 33.

43. STEVENSON and PARSLOE, *op. cit.*

Chapter nine
COMMUNITY CARE – THE FAMILY

INTRODUCTION

When planning the provision of any social service three fundamental questions have to be asked. What is the need? How is it to be met? Who is to provide?

The first and second questions were discussed in Chapters 5–8 which dealt with particular need and services, and a wider examination of need is to be found in Chapter 12. Chapters 5–8 paid special attention to developments in the statutory services. But there are other sources of help which are both more numerous and of longer standing. They are first, the family, second, the community expressed through voluntary organisations, volunteers and the wider network of neighbours and friends and, third, the elderly themselves. These three will be examined in this and the next two chapters.

It has already been suggested in Chapter 4 that community care is provided in many different ways. As far as the elderly are concerned there is no doubt that the main provider is the family and is likely to remain so in the future [doc 38]. Abrams comments that even the 'classic' English community study by Young and Willmott (1957) 'is of course almost exclusively a study of care among kin – although it is hardly ever read that way' [doc 38].

It is now proposed to look first at the rise of the welfare state and its effect on the family (in particular the extended family) and the three-generation household. Then some factors which are changing the pattern of family care will be discussed. Evidence will be presented about the degree of contact the elderly have with relatives and the extent of family care. Finally, questions will be asked about how families can be supported in their caring role.

THE RISE OF THE WELFARE STATE AND ITS EFFECT ON THE FAMILY

Before examining the part that families play in providing help for the elderly some consideration must be given to the debate about the rise of the welfare state and the alleged consequent decline of the family as a caring group.

If it is accepted that the welfare state is a 'state which has a policy of collective responsibility for individual well-being',[1] with social services provided on behalf of society, then, some have argued, the state must have taken over at least part of the role of the family. *The Times* in a leader (28.6.68) said: 'There is a widespread belief that as the welfare state has developed so the old sense of family responsibility has declined', but then went on to refute this view. Fletcher in *The Family and Marriage in Britain*, though not holding this view himself, also reports that some believe that 'since much is now publicly provided for old people . . . responsibility on the part of their families for the care of the aged has fallen away'.[2] Shanas *et al.* argue that the relationship between the social services and the family must be regarded as central to the theoretical disputes about the rise of the welfare state.[3]

Wright and Randal attempt to summarise the position of the family in pre-industrial England and give some reasons why the state has taken over some (but not all) of the functions of the family.[4] But after weighing the evidence they conclude that, in spite of all the forecasts about its imminent dissolution, the family continues to exist. They also examine some of the alternatives to the family, but say that it is too early to say whether or not they do in fact offer a realistic alternative.

The conclusion of an extensive examination of the family and the state by Moroney is 'on balance, that the evidence does not support the view that the modern family is giving up its caring function, or transferring its traditional responsibilities to the state'.[5]

The difficulty in trying to make comparisons with the past lies in the lack of available data. Great care must be exercised in drawing conclusions when the picture of past conditions is so hazy. Most of such evidence as there is about family care of old people relates to two separate concepts, the extended family and the three-generation household.

THE EXTENDED FAMILY AND THE THREE-GENERATION HOUSEHOLD

The extended family is not easy to define. Stacey attempts this definition: 'The extended family has generally been used for a persistent group of relatives, wider than the elementary family. Empirical evidence suggests that the numbers and categories of kin included in such social groups are highly variable. It is not therefore susceptible of precise definition.'[6]

A more commonly used definition is that used by Rosser and Harris: 'Any persistent kinship grouping of persons related by descent, marriage or adoption, which is wider than the elementary family, in that it characteristically spans three generations from grandparents to grandchildren.'[7] Many sociological studies, especially Young and Willmott's *Family and Kinship in East London*, have stressed the importance of the extended family in exercising a mutual caring role.[8]

The second concept which is held to have a bearing on the family–old person relationship is the three-generation household. Much discussion has centred on the living arrangements of families and it is often assumed that the common pattern used to be one of three generations living as one household. The further assumption is then made that if people live under the same roof they will care for one another. Whether many families did live like this is uncertain. There certainly have been many statements made that the three-generation household was fairly common. For example Cullingworth states: 'The increasing break-up of three-generation households into two separate units . . . involves the provision of two or even three dwellings for every one that would have been required 50 years ago.'[9] Beyer and Nierstrasz likewise talk about 'the days when the three-generation household was the norm'.[10]

But recent research casts doubt on whether the three-generation household ever existed to any extent, although there is no doubt that the *size* of households has declined. In 1961 12 per cent of all households in Great Britain were one person, but in 1976 they represented 21 per cent. Hole and Pountney in *Trends in Population, Housing and Occupancy Rates 1861–1961*, suggest that the larger households in Victorian times were due partly to a large number of children and partly to apprentices, domestic servants and lodgers. They say: 'Considerable doubt has been thrown on the popular conception of the Victorian household . . . it seems that a household consisting only of parents and children was as typical then as it is today.' They later conclude that the typical household was not an extended family, but one consisting of parent(s) and children only.

Laslett in *Household and Family in Past Time* comes to a similar conclusion. He suggests that the nuclear family was the normal arrangement even before industrialisation. He points out how few old people survived to old age anyway, making the three-generation household a physical impossibility in many cases. His explanation of the myth of this type of household is that it was probably due to a cherished ideology:

The wish to believe in the large and extended household as the ordinary institution of an earlier England and an earlier Europe, or as a standard feature of an earlier non-industrial world, is indeed a matter of ideology. . . . It came into being, and has been nurtured by a wish to be able to believe in a doctrine of familial history which until now has scarcely begun to be investigated in the surviving records of behaviour.

It is possible to obtain figures of three-generation households at the present time. In a recent study Hunt found that 12.5 per cent of elderly people live with the next generation.[11] This figure compares with that of 8 per cent found in the 1980 GHS[12]

CHANGING FACTORS

However, there are some qualifications arising out of all the research which must now be considered. These qualifications revolve around two points: whether close links are always desirable and whether this situation is likely to continue.

The first question is whether the close links which can obtain without families living in the same household are always desirable. For example there is the question of standards of care. Townsend and Wedderburn hint at this when they say: 'Uneducated expressions of love and loyalty are crucially important in many of life's situations, but not all. We have too little information on the quality of care provided for old people by their families at home.'[13] Willmott and Young found that 'a good deal of trouble arises because the generations so often have to live under the same roof', pointing out that this is often because there is no suitable accommodation nearby.[14] Brandon in *Seventy Plus* describes the tensions when a family of three generations live together.[15] Pruner, concluding that the family is as sound and as extended as ever, claims that separate households do not mean the end of family ties and that living together is not necessarily a sign of family stability but can involve strain.[16]

There is also the point raised by Fletcher that the closeness of family ties may not be as satisfactory as a greater degree of independence. He argues that 'the closeness of kinship ties in earlier times was largely a matter of necessity, and it entailed many elements of individual constraint'.[17] He went on to maintain that: 'Close kinship relationships have their value but they can also be limiting, confining, frustrating, so that the loosening of these ties, for some people at any rate, may constitute a desirable improvement.'[18]

The second question is whether family links are likely to continue. Pessimists point to demographic changes such as the reduction in family size which will mean that the elderly will have fewer children to turn to, the non-availability of the family when everyone is out of the house all day at school or work, the emergence of the four-generation household and the increased mobility of families. Yet a closer examination of all these factors shows that the position is not only not as bleak as might be supposed but there are other factors emerging that potentially may lead to more help being available.

Taking first the reduction in family size the most striking point is that it was between 1860 and 1910 that the average number of children born to a woman dropped most dramatically (from an average of 7 to one of 3). Since then the numbers have altered little. They dropped to 2.4 for women married in 1920 and 2.1 for women married in 1930. But the figure remained at 2.1 in 1940 and rose to 2.3 in 1950.[19] Subsequent numbers, as far as can be ascertained where families have been completed, seem to be just over 2 children per married woman. This shows that smaller families are not a new phenomenon but have been in evidence since around the beginning of the century.

What is more significant is that today more children survive. A mother having seven children in 1860 would not expect that number to be still alive when she was old. There has been a remarkable decline in the infant mortality rate. This is most pronounced for infants under one year, but still appreciable for all ages of childhood as the Court Report (1976) on Child Health Services, *Fit for the Future*, showed. It is now the exception rather than the rule for a mother not to have her children survive to adult life.

Added to this is the fact that children live longer and therefore are more likely to be alive when their parents are old. The expectation of life at birth for a man in 1891–1900 was 44.1 years and for a woman 47.8. In 1950–52 it was 66.5 for a man and 71.5 for a woman. In

1979 it was 70.2 for a man and 76.2 for a woman. This certainly means that there will be an increasing number of elderly people living. But it also means that there will be more in middle and early old age who are able to assist their own parents as they move into extreme old age.

The alleged diminution in the pool of family care is also a more complex matter than would appear at first sight. On the one hand there are trends to suggest that sources of family help are diminishing. There are fewer unmarried women to remain at home to care for aged relatives. There are also fewer married women at home because many more now go out to work. In 1921 8.7 per cent of married women worked,[20] but by 1961 this was up to 29.7 per cent[21] and in the *GHS 1982* this had risen to 50 per cent. So a lower proportion of potential carers will be available than in the past. On the other hand the decline in the number of single women means that more are marrying and therefore probably will have children to support them when they are elderly. And while there is a great increase in the number of married women working, many part-time, their greater financial independence may well enable them to buy in help for their elderly parents or give assistance with labour-saving devices.

Much of the discussion ignores the role of husbands (and men) as carers. A shorter working week, the increased possibility of flexible working hours and the greater sharing of tasks may all contribute to more men being able to help. The pattern of family life which seems to be emerging is increasingly based, if not on equality between husbands and wives, on 'at least something approaching symmetry', as Young and Willmott have argued in *The Symmetrical Family*.[22]

The emergence of the four-generation family must also be taken into account. The reduction of the age gap between generations may mean that a grandparent is far from being a dependant. Cullingworth describing his own findings says: 'And "Mum" differs from the stereotype of a frail grey-haired old lady spending her last remaining years in a lonely, dreary way . . . on the contrary, the majority of the Mums referred to by the families we interviewed were agile middle-aged women who went out to work full-time.'[23]

And a correspondent to a women's magazine wrote: 'I got home at 1.30 a.m. and tried to creep quietly past my mother's open bedroom door but she called to me and said that she had been just a bit worried for me. But I'm not a naughty girl. I have seven grandchildren and Mum is 93!' A four-generation family can mean that a grandmother in her 60s is torn in two directions because her life is divided between the demands of her mother and her own children who may expect help with grandchildren.

Family ties are also affected by increased mobility. Willmott and Young found that in Woodford couples took it for granted that the husband's job was the first consideration.[24] In 1977 nearly one-third of the population over 16 in Great Britain had moved in the last five years. However, a closer look at the figures reveals that of the 31 per cent of people who moved the majority (22%) moved only a fairly short distance.[25] Abrams found that nearly two-thirds of his sample of elderly people over 75 lived in the same dwellings, the same street or neighbourhood as their sons and daughters or only five to six miles away.[26]

Another factor which may affect the future and influence whether families continue to exercise a caring role, is the views of the elderly themselves. Age Concern found that the expectation that children will look after their elderly parents was not accepted to any great extent. Of the elderly, 67 per cent felt that 'old people should not expect their children to look after them' and elderly parents were most likely to agree strongly with that statement.[27] But when they speak of 'looking after' they may mean 'having them living in the same house'.

What is known about extended families and three-generation households does not provide enough evidence of greater family care in the past to justify the theory that the welfare state has caused a decline in family care. Perhaps the four factors mentioned in this section are the real reasons for any changes in family care rather than any theory about the consequences of the rise of the welfare state or the supposed breakdown of the extended family and the three-generation household.

CONTACT WITH RELATIVES

Most social surveys find that elderly people have frequent contact with a relative. Willmott and Young found that 56 per cent of their sample in Woodford had seen a relative the previous day and in Bethnal Green it was 58 per cent.[28] And surveys of other areas which were not tight-knit communities in the sense that Bethnal Green was (and probably still is) show that family links are still very much alive (e.g. Britton,[29] Tinker,[30] Hunt[31]).

With children

In most cases the contact was with a child. This is as true now as it was in the earlier sociological studies such as those by Willmott and Young. In 1978 Hunt said that visits from daughters/daughters-in-law and sons/sons-in-law easily outstripped those of other relatives.[32] Abrams in 1978 said that three-quarters of those with children saw them once a week or more often.[33]

The general impression is that nothing really makes up for the loss of a member of the immediate family. Whether it was the death of a spouse, the loss of children (through death or emigration) or the pain caused in the rare cases where a child did not visit, the sadness is obvious.

It must also be remembered that some old people either will have no children or will have outlived them. Abrams found that 30 per cent of his sample of the over 75s had had no children.[34]

With other relatives

Nevertheless, old people do compensate for the lack, or the loss, of children. Willmott and Young commented on the adaptability of the family: 'Almost everyone succeeds, somehow or other, in surrounding himself with a family or its atmosphere' they claim.[35] Shanas *et al.* argued that:

An individual's relationships adjust to variations in family structure. One of the functions of kinship associations is to provide replacements for intimate kin lost by death or migration. . . . Thus old people who have never married tend to maintain much closer relationships with their brothers and sisters than those who marry and have children. Persons without children tend to resume closer associations with siblings upon the death of a spouse, but interestingly, not as close as single persons. Widowed persons tend to have closer contacts than married persons with their married children.[36]

It seems that few people claim to have no living close relatives. Brothers, sisters, nieces and nephews can take the place of children and grandchildren when someone has been childless.

EVIDENCE ABOUT CARE BY THE FAMILY

Research confirms the evidence that social services do not undermine self-help or responsibility. The family still plays a major role in meeting the needs of the elderly.

Abel-Smith and Pinker, who looked at the elderly in institutions from 1911 to 1951, said: 'At the very least our conclusions do not support theories of increasing family neglect.'[37] In 1957 Townsend published his famous study of Bethnal Green, *The Family Life of Old*

People.[38] Although it was based only on just over 200 interviews it evoked a great deal of discussion about the extended family life of the East End. Townsend came to two, as he put it, inescapable conclusions. They were firstly that old people, particularly women, with daughters and other female relatives living near them, make least claim on the services of the state. Secondly, isolated old people make disproportionately heavy claims. In the same year Young and Willmott published their study of Bethnal Green, *Family and Kinship in East London,*[39] based on a sample of 1,000 families. This showed a very close family network based on the mother, with a great deal of mutual help between her and her daughters. Both these studies were based on working-class areas and they showed considerable dependence and mutual aid between the elderly and their families (especially through the female side of the family).

Willmott and Young then turned their attention to Woodford, where they found looser ties than in Bethnal Green but still quite close contact.[40] Some of the elderly had followed their families out from the East End to Woodford and either lived with them or had managed to buy a house very near or, even in some cases, next door. 'Kinship may mean less in the suburb at other stages in life, but in old age, when the need arises, the family is once more the main source of support.'[41]

An interesting study by Barley in 1961 looked at 73 old people both before and after they retired. One aspect was support from families and the conclusion was: 'The evidence of the present survey strongly supports Townsend's suggestion that, far from weakening, family ties are as important as they ever were.' Two years later another study of a working-class area was published. Willmott in *The Evolution of a Community* suggested that the concept of family support and the extended family was equally valid in Dagenham.[42] In fact his findings were remarkably similar to the studies of Bethnal Green. He also claimed that there would be still more extended families on the estate, and fewer parents left alone, if all the sons and daughters who wanted to stay had been free to do so. The inference was that housing policy was not helpful in keeping families together.

The next important study was part of a cross-national survey of about 2,500 old people in each of three countries (United States, Denmark and Britain). The findings which related specifically to Britain were published by Townsend and Wedderburn in *The Aged in the Welfare State*. The aim of the study was to find out how effective social services were in meeting the needs of the aged, to find

127

out whether it was true that certain functions formerly performed by the family had been taken over by the social services and to examine new needs in view of changing circumstances. Their conclusion was that: 'There is little evidence of health and welfare services being "misused" or "undermining" family responsibilities. Those who benefit from the services are mainly infirm or incapacitated persons who lack a family or have none within reach. This suggests that the family does in fact play a positive role for many old people, and a considerable body of data support this suggestion.'[43]

In Swansea, Rosser and Harris in 1965 based their research on some 2,000 families. Little difference was found between the families studied here and those of Bethnal Green. The authors stated that industrialisation 'has not prevented the maintenance of high levels of contact and the interchange of services between related households'.[44] Nor was there any significant difference between those whose origin was Welsh or non-Welsh or between social classes.

A new element was introduced into the subject in 1966 when Hubert published his study of middle-class families in Highgate. He suggested that ties were strong between the elderly and families in this area despite the distances separating them. While there was not the same frequency of contact the links were still strong. Comparing a group of American pensioners with some English ones Bracey summarised the situation: 'We have uncovered virtually no evidence of real neglect of old people by their children.'[45] The finding that the closer children lived to their parents the more complete the assistance they were able to give in time of need is similar to that of the Tinker granny annexe study.[46]

Jackson in 1968 had come to a similar conclusion based on a series of studies in northern England.[47] In the same year Shanas *et al.* published the comprehensive survey referred to above. They found that while substantial numbers experienced problems they were far more integrated into society than is often assumed by the general public or, they claimed, by sociological theorists. Again the role of the family as a supplier of services was dominant in all three countries. Most of the literature stressed the importance of the mother–daughter link. But Bell, in his study of 120 middle-class families, found that there was also a strong father–son link.[48] Finally, Hunt (1978) has confirmed the extent of family help [doc 39].

Is there evidence of neglect by families? Isaacs in 1969 at the Conference of the Housing Centre Trust claimed that: 'It was rare indeed for an old person to be neglected by their family.' In 1971 he published the results of a sample of 280 elderly patients admitted to a Glasgow hospital in the *British Medical Journal*. He found that only 1 per cent could be considered to have been neglected by their families. However, there are from time to time allegations of 'granny bashing' and a doctor recently asked nurses in particular to be aware of the problems and report anything suspicious.

What cannot be assessed simply from measuring frequency of contact and the number of tasks undertaken is the depth of the relationship. There is no doubt, however, from the research cited above that the great majority of families do care about their elderly relatives and do help them. The evidence clearly does not support the theory mentioned at the beginning of this chapter that the family is declining as a caring group because of the provisions of the welfare state.

THE NEED TO SUPPORT THE FAMILY

There has been a growing recognition during the last few years of the vital role families play in caring for their relatives. It is significant that the terms of reference of a committee which was to have a marked effect on social services (the Seebohm Committee) had as one of its objectives in 1965 'to secure an effective family service'.

All the major political parties have been committed to maintaining and sustaining the family. In a fascinating analysis in *The Times* (1.8.78) of party manifestos from 1918 to 1974 Bain shows how alike all of them are in the attention paid to the family. The family is also the subject of an independent Study Commission set up under the chairmanship of Sir Campbell Adamson and with financial support from the Leverhulme Trust.

What is less likely to be discovered is much information about what family care of the elderly actually means in terms of financial, emotional and other costs. Work now sponsored by the DHSS is expected to provide some information. In the meantime it has been largely left to the medical profession and to particular groups to speak out about the stresses involved. Isaacs, Livingstone and Neville in *Survival of the Unfittest* say in their conclusions: 'Relief must be provided to aged spouses, daughters and others enmeshed in the home care of the severely disabled and the mentally disturbed.'[49] Another geriatrician, Millard, says:

The cry goes up that the elderly become long-stay and need to be looked after because their relatives do not care. This is wrong, for in most instances the relatives have cared and we as a community have not; most of my problems [in a hospital] come in those families that have taken on the care of the elderly relatives in their own homes (too soon and perhaps misguidedly) and have then soldiered on for years on the broken nights' sleep, no holidays and in some cases no nights out until they can take it no longer; and it is often not until the daughter or daughter-in-law has a nervous breakdown that anyone gives them help ('The Care of the Elderly', *County Councils Gazette*, Jan. 1971, p. 6).

It is significant that Millard refers to the 'daughter or daughter-in-law' because most studies such as Hunt's of the Home Help Service show that it is the women on whom the burden usually falls. In this survey it was found that 14.7 per cent of home helps were responsible to some extent for the care of at least one elderly or infirm person other than the patients they attended. This compared with 9.9 per cent of all working women.[50] Groups such as the National Council for the Single Woman and Her Dependants have produced evidence of the extent of caring that their members give to elderly relatives.

Land in the *Journal of Social Policy* (July 1978) claims that: 'It is clear then that men are not expected to look after themselves as much as women are and that they are accordingly given more help from publicly provided support services. Neither is it assumed that they will be able to look after elderly or infirm relatives.'

However, Moroney and others have pointed out that the family is changing 'and it is of little value to suggest a return to the past'.[51] And Johnson argues that each family and its particular solution may be different [doc 40].

What is needed is a realistic assessment of how families willing to care for an elderly person can be supported. I have stressed elsewhere that: 'Making it easier for families to move closer or enlarge their homes are two ways. Another is to give adequate professional support, such as extra nursing help, incontinence services and holiday relief, to families who want to care for a disabled member.'

A similar view has been expressed by Utting, Chief Social Work Officer at the DHSS, who said at an Age Concern conference in 1977: 'There may therefore be a special value to a state service that enables family and friends to provide better care, or that supports them during periods of stress and difficulty.'

Pruner elaborates this point and also stresses the need for wider support.[52] As Young and Willmott expressed it: 'The family is not a society on its own, merely part of the wider society, and, if it is to perform its proper function within its own sphere, the family needs the support which only the wider society can give.'[53] And as the DHSS concluded in *A Happier Old Age*: 'Although family links are irreplaceable we cannot assume that the family can carry the whole responsibility for caring for the growing numbers of very old people. We may therefore need to look increasingly to the wider community to give more support of the kind traditionally expected of the family.'[54]

It is with this wider community that the next chapter is concerned.

REFERENCES

1. CLEGG, see Ch. 4 note 29.
2. FLETCHER, R., *The Family and Marriage in Britain*, Penguin, 1966, p. 160.
3. SHANAS *et al.*, see Ch. 3 note 7.
4. WRIGHT, F. and RANDAL, F., *Basic Sociology*, Macdonald and Evans, 1970.
5. MORONEY, R., *The Family and the State*, Longman, 1976, p. x.
6. STACEY, M., *Comparability in Social Research*, Heinemann, 1969, p. 36.
7. ROSSER, C. and HARRIS, C., *Family and Social Change*, Routledge and Kegan Paul, 1965, p. 32.
8. YOUNG, M. and WILLMOTT, P., *Family and Kinship in East London*, Penguin, 1957.
9. CULLINGWORTH, J. B., *Housing Needs and Planning Policy*, Routledge and Kegan Paul, 1960, p. 5.
10. BEYER and NIERSTRASZ, see Ch. 3 note 51, p. 11.
11. HUNT, see Ch. 2 note 3, p. 16.
12. CSO, *Social Trends* (No. 13), see Ch. 2 note 12, p. 25.
13. TOWNSEND and WEDDERBURN, see Ch. 3 note 6, p. 43.
14. WILLMOTT and YOUNG, see Ch. 3 note 5, p. 109.
15. BRANDON, see Ch. 3 note 39, p. 8.
16. PRUNER, see Ch. 3 note 31, p. 129.
17. FLETCHER, *op. cit.*, p. 170.
18. *Ibid.*, p. 171.
19. MORONEY, *op. cit.*, p. 18.
20. *Ibid.*, p. 19.
21. CSO, *Social Trends* (No. 11), see Ch. 8 note 19, p. 72.
22. YOUNG, M. and WILLMOTT, P., *The Symmetrical Family*, Routledge and Kegan Paul, 1973.
23. CULLINGWORTH, *op. cit.*

24. WILLMOTT and YOUNG, see Ch. 3 note 5, p. 36.
25. CSO, *Social Trends* (No. 9), see Ch. 2 note 12, p. 153.
26. ABRAMS, see Ch. 2 note 4, p. 21.
27. Age Concern, *The Attitudes of the Retired and Elderly*, see Ch. 3 note 48, p. 59.
28. WILLMOTT and YOUNG, see Ch. 3 note 5, p. 43.
29. BRITTON, R., *Housing and Related Benefits*, Age Concern, 1974.
30. TINKER, see Ch. 7 note 27.
31. HUNT, see Ch. 2 note 3.
32. *Ibid.*, p. 96.
33. ABRAMS, see Ch. 2 note 4, p. 22.
34. *Ibid.*, p. 19.
35. WILLMOTT and YOUNG, see Ch. 3 note 5, p. 57.
36. SHANAS *et al.*, see Ch. 3 note 7, p. 166.
37. FLETCHER, *op. cit.*, p. 162.
38. TOWNSEND, see Ch. 3 note 4.
39. YOUNG and WILLMOTT, *Family and Kinship*.
40. WILLMOTT and YOUNG, see Ch. 3 note 5.
41. *Ibid.*, p. 51.
42. WILLMOTT, P., *The Evolution of a Community*, Routledge and Kegan Paul, 1963.
43. TOWNSEND and WEDDERBURN, see Ch. 3 note 6, p. 135.
44. ROSSER and HARRIS, *op. cit.*, pp. 291–92.
45. BRACEY, see Ch. 3 note 3, p. 44.
46. TINKER, see Ch. 7 note 27.
47. JACKSON, B., *Working Class Community*, Routledge and Kegan Paul, 1968.
48. BELL, C. R., *Middle Class Families*, Routledge and Kegan Paul, 1969.
49. ISAACS, LIVINGSTONE and NEVILLE, see Ch. 3 note 13, p. 102.
50. HUNT, see Ch. 4 note 11, p. 39.
51. MORONEY, *op. cit.*, p. 9.
52. PRUNER, see Ch. 3 note 31, pp. 135–37.
53. YOUNG and WILLMOTT, *Family and Kinship*.
54. DHSS, *A Happier Old Age*, see Ch. 3 note 61, p. 6.

Chapter ten
COMMUNITY CARE – SUPPORT FROM THE WIDER COMMUNITY

INTRODUCTION

In the last chapter it was suggested that, if family support is lacking, the elderly may turn to 'the wider community'.[1] But what do we mean by 'the wider community'? And if it is possible to define this group what is its role and what are its limitations?

Examining the literature it would appear that there are three seemingly distinct groups: voluntary organisations, volunteers and friends/neighbours. Each of these will be considered in turn.

VOLUNTARY ORGANISATIONS

Type

A voluntary organisation is defined by Clegg as: 'Any organisation which relies for its funds at least in part on voluntary subscription.... It is to be distinguished from (a) statutory authorities and (b) businesses run for profit.'[2] It is therefore not a statutory body like a local authority nor a commercial organisation such as those which run private nursing homes for the elderly. In the context of voluntary bodies concerned with the welfare of the elderly many would be known as charities whose prime purpose was to give 'charity', money, goods or services, to the poor.

The Wolfenden Committee, which was set up by the Joseph Rowntree Memorial Trust and the Carnegie United Kingdom Trust specifically to look at the role and functions of voluntary organisations, did not find it easy to establish a satisfactory definition: 'We decided that as a general guideline common sense or common parlance must prevail over verbal consistency or logical precision and that we would take as the centre or focus of our review voluntary organisations dealing with the personal social services and what is generally known as the "environment".'[3]

Many of the early voluntary organisations, such as almshouses, were concerned primarily with providing for the elderly and so are many (e.g. Age Concern and Task Force) of those established more recently. The different origins of these groups give an indication of their strengths and weaknesses today.

Sometimes a benefactor has provided money for a very specific purpose. For example, an almshouse was established in Reading in 1634 for 'six aged and impotent men, without wives'. Some of the oldest charities were set up to provide money, fuel or food for such elderly people as satisfied certain conditions, usually relating to age, sex, place of birth or area of residence. These charities are often administered by churches which may interpret their brief widely. In place of the specified bag of fuel, money may be given to help pay the fuel bills. The modern counterparts, though often of a more transitory nature, are organisations giving food parcels to the elderly at Christmas, harvest or other special times.

A second type of voluntary organisation is that set up to further some particular cause or help some particular group and raises the necessary funds for it (e.g. Help the Aged).

A third type is the body which has one major objective but which also engages in voluntary social service. The churches, for example, have worship as their primary purpose, but they also provide many services for the elderly in such ways as sponsoring housing associations, opening their crypts or providing food and shelter for those in need (many of whom are elderly).

A fourth type is the charitable trust set up with broad aims and little or no restriction on who may benefit. This gives the trustees considerable freedom to seek out and support worthwhile and often pioneering causes. The Nuffield Trust, which partly funds the NCCOP, and the Wolfson and Rowntree Trusts are good examples of this type.

An interesting new development is the self-help organisation, like the Link groups sponsored by Age Concern which link people offering various kinds of help (see Ch. 5).

Some of these voluntary organisations are tiny charities while others, such as the City Parochial Foundation, handle millions of pounds a year. But whatever their size there is need to see what they do for the elderly in the widest context. In order to do that one needs to look at their functions and their problems.

Functions

Throughout the centuries individuals and groups have responded in various ways to the social conditions of their time. Some have worked through the state and tried to get services provided publicly. Others have set out, either alone or with others, to provide the service themselves. For the elderly this voluntary provision has embraced housing, residential homes, hospitals, pensions and many other kinds of service.

There has never been a time when it was foreseen that the state would take over total provision. Indeed Beveridge in his report, which formed the basis for much of post-Second World War provision went out of his way to stress the need for voluntary action alongside that of the state.[4] Subsequent investigations such as that by the Seebohm Committee[5] and by Murray[6] have endorsed this view.

The Wolfenden Committee came to a similar conclusion: 'There is widespread voluntary involvement in caring for the elderly, for children and for the handicapped. Some of this amounts to filling gaps in statutory provision but much of it is different in kind from statutory provision.[7] They went on to give evidence that, rather than declining, the amount and the scale of voluntary provision was growing.[8]

What then is the special contribution of voluntary organisations to the care of the elderly? There are a number of functions that can be identified.

Filling gaps and supplementing services   In a number of cases a voluntary body provides a service, or part of a service, which the state does not or cannot provide. Meals on wheels is probably one of the best known examples. Another is the loaning of medical equipment for old people at home by the Red Cross and the provision by them of many services for the elderly (and others) in hospital. These often include a mobile library and shop.

Giving a choice   When a voluntary body gives a service slightly different from that provided by the state this in theory offers choice. The role of voluntary bodies in extending choices was an important theme in the Wolfenden Report.[9] The various types of accommodation, for example, provided by voluntary bodies range from nursing homes, old people's homes and hostels to self-contained flats and bungalows. This should enable old people to choose what suits their wishes and their state of dependency. Voluntary bodies also offer choice to the workers, though this is less often noticed. Social workers, who wish to specialise in the elderly, may feel happier in an organisation concerned just with this one age group than in a local authority team organised on a generic basis.

Pioneering and experimenting   Many social services for the elderly have been started on an experimental basis by a voluntary body. Chiropody, meals on wheels and good neighbour schemes are three examples. Sometimes it may be more appropriate for the service to be provided by a non-statutory organisation. Age Concern has been pioneering methods of informing the elderly about their rights to statutory benefits and 'persuading them to accept services; or hopefully, ways of establishing what services the elderly really want and involving the elderly client in the detailed provision of services'.[10] A word of warning was sounded by the Younghusband Report in suggesting that an evaluation of some services already provided, might be more appropriate than fresh experiments.

But pioneering and experimenting is not necessarily the prerogative of voluntary organisations. Sometimes the two sorts of body may be trying similar new schemes alongside each other. This was the case with sheltered housing in the 1950s and early 1960s.

Harnessing individual and community enthusiasm   Many voluntary bodies seem able to attract voluntary help through the personal appeal of the organisation concerned. Murray in *Voluntary Organisation and Social Welfare* pays tribute to the great benefit which the community derives from the involvement of large numbers of enthusiasts in voluntary activities.[11] The many local branches of Age Concern, the numerous people involved in Help the Aged and the young volunteers who work for Task Force are living examples of the commitment of many thousands of people of all ages to the welfare of the elderly. However, this is not to say that statutory bodies cannot harness local enthusiasm in this way. There is already some evidence that some social service departments are in fact beginning to do so.

Providing information and doing research   Another traditional role of voluntary bodies has been the collection of information and the presentation of research findings. At the end of the last century voluntary bodies led the way in recording and analysing social conditions. This role has been continued in this century and has been officially blessed by the Goodman Committee which was set up to examine the effect of charity law and practice on voluntary organisations.[12] In their report *Charity Law and Voluntary Organisation* they say: 'Research has been recognised as a charitable object provided that it can be shown that the research is of educational value to the researcher and its fruits are disseminated to the public generally.'[13]

In the 1960s and 1970s there has been a more sustained attempt to do research on a number of different fronts. Age Concern have included in their activities the sponsoring of research by outside academics and by their own staff (e.g. the Profiles Series). They have also asked specialists to write short accounts of their own research and have published these in an easy-to-read form (e.g. Karn). The NCCOP have in the past acted as a funding body for much research, but have increasingly turned their attention to doing it themselves and in some cases have sought outside funding.

Some excellent examples of the dissemination of research, which is a much neglected area of social policy, have come from these voluntary bodies. The directory, *Old Age: A register of social research*, produced annually by the NCCOP brings together information about many current projects and enables researchers to learn about research other than their own.[14]

Acting as pressure groups Many voluntary bodies attempt to influence policy by acting as a lobby on special issues. When they are closely involved with the group they represent, like Age Concern who based their *Manifesto* on interviews with old people, their views may carry considerable weight.

The Aves Committee which looked at the *Voluntary Worker in the Social Services* cited Age Concern (then called the National Old People's Welfare Council) as a body recognising a responsibility to involve the public 'in seeing where action is needed and bringing pressure to bear upon the authorities to make more adequate provision'.[15]

Giving advice Not all elderly people like to go for advice to official agencies. They do not for example use housing advice centres to any great extent. Voluntary bodies (such as the CAB) are often more acceptable as they are thought to be one step away from the agencies providing the services.

The Goodman Committee considered that the giving of advice in appropriate cases was a charitable objective.[16] But the Wolfenden Committee felt that 'the relationship between casework for individuals and wider ranging pressure group activities is a delicate one for organisations in this field'.[17]

Others It could be argued that, apart from the functions just mentioned, voluntary organisations have other advantages. It is said that they save taxpayers' money, that their freedom makes them more flexible than statutory agencies and that they perform a valuable role in supporting the informal caring system.

The flexible approach may be useful when the elderly person does not fit exactly into the rules for a particular state service. For example a local authority may exclude owner-occupiers from council accommodation while a voluntary body such as a housing association may feel able to accept them. It is also argued that flexibility may be more possible for bodies not subject to public election and the vagaries of party politics.

Some problems

Among the problems associated with voluntary organisations are the following:

What is the role of voluntary organisations vis-à-vis *statutory bodies?* The question of which services can best be provided by voluntary bodies and which by statutory authorities is particularly difficult to determine. Jefferys notes that in fact the present division relates not to different sorts of needs but to which body first diagnosed the need and suggested the service.[18] The Wolfenden Committee expressed the view that voluntary action should now 'best be seen in terms of the ways in which it complements, supports, extends and influences the informal and statutory systems'.[19] They give more specific examples relating to central government in Chapter 4 and local authorities in Chapter 5.

Are there variable standards? When there are a number of different voluntary bodies working in the same field standards may be uneven. Such variation was seen by the Wolfenden Committee as a major weakness of voluntary bodies.[20] However, standards also differ between local authorities.

A reason for the variation in provision for the elderly by voluntary bodies is that so much depends on the energy and enthusiasm of individual people and committees. In an interesting study of the factors affecting the location of voluntary organisations, Hatch and

Mocroft conclude that one of the most important is high social class which seems to lead to a greater degree of provision.[21]

To whom is a voluntary body responsible? Age Concern in *Voluntary Organisations and the Retired and the Elderly* alleged that voluntary bodies are often responsible only to a small self-selected group of people and that they are often not accountable to the people they attempt to serve.[22] They compared this with social service departments which are responsible to elected councillors. Two of the characteristics which differentiate statutory bodies from voluntary organisations are that they must work within legally authorised limits and that they are accountable for the expenditure of public money.

These points were considered by the Goodman Committee which looked particularly at controls over fund raising and the wider question of the accountability of charities.[23] The Wolfenden Committee, taking into account also the evidence of the Goodman Committee, did not feel that the restricted accountability normally leads to serious problems, although they thought that some smaller organisations need advice and help on how to keep and present accounts.[24]

Are there overlaps? Critics of voluntary bodies sometimes point to the number of voluntary organisations apparently working in the same field and suggest that there is duplication. Jefferys, for example, claimed that the proliferation of voluntary societies reduced the time available for voluntary social service to the elderly and the handicapped.[25] But the Wolfenden Committee suggested that there may well be valid reasons why one organisation is more appropriate than another 'even if the outside world finds them almost indistinguishable'.[26]

In the case of the elderly three of the major national organisations are Age Concern, Help the Aged, and the NCCOP. A closer look at them shows two things. First their aims and the way they carry these out are different. Age Concern claim that: 'It is likely that the variety of voluntary organisations – while certainly a source of difficulty – is also one of their greatest strengths. It is impossible to believe that all the people who wish to help the elderly could work together under one organisation.'[27]

Second, these voluntary bodies have in fact combined for various purposes when the circumstances seemed appropriate. In 1976 68 organisations with an interest in the elderly formed Age Action Year

1976 to press jointly for certain specific objectives. This sort of co-operation was endorsed by the Goodman Committee which urged persuasion rather than legal means to encourage it.[28] They also found, on investigation, that there were sometimes quite valid reasons for the lack of co-operation.[29]

Do they take the heat out of problems?   It is argued that even the existence of a voluntary body, in however small a way, may give the impression that a need is being met. The voluntary body may be making only a minimal provision, but there is the feeling that something is being done and that therefore others (perhaps the state) need not act. This allegation is very difficult to prove, but it is only fair to point out that some voluntary bodies are aware of the danger.

Do they have a charitable image?   Some voluntary organisations founded as charities in previous centuries are said to have a lingering image of providing for the 'undeserving poor'. But this image may not be attached only to voluntary bodies since one reason why some old people do not claim the statutory benefits to which they are entitled seems to be the feeling that they are accepting 'charity'.

What about lack of resources?   The services that voluntary organisa-tions can provide and their independence is partly affected by the amount of money they can raise. Money comes largely from voluntary and statutory sources and also from the charitable foundations. For example the NCCOP receives grants from the Nuffield Foundation.

The Wolfenden Committee tried to obtain data from various sources on trends in voluntary giving since 1970. Listing the income of the largest 50 fund-raising charities in 1970–75 they found that 2 were exclusively for the elderly – Help the Aged with a total income in 1975 of £5.6 million and Methodist Homes for the Aged with £1.2 million.[30] However, they also found that the deterioration of the economic situation since 1974 had been accompanied by a sharp decline in voluntary giving. But they did not find any evidence that the voluntary sector was in danger of financial collapse.[31] In fact, a large part of the income of voluntary organisations now comes from non-voluntary sources, much of it from government departments. Since 1973 there has been a special part of a government department, the Voluntary Services Unit at the Home Office, dealing with voluntary bodies. Not everyone, however, is happy with this dependence on statutory funding.

Does what is provided depend more on the personal appeal of the voluntary organisation rather than the value of its work? Voluntary organisations concerned with the elderly, children and the blind attract a good deal of support because there is much public sympathy for these groups. The elderly are fortunate in coming into this category for there is evidence that some organisations operating in difficult or contentious fields find virtually no public response. The Wolfenden Committee described 'unpopular causes' which 'seem to attract less support from the public than do children and the elderly'.[32]

Conclusion

Despite the problems of voluntary organisations there are both positive and negative reasons for the continuation of their role in making provision for the elderly. What is essential is for them to be constantly questioning and redefining their roles. The main conclusion of most reports on community care (e.g. the Younghusband 1959 Report on social workers, MOH 1963 and 1966 Health and Welfare Plans and also the Wolfenden Report, 1978) has been in favour of co-existence. But this does not necessarily always result in a close and co-operative relationship. There may well be tensions.

VOLUNTEERS

Introduction

Visiting an old person sounds a useful activity and seems to appeal to volunteers of every age. But who are these voluntary workers and what is their role? These were two of the questions examined by a committee which was set up by the National Council of Social Service (NCSS) and the National Institute of Social Work Training in 1966 under the chairmanship of Geraldine Aves. Its task was 'to enquire into the role of voluntary workers in the social services and in particular to consider their need for preparation or training and their relationship with professional social workers'. They reported in 1969. They did not find it possible to formulate any neat definition because, among other things, they did not want to rule out token payments and they concluded 'that there was no merit in attempting to restrict the term in any precise way'.[33]

The Aves Committee obtained information about approximately 800 volunteers as well as investigating a number of voluntary bodies such as the NOPWC. Many of these volunteers were involved with the elderly. Following this report there have been a number of research studies concerned with volunteers. Shenfield and Allen in *The Organisation of Voluntary Service* studied domiciliary visiting of the elderly by volunteers.[34] They included a profile of 100 voluntary visitors and 126 old people being visited. In 1973 Kettle and Hart in *Health of the Elderly Project* reported on an experiment in the voluntary visiting of old people in Newcastle upon Tyne.[35] Hadley, Webb and Farrell looked particularly at young volunteers working with old people in *Across the Generations*.[36] This included a survey of 86 old people and 145 volunteers in 4 areas. In 1977 came a useful review of existing research and a discussion on how volunteers were organised by Leat and Darvill called *Voluntary Visiting of the Elderly*.[37]

In 1978 two research studies were published. One, based on interviews with over 2,000 people provided information for the Wolfenden Committee. It was by Hatch and called *Voluntary Work: a Report of a Survey*.[38] In this it was found that the largest group (35%) of volunteers helped the elderly. The other study by Holme and Maizels, *Social Workers and Volunteers* was primarily concerned with the use of volunteers by social workers.[39] They surveyed 1,423 local authority social workers. Another important source of information is the Volunteer Centre which was set up in 1973 with funds from trusts and central government to promote and encourage the use of voluntary workers. There is then a wealth of material to draw on and nearly all of it is concerned with the elderly – some exclusively.

The contribution of the volunteer

Volunteers can add greatly to the well-being of the elderly, but what is their special contribution?

Supplementing the statutory services In her study of Buckinghamshire Jefferys found that there seemed to be a view that paid staff are always preoccupied with meeting material requirements while voluntary workers provide intangible services such as friendship.[40] In practice she found that quite often the reverse happened with paid staff giving friendship as well as professional help, and volunteers giving very practical help as well as friendship. In general, however, the role of the volunteer is seen as providing something that paid workers for various reasons, such as lack of resources or time, cannot offer. It is important to consider exactly what this may mean. South Camden Health District, for example, have issued clear notes to voluntary organisers which state that 'work done by volunteers should be complementary to the work of the staff. They should not do work which should be paid, nor should they be used to combat staff shortages or financial restraints, or supply services which should be statutory.' The Aves Committee were equally clear that volunteers should not be used as substitutes for paid professionals.[41]

Continuity Since statutory workers move, especially in order to gain promotion, the volunteer may be in contact with an old person over a longer period of time. This will not, of course, always be the case since the younger volunteers also move frequently. But the advantage of continuity is that the old person has no difficulty in knowing who to contact. In one scheme in Norfolk each village had one person as its representative and they liaised with helpers in the village and kept track of who needed support and when.

Less identification with authority Many people, the elderly included, seem reluctant to go to official sources for advice. They seem more likely to go to an organisation, such as the CAB, which is staffed almost entirely by volunteers. As Age Concern puts it: 'Volunteers may also offer, particularly when it comes to problems of welfare rights, a very useful independence from the relevant Government departments. They can therefore, if well-equipped with information, help claimants who might otherwise be reluctant to press for their rights.'[42]

Helping elderly people keep in touch with the outside world Elderly people in institutional care are surrounded by officials of various kinds and all of these occupy some part in the hierarchy. A volunteer coming in from outside represents a different perspective. As Bamford, reviewing Holme and Maizels,[43] comments: 'What does emerge from the survey is a sense of the imaginative ways in which volunteers can be used in other settings than field work. In day-care centres, and especially in homes for the elderly, volunteers can make a significant contribution to raising the quality of life by bringing new stimulation into what is sometimes a passive environment.' A similar conclusion was reached in a study by the Volunteer Centre, *Creative Partnerships*, where Chapter xi gives details of voluntary involvement in a local authority old people's home and a geriatric hospital in Leicestershire.

Types of help

In *Health of the Elderly Project* one outstanding finding was the variety of help given by volunteers to the elderly.[44] The Aves Committee thought that three sorts of activity were particularly useful. Work of a mainly practical kind was one, and many elderly people benefit from volunteers who decorate, do repairs, garden and cook for them. Another activity was work for which special skill or knowledge is required. Home nursing, first-aid and advice and information come into this category. The third area was work involving personal relationships. The Aves Committee felt that if volunteers worked under the guidance, and with the support of, professionals, they need not limit their activities to practical tasks. Morris had also felt that personal contact, particularly if it was unhurried, was particularly valuable for the elderly.[45]

Who volunteers?

Before considering some of the problems about volunteers it is pertinent to examine who it is who help the elderly. Hatch in his study of volunteers found from the *GHS* that in 1973 8 per cent of a national sample had undertaken some form of voluntary work in the preceding 4 weeks.[46] In his own survey for the Wolfenden Committee he found that of a sample of 2,114 people, 15 per cent had taken part in some form of voluntary work in the previous 15 months.[47]

The image of the typical volunteer as a middle-aged middle-class married woman still has some truth in it the Aves Committee found. But they also noted that men were 'playing a much greater part than was sometimes realised'.[48] However, in the study of social workers and their volunteers it was found that women were more likely than men to have helped the elderly.[49] And the existence of Task Force shows how much help the young give to the elderly. Commenting on this the Aves Committee said: 'In their work with old people the ability of young volunteers to bridge the generation gap seems particularly valuable.'[50]

As for the motives of volunteers these seem very mixed and range from a genuine desire to help others, or the wish to further a particular cause and the satisfaction of their own personal needs. Both the Aves and Wolfenden Committees agreed that motives were mixed. The Aves Committee felt that most volunteers worked to meet some need, or combination of needs, and the Wolfenden Committee felt that most of them would not understand about introspection or self-examination about motives. Leat in *Why Volunteers? – ten points of view* (1978) produced an interesting list of reasons.

Some problems

The need to define the role of the volunteer What seems to emerge from studies of volunteers are two clear recommendations. First that the respective roles of paid and voluntary workers should be clearly defined. After consultation with the unions and statutory services the Volunteer Centre produced *Guidelines for Relationships between Volunteers and Paid Non-Professional Workers*. But even after this the view was expressed in the Consultative Document on the voluntary sector that 'it is possible that more precise guidance is needed'.[51]

The second recommendation arising from the research studies is that these definitions must be kept under constant review because the roles decided upon may change. The Aves Committee Report concluded: 'There are some areas in which it is not possible to draw precise boundaries between the functions appropriate to either type of worker; though it is always necessary for each to be aware of what the other is doing in relation to a particular client.'[52] Ten years later this consistent finding was reiterated by Holme and Maizels: 'Taking into account the fact that, in our view, there are no fixed or settled roles for either professionals or volunteers and that any definition of the roles must be transient, this aim can only be to ensure the proper use of their respective contributions and a corresponding standard of service.'[53]

Relations with statutory bodies Although many voluntary workers work for voluntary organisations some work under the umbrella of statutory bodies. When this is the case the role of the voluntary worker needs to be defined and help and support given where necessary by statutory workers. But as Moore points out volunteers are sometimes in a good position to support each other.[54] In an organisation like Contact, which arranges weekend activities for the elderly, volunteers have a limited commitment and are able to share responsibility for this.

Some very practical suggestions about the role of volunteers in social work teams are now being put forward – for example there is an experimental scheme in Norwich for linking volunteers to an area team. It is claimed that their involvement has enabled a number of families to remove elderly relatives from Part III accommodation. Elderly people have been offered a choice of options including day-care places in residential homes with some volunteers providing transport.

In practice, fewer than three in five local authority social workers with case-loads are using the services of volunteers for their clients and there is some evidence that in some cases there may be mutual distrust.[55] One commentator stated: 'The critical views of some professionals about volunteers, as expressed to the committee [Aves] were matched only by the serious doubts of some voluntary workers about professional workers.' Another source of possible conflict is when statutory workers are on strike.

Training and organisation   It is not enough for volunteers to know what their tasks are. They must also know how to go about them, what the limits of their job are and in what circumstances they should call on professional help. This particularly entails a knowledge of the needs of the elderly and of the services that can be called in to help them. The Aves Committee made detailed recommendations in regard to training, and Hobman has made the useful point that time should be given in the training of professionals to the study of the voluntary contribution.[56]

Some feel that a paid organiser is necessary. Morris, commenting on old people's welfare organisations, felt that either a central bureau or at least a single person was needed to recruit and place volunteers, as well as to collect information about openings and to receive offers of help.[57] Age Concern felt that one of the main jobs of a paid organiser was to prepare and support volunteers.[58] On the other hand, the Aves Committee found that not all volunteers felt the need for an organiser, so perhaps this will depend upon the task and circumstances as well as the scale of the operation.[59]

Evaluation   'There is something almost improper about suggesting that voluntary social work ought to be evaluated. It is rather like proposing to measure the efficiency of concern or goodwill, when the most important thing is that they do or do not exist.' So wrote two researchers who had just completed a study of old people and young volunteers (*New Society*, 7.11.74, pp. 356–8). Yet evaluation there must be if money and effort are to be put into this form of helping the elderly. Leat and Darvill considered that schemes may be evaluated 'from at least three (sometimes conflicting) viewpoints – the elderly, the volunteers and the professionals; from each viewpoint it will be possible to specify a number of different criteria of success'.[60] Kelly and Power have attempted to analyse for the Volunteer Centre some of the difficulties involved. Shenfield has suggested some ways in which the effectiveness of visiting the elderly can be assessed [doc 41]. Despite the difficulties some researchers have attempted to evaluate the work of volunteers and the results are almost entirely favourable. Shenfield found that, if the results of her research are typical, large numbers of old people were being visited regularly and with considerable devotion. Nevertheless, by her criteria [doc 41] for over a fifth of the old people the visiting which they were receiving was not apparently appropriate to their needs, and for 10 per cent the visiting seemed unnecessary and valueless.[61] Hadley, Webb and Farrell found an overall success rate which they considered quite respectable, although they suggested that refining the methods of selecting and matching clients and volunteers would raise the quality of the work.[62] Looking at the evaluation from the point of view of social workers, Holme and Maizels said: 'Generally social workers have a consistently favourable view of their experiences with volunteers, irrespective of the type of relationship they have with them.'[63]

The volunteer then, like the voluntary body, has a distinctive contribution to make to the care of the elderly. But as the Aves Committee and others have observed it is difficult to differentiate between the role of the volunteer and that of the involved citizen. The Aves Committee went as far as to declare: 'We wish to make it abundantly clear at the outset that nothing we have to say about voluntary workers, their recruitment or their training, is intended to detract from the spontaneous contribution of the neighbour; indeed quite the contrary.[64]

FRIENDS AND NEIGHBOURS

Who are they?

When studies are done of informal networks of caring, more often than not the local caring group for an old person turns out to be their family. Neighbours, too, although considered as a separate category, may also be relatives. Evidence has already been given (in Ch. 9) of the numbers of old people living near their relatives and it has also been seen how close some of their children live. It is clear from most of the studies that neighbours are not necessarily the people who actually live next door although many of them appear to live quite close. Neighbourly help that is spontaneous and unorganised is easier if people have some sort of link and physical proximity may be the most important determinant. People who feel that they belong to a physical community may feel a sense of responsibility to one another, and it is interesting that in Cheeseman, Lansley and Wilson's study of neighbourhood care of the elderly the help given by local shopkeepers and tradesmen is described.[65]

But a community which has physical boundaries may not be the only friendship network. Friends from many different groups – churches, former workmates, adult classes and clubs of various kinds form quite a different system from the world of clubs where elderly people meet only people of their own age.

Evidence about help

In addition to the evidence already cited in the previous section many studies of the elderly say something about care by neighbours and friends. In the cross-national survey of old people in Great Britain, the USA and Denmark, considerable help had been recorded from neighbours and friends.[66]

In an interesting study of old people who had moved to the seaside resorts of Bexhill and Clacton, Karn found that the statutory health and social services were not seen as a major source of help. The most important group of people whom the elderly would call on for help were neighbours.[67] But it must be remembered that only 53 per cent of retired people in Clacton and 70 per cent in Bexhill had children. They had also all moved away from their original homes where any children they had might have lived near them. This heavy reliance on neighbours and friends, Karn found, posed problems in an area where the neighbours and friends were also very likely to be old.

Hunt's recent study also found some disquieting factors about help from neighbours. Although nearly three-quarters of the sample got on very well with all their neighbours, not all felt that they would be able to ask their neighbours for help in an emergency. In answer to the question: 'If ever you needed help urgently, how many of your neighbours would you feel able to ask?', 10 per cent said they would not feel able to ask any.[68] The most vulnerable group, the bedfast and housebound, were the least likely to feel able to ask neighbours for help.

Formal neighbouring schemes

Age Concern claim that the terms 'good neighbour', 'neighbourly care' and 'neighbourhood groups' 'appear to be emotive and confusing expressions, with different meanings for different people'.[69] They then attempted two broad definitions which could be established from the way the terms were already in use, i.e. the one-to-one relationship of a person helping a neighbour in a completely spontaneous way and a group of people arranging to help individual people – that is, community organised on a regular basis. They categorised schemes into:

1. Paid help: person-to-person;
2. Voluntary help: person-to-person;
3. Paid help: one person responsible for a group;
4. Voluntary help: one person responsible for a group;
5. Paid group help for individuals;
6. Voluntary group help for individuals.

Four years later they presented a practical account of four schemes in a neighbourhood care workshop and discussed another element, the role of the community development worker.

Neighbourhood care schemes on some sort of organised basis have been in existence for many years, often under the auspices of a church. The Fish Scheme which began in Oxfordshire is one of the best known. National campaigns have also been sponsored. For example in 1967 church members of all denominations combined with non-churchgoers in the People Next Door Campaign aimed at giving service of the good neighbour type.[70]

One interesting scheme in Nottingham, 1965–69, was funded by the NCCOP and later written up and evaluated. By breaking down into very small local schemes people were drawn in who it was thought would not have taken part in a city-based scheme.[71] More ambitious good neighbour schemes were launched by David Ennals, Minister of State at the DHSS, in 1976. A report on some good neighbour schemes, *Limited Liability?*, attempts to look objectively at the contemporary evidence and contains useful case studies. It points out both the advantages and some problems [doc 42]. It is significant that there should be so much more evidence about voluntary organisations and volunteers than about the help given by friends and neighbours to the elderly. The Wolfenden Committee suggested that it is so much taken for granted that it is scarcely mentioned in discussion about the provision of social services [doc 43]. This point will be taken up later (Ch. 12) in the discussion about the meaning of community care.

REFERENCES

1. DHSS, *A Happier Old Age*, see Ch. 3 note 61, p. 61.
2. CLEGG, see Ch. 4 note 29, p. 110.
3. WOLFENDEN, LORD, *The Future of Voluntary Organisations* (the Wolfenden Committee), Croom Helm, 1978, pp. 11–12.
4. BEVERIDGE, see Ch. 5 note 1, pp. 6–7.
5. HOME OFFICE *et al.*, Seebohm Committee, see Ch. 4 note 5, pp. 152–54.
6. MURRAY, G-J., *Voluntary Organisations and Social Welfare*, Oliver and Boyd, 1968, p. 132.
7. WOLFENDEN, *op. cit.*, p. 59.
8. *Ibid.*, pp. 183–84.
9. *Ibid.*, p. 27.
10. AGE CONCERN, *Voluntary Organisations and the Retired and the Elderly*, Age Concern, 1973, p. 5.
11. MURRAY, *op. cit.*
12. GOODMAN, LORD, *Charity Law and Voluntary Organisations*, report of a committee set up by the NCSS, Bedford Square Press, 1976.
13. *Ibid.*, p. 27.
14. NCCOP, *Old Age*, see Ch. 3 note 54.
15. NCSS and NATIONAL INSTITUTE FOR SOCIAL WORK TRAINING, *The Voluntary Worker in the Social Services* (the Aves Committee), Bedford Square Press, 1969, p. 28.
16. GOODMAN, *op. cit.*, p. 32.
17. WOLFENDEN, *op. cit.*, p. 49.
18. JEFFERYS, M., *An Anatomy of Social Welfare Services*, Michael Joseph, 1965.
19. WOLFENDEN, *op. cit.*, p. 26.
20. *Ibid.*, p. 88.
21. HATCH, S. and MOCROFT, I., 'Factors affecting the location of voluntary organisation branches', *Policy and Politics*, 6 (No. 2), 1977, p. 163.
22. AGE CONCERN, *op. cit.*, p. 4.
23. GOODMAN, *op. cit.*, Ch. 7, part 8.

24. WOLFENDEN, *op. cit.*, p. 148.
25. JEFFERYS, *op. cit.*, pp. 323–24.
26. WOLFENDEN, *op. cit.*, p. 191.
27. AGE CONCERN, *op. cit.*, p. 6.
28. GOODMAN, *op. cit.*, p. 99.
29. *Ibid.*, p. 96.
30. WOLFENDEN, *op. cit.*, pp. 259–71.
31. *Ibid.*, p. 193.
32. *Ibid.*, pp. 97–98.
33. NCSS, Aves Committee, *op. cit.*, p. 19.
34. SHENFIELD, B. E. with ALLEN, I., *The Organisation of Voluntary Service*, PEP (Broadsheet 533), 1972.
35. KETTLE, D. and HART, L., *Health of the Elderly Project: an experiment in the voluntary visiting of old people*, King Edward Hospital Fund and Young Volunteer Force Foundation, 1973.
36. HADLEY, R., WEBB, A. and FARRELL, C., *Across the Generations. Old People and Young Volunteers*, Allen and Unwin, 1975.
37. LEAT, D. and DARVILL, G., *Voluntary Visiting of the Elderly*, the Volunteer Centre, 1977.
38. HATCH, S., *Voluntary Work*, the Volunteer Centre, 1978.
39. HOLME, A. and MAIZELS, J., *Social Workers and Volunteers*, BASW, 1978.
40. JEFFERYS, *op. cit.*, p. 294.
41. NCSS, Aves Committee, *op. cit.*, p. 195.
42. AGE CONCERN, *op. cit.*, p. 6.
43. HOLME and MAIZELS, *op. cit.*
44. KETTLE and HART, *op. cit.*
45. MORRIS, M., *Voluntary Work in the Welfare State*, Routledge and Kegan Paul, 1969, p. 227.
46. HATCH, *op. cit.*, p. 5.
47. *Ibid.*, p. 2.
48. NCSS, Aves Committee, *op. cit.*, p. 33.
49. HOLME and MAIZELS, *op. cit.*, p. 145.
50. NCSS, Aves Committee, *op. cit.*, p. 26.
51. HOME OFFICE, *The Government and the Voluntary Sector*, a Consultative Document, Home Office, 1978, p. 31.
52. NCSS, Aves Committee, *op. cit.*, p. 180.
53. HOLME and MAIZELS, *op. cit.*, p. 185.
54. MOORE, S., *Working for Free*, Pan, 1977.
55. HOLME and MAIZELS, *op. cit.*
56. HOBMAN, D., *Who Cares? A guide to voluntary and full-time work*, Mowbrays, 1971, p. 86.

The elderly in modern society

57. MORRIS, *op. cit.*, pp. 232–33.
58. AGE CONCERN, *op. cit.*, p. 5.
59. NCSS, Aves Committee, *op. cit.*, p. 93.
60. LEAT and DARVILL, *op. cit.*, p. 161.
61. SHENFIELD with ALLEN, *op. cit.*, p. 163.
62. HADLEY, WEBB and FARRELL, *op. cit.*, Ch. 8.
63. HOLME and MAIZELS, *op. cit.*, p. 106.
64. NCSS, Aves Committee, *op. cit.*, p. 19.
65. CHEESEMAN, D., LANSLEY, J. and WILSON, J., *Neighbourhood Care and Old People*, NCSS, 1972, p. 75.
66. SHANAS *et al.*, see Ch. 3 note 7.
67. KARN, V., *Retiring to the Seaside*, Routledge and Kegan Paul, 1977, p. 99.
68. HUNT, see Ch. 2 note 3, p. 108.
69. AGE CONCERN, *Good Neighbours*, Age Concern, 1972, p. 1.
70. MORRIS, *op. cit.*, p. 183.
71. CHEESEMAN, LANSLEY and WILSON, *op. cit.*, p. 69.

Part three
ASSESSMENT

Chapter eleven
THE CONTRIBUTION OF THE ELDERLY

INTRODUCTION

In the last two chapters attention has been focused on the help given to those elderly people who need some outside support. The main sources of help apart from the statutory services, were described. In this chapter attention is turned to the help which the elderly themselves give to others. This is set in the context of a discussion of the theory of the exchange relationship and of the stigma and dependency which are often associated with services provided for the elderly. The help given by the elderly both to their own families and to others is examined. Then the wider role of the elderly in policy making is assessed.

Writers about the elderly tend to consider them almost exclusively as consumers of social services. But what is their role as contributors? Apart from their input to the statutory services in the past through the system of rates and taxes, what they give through voluntary service as they become older is seldom mentioned in the literature.

THE EXCHANGE RELATIONSHIP

The exchange relationship can be defined as an encounter in which both giving and receiving takes place. It is nearly always assumed that it is more prestigious to give than to receive and that there is a clear economic and social distinction between the giver and the receiver. Often there is stigma attached to receiving and, when the elderly are in this position, they are usually considered to be in a state of dependency. These concepts of the exchange relationship, dependency and stigma will now be considered briefly.

One of the most comprehensive analyses of the exchange relationship, as it relates to social policy, is given by Pinker[1] who also comments on the theories of Titmuss.[2,3] This study is not concerned with the wider applications of the theory but only with those that relate specifically to the social services as a whole as they affect the position of the individual. Whether people do in fact see themselves as involved in this way is of course another matter.

There is first the distinction between the exchange relationship in economic matters and that in social matters. Pinker points out that people know where they stand in an economic exchange relationship because money confers a recognised right to buy goods and services.[4] In social relationships the rate of exchange is not so clearly agreed.

Secondly, there is the exchange relationship which applies to all the social services. The theory is that people pay a contribution in some way (e.g. taxes, rates, etc.) and therefore should feel as entitled to social services as they do to goods and services in an economic exchange. Pinker claims that this is unrealistic: 'The idea of paying taxes or holding authentic claims by virtue of citizenship remains largely an intellectual conceit of the social scientist . . . consequently most applicants for social services remain paupers at heart.'[5]

Thirdly, there is the exchange relationship involved in a specific (or particular) service. Forder states that it is, for example, the basis of schemes of national insurance.[6] People who are currently at work pay into a scheme which supports older people in the expectation that a similar exchange will take place when they themselves reach old age.

Fourthly, there is the exchange relationship on an individual basis. Services may be exchanged between individuals or between small groups such as families. Sometimes there may be a real expectation that another service will be conferred in return, while at other times it may be given as a 'gift'. But, as Titmuss points out in *The Gift Relationship*, motives may often be mixed.[7]

The position of the elderly is special because of a number of factors which can make them feel that they are receivers rather than givers. Firstly, for many, there is a sudden ending of employment and of being productive members of the community (see Ch. 5). This is a point put forcibly by Johnson [doc 44]. Parsons suggests that many elderly in pre-industrial society did not actually retire. However, it is equally true that many did not survive to old age either. People like farmers are able to 'taper off' in their particular professions. Although this is still possible for some, for the majority the attainment of the age of 60 or 65 means the automatic end to their lifetime as an economic contributor to society. O'Keefe, however, has pointed out that there may be differences between social classes. He argues that those in middle-class professions often do retain some status – the doctor keeps his title on retirement. But the working-class majority hold neither the 'power to strike nor the significant remnants of social acclaim and distinction that accrue to the middle-class elderly'.[8]

Secondly, there is the current psychological atmosphere in which the elderly are regarded as being beyond the point when they have anything to contribute. It is part of what Hobman calls the false sentimentality about old age. The old, he declares, are 'frequently required to adopt a somewhat passive role and to express a sense of gratitutde for what is provided'.[9] Another aspect of this is the problem of the elderly in a youth-centred society. However, Faulkner in a letter to *The Times* (5.12.72) says that the loss of role and identity can be retarded by keeping retired people within the community, not as passive observers but as active participants.

Thirdly, the emphasis on receiving is underscored because in economic matters most old people are dependent on a state pension for their main source of income. Fourthly, Pinker argues that the growth of selective social services differentiates the recipients much more clearly than those social services which are universal and do not single out those who receive.[10]

All these factors contribute to the elderly being looked on usually as a dependent group, if dependency is defined as being in a subordinate relationship. Whether the elderly are more or less dependent than in the past is arguable. Some maintain that a state pension lessens the dependence of the elderly on their families while others hold the view that the elderly are now more dependent on social services.

There is no doubt that the elderly themselves wish to be independent, although there are many different interpretations of independence. Hunt found that it is often thought of in economic terms.[11] For the working elderly it seemed to mean not being dependent on a supplementary pension, while for the non-workers it meant being independent of the constraints of employment. Most surveys of the elderly find that the majority do not want to be dependent on other people. Even the elderly people who lived close to their own families in granny annexes stressed the importance of being 'independent'.[12]

Equally important is the feeling of having something useful to do. Age Concern in *Attitudes of the Retired and Elderly*[13] noted that over half the elderly in their study felt that no one relied on them. It seemed that not being relied on by anyone was part of the poor health–loneliness–social isolation syndrome. A sense of purpose in life was held by Dame Eileen Younghusband, writing from both professional and personal experience, to be one of the main sources of morale. She felt that creating situations which strengthened morale was of crucial importance.

Colthorn in *Living Longer* judged that the most acute problem of the elderly was the feeling of being unwanted and of having no place in the life of the community.[14] She went on to quote Mochansky, a Russian physician, who had analysed the emotional effect of the 17 months siege of Leningrad. He attributed the lack of breakdowns 'to the fact that everyone from the smallest child to the oldest inhabitant had a job to do. The fact that they were busy meant that they were mentally healthy and if "something to do" is a prerequisite for mental health, both industrialist and social worker must combine to provide this for the elderly.'[15]

If people feel that they have no role and they also feel dependent this may engender a sense of stigma. Forder suggests that one reason why stigma is attached to being a beneficiary of services is that the welfare state is not a mutual benefit association and is not based on an equal exchange of services.[16] It is possible that those who contribute the least may be in need of the greatest number of services and vice versa. Pinker, however, suggests that it is possible to use the social services as a device for restoring and compensating those individuals who have previously been stigmatised by the economic market.[17] But he also points out that an individual may be less conscious of any stigma if he receives help from a number of different sources, rather than being dependent on a single source.[18]

Is there any evidence that the elderly wish to reverse the process of dependency and be more equal contributors to society? While it is unwise to generalise, one of the leading groups concerned with the elderly (Age Concern) said that it spoke for the majority when it declared in its *Manifesto* the need for a change of attitudes by society:

It is therefore urgently necessary to educate the public mind in its attitude towards the elderly in order to banish once and for all, the widely held image of the old as passive, poor and pitiful second-class citizens. The elderly themselves need to be convinced of their value and usefulness – they, like everyone else, are subject to social and psychological pressures and have been conditioned to accept the estimate of their comparative worthlessness and insignificance. By the realisation of their rights and responsibilities as participating members of society, and by re-charging their own powers of self-reliance and self-help, they will be better equipped to assert their own claims to equal consideration.[19]

Titmuss said that people have a social and biological need to help.[20] Gilholme had made a similar point in *The Emotional Needs of the Retired and Elderly* when she said: 'The desire to contribute does not necessarily diminish with age, though it becomes more difficult to realise.' But then went on to add another important point. 'How can we be so shortsighted as to allow time to go wasted when it could be so willingly given?'[21] It may therefore be right to take account of the needs of the elderly to contribute, not only from the point of view of their own welfare but also of their use to society.

FACTORS AFFECTING THE ABILITY OF THE ELDERLY TO GIVE

Whether the elderly wish not only to remain independent but to give help in some form to others depends on a number of different things. These include their abilities, how they choose to use their time, the opportunities given by society and the general concept of retirement.

Abilities

One of the most comprehensive discussions of the abilities of the elderly occurs in Jones, *Liberation of the Elders*. In this Jones shows how so-called objective tests are a less true measure of ability than the evidence coming from new interests, and the right kind of opportunity to learn.[22] He points out that: 'It is not only an impoverished education which leads to an under-exploitation of potential; the circumstances of adult life, particularly the work undertaken, can compound and encourage the narrowing of interests.' Thus, someone in a clerical job may find that manipulative skills are left unused. Worse still, many women after years at home have become narrow in their interests. He gives evidence that where opportunities for gaining new skills are offered, older people rapidly and thoroughly acquire new knowledge. He concludes that the majority of people can master new materials irrespective of their age, and that what prevents many from doing this is the limited expectations which they have of themselves and which others have of them.[23]

Use of time and leisure activities

Comparing participation in social and cultural activities by age there was in 1977 a clear pattern that the elderly took less part in nearly every activity.[24] In open-air activities, cultural entertainments, social activities, home-based activities and betting and gambling the elderly participated less in each of the 30 listed pursuits, with the exception of outings and social and voluntary work in which the elderly took as much part as other groups. More older men and women went to church than other age groups.

In Hunt's survey of elderly people at home she found that pets, church and hobbies such as knitting and needlework for women and gardening for men were the main leisure activites.[25] Figures produced by the BBC show that the elderly watch more television than any other age group, with the exception of the 5–14 year olds.

Abrams, however, has shown that averages conceal wide differences and that for both 'passive' (e.g. watching television) and 'active' occupations (e.g. walking) there were sizeable minorities falling into extreme categories. The key to this variety in the use of time and in behaviour by those reaching pensionable age lay, he felt, primarily in social class differences, and this was particularly so with men. While the average AB man on retirement reduced his paid work time and also reduced the hours he spent on passive leisure activities, the average DE man cut out paid employment almost entirely and increased the time spent on passive leisure activities. The transition for women on reaching old age was less dramatic because for all social classes there were still the same household activities to be undertaken.

Abrams concludes that 'a strong case can be made out on grounds of general social well-being for introducing working class men and women in middle age, and even earlier, to the skills, interests and values that are now enjoyed by middle class people' (*New Society*, 21.12.78, p. 686). He thinks that the differences in life style helps account for the fact that on average middle-class men outlive their working-class fellows by anything up to 10 years.

Opportunities given by society

While some old people will wish to relax in their retirement and to remain as uninvolved as they were in earlier years, others may wish to further their own education, to take up or develop former interests or to contribute to the life of the community.

For some opportunities looked for are educational, and Glendenning writing of lifelong education and the over 60s states that only recently have we begun to pay serious attention to the educational needs and potential of the over 60s. He marshals the evidence about mental functioning being only minimally related to age. He says: 'It has become increasingly clear that mental health can be considerably improved after retirement if a sense of purpose and of belonging to the whole community can be found. Lifelong education is only one of the ways in which this can be achieved.'[26]

For others the opportunities wanted are the chance to do really worthwhile things for the community, but 'not pastimes or diversional therapy to fill in time till death comes'.[27] Age Concern in their *Manifesto* declared that there was scope for the energetic and outward-looking retired to create a self-help network because people respond readily to the examples and initiatives of their own generation. What is needed is the creation of a favourable atmosphere for mutual encouragement. The *Manifesto* stated that: 'It is not "natural" that individuals should be discouraged, and even precluded, from exploring and developing their full potential simply because of their chronological age and because society no longer expects this of them.'[28]

Retirement and its meaning

When Vic Feather retired as General Secretary of the Trades Union Congress he is reported to have analysed the theme of his retirement cards. The predominant motif was the setting sun closely followed by pictures of 'a decrepit old man sitting in an armchair with, beside him, his faithful hound, its head resting on his knee. From the soulful expression in its eyes the sentiment was clear. If only the dog could speak, it would be saying, "you've had it, chum".'[29] This conventional view of retirement is bound up, as some of the Age Concern Manifesto Groups found, with the larger question of whether retirement is a separate phase in the human life span. The groups accepted that the word 'retirement' implies some form of planned withdrawal from constant occupation, but the majority view was that elderly people are conditioned by society as to what they can be and do in retirement.

Reflecting the views of over 8,000 elderly people the Manifesto Group said over and over again that two of the main disadvantages of retirement are loss of status and difficulty in adjusting to a lack of a definite role in society.[30] However, several groups felt that the present climate of opinion was more enlightened than 20 years ago and that the next generation of retired would be more active and take a more positive approach to retirement.[31]

Part of this positive approach could be an active preparation for retirement. An organisation which is particularly concerned with this is the Pre-Retirement Association. They suggest that everyone about to retire should have adequate opportunity and facilities for preparing for this phase of their life.

SOME CONSTRAINTS, INCLUDING SOCIAL ISOLATION

Though the elderly may have both the time and the ability to give help to others there may be other constraints over the degree to which they are able to do so. In a survey of 2,700 people of pensionable age 61 per cent said they had difficulty in committing themselves to arrangements in advance either because of the state of their health or that of their spouse or because they had someone else that they looked after.[32]

Table 8. Elderly households:* use of car and telephone, in England, 1976 (%)

	Age of head of household			All elderly	All house-holds
	65–74	75–84	85+		
Percentage with use of:					
Both car and telephone	22	12	7	18	37
Car only	13	5	6	10	19
Telephone only	21	27	28	23	13
Neither car nor telephone	44	57	59	49	31
Total	100	100‡	100	100	100
Percentage with use of a car:					
Male head	45	25	17	39	65
Female head	18	10	11	14	20
All households	35	16	12	28	56
Sample size† (numbers)	894	776	141	1,811	6,695

* An elderly household has a head who is aged 65 or over or who is the husband of a woman aged 65 or over. The group 65–74 includes married couples where the wife is aged 65 or over but the husband is aged under 65.

† These figures show the actual number of interviews, but as age groups were sampled with different probabilities percentages are based on numbers which have been weighted to restore true proportions.

‡ Figures have been rounded up.

Source: From CSO *Social Trends* (No. 9), Table 10.12, p. 165.

The elderly in modern society

There are also practical constraints relating to their ability to help other people, such as whether they can be contacted readily and, in some cases, how mobile they are.

Table 8 shows that elderly households are less likely to have the use of a telephone or car than other households. Nearly half all elderly people in 1976 had neither telephone nor car compared with less than one-third of all households. Table 8 also shows that the older the person the less likely he or she is to have either telephone or car. Where the head of an elderly household is a woman there is a greater likelihood that she will be without the use of a car.

In Hunt's survey, *The Elderly at Home*, it is clear that those who lived alone were worse off than those who lived with others so far as the telephone was concerned. Whereas 55.6 per cent of all elderly people had no telephone 64.2 per cent of those living alone had none. She commented: 'It is particularly disquieting that only just over one-third of those living alone have a telephone.'[33]

Social isolation

It is often thought that isolation and loneliness are common problems in old age and that they are both a cause and a result of the lack of a contribution to society by elderly people. Shanas *et al.*, however, state that the concept of isolation is by no means straight-forward.[34] To some it means 'lack of communion between man and his fellow'. The individual may be immersed in social activities but unable to communicate his feelings and experience. Others see isolation as lack of integration into a particular group. Shanas *et al.*, consider the isolation of the elderly from society in four separate ways:
'1. By comparison with their contemporaries – peer-contrasted isolation.
2. By comparison with younger people – generation-contrasted isolation.
3. By comparison with the social relationships and activities enjoyed by [other younger or middle-aged people] – age-related isolation.
4. By comparison with the preceding generation of old people – preceding cohort isolation.'[35]

Isolation is clearly extremely difficult to analyse. It may be objective (e.g. social contacts can be counted) or it can be subjective (people can be asked about their feelings). Most studies of social isolation such as Townsend,[36] Tunstall[37] and Shanas *et al.*[38] have been concerned primarily with the first of the four types of isolation mentioned above. In these three studies approximately the same method of measuring was used and this involved collecting information about social activities as a way of estimating the number of 'social contacts'. Approximately one-fifth of the samples were isolated or extremely isolated and they were more likely to be women and have no children. However, isolation does not necessarily increase with age, although Abrams, using a different method of scoring, did find a slightly higher percentage of the over 75s who were isolated than the 65–74 year olds.[39]

Loneliness

There is a conceptual distinction between isolation and loneliness. Isolation relates to *circumstances* (which can usually be measured, however crudely), whereas loneliness relates to feelings (often about those circumstances). A common dictionary definition of isolation is 'apart or alone'. One of the most important findings of all the recent studies of the elderly has been that loneliness appears to have little relation to lack of contact with relatives, friends, clubs or other social activities. That isolation and loneliness are not synonymous was one of the most important findings of the cross-national survey in 1968.[40] Tunstall made important distinctions between living alone, social isolation, loneliness and anomie (a feeling of 'normlessness' or pointlessness).[41] In the study of sheltered housing tenants in Hanover Housing Association schemes it was also concluded that there seemed to be little association between lack of social contact and loneliness.[42] Hadley and Webb in *Social Isolation and Old People* came to a similar conclusion.[43]

A group of social workers from BASW pointed to two main factors in loneliness.[44] These were the lack of a close relationship with another person and the emotional trauma caused by the loss of a life companion.

A national study found that 7 per cent of the elderly felt lonely often, 21 per cent sometimes and 72 per cent rarely or never.[45]

Not all the socially isolated in the various samples were lonely by any means. Some seemed to enjoy things as they were and enjoyed being alone. Sainsbury found exactly the same among the disabled. 'Even the most isolated and severely incapacitated persons felt a passionate attachment to their life at home.'[46] Abrams concluded:

It is no longer assumed that there is a simple one-to-one relationship between isolation and loneliness, that all those who live alone and have

comparatively few contacts with the outside world at a face-to-face level
automatically feel lonely, unhappy and dissatisfied with their lives. Some
isolates are happy, satisfied with their lives and feel far from lonely; and at
the same time some of those leading highly gregarious lives are not immune
from a sense of loneliness and depression.[47]

HELP GIVEN BY THE ELDERLY

Evidence has already been presented in Chapters 9 and 10 about the
extent of help which the elderly receive from their families, from
their neighbours and from the wider community. But the elderly
also give help to these groups and this will now be examined.

To families

Because there have been few systematic studies in the past of help
given by the elderly it is impossible to make comparisons. Most of
the studies about to be referred to only touch on the subject in
passing and do not have it as their main focus. Those who look back
with nostalgia claim that the old kept a role right to the end; though
it is to be hoped that it was not quite such a macabre one as that
described by Simmons:

Even with their bent and nearly broken bodies the few surviving old people
could be prized for their nimble fingers and ready wits – and above all for
their knowledge, skills and experience . . .
  Old women too feeble to travel stayed indoors, attended household
chores, repaired garments, tanned leather . . . and shredded with their very
worn teeth the sinew of dried caribou and narwhat. While a Chippewa family
slept at night with their feet towards the coals, an old man kept watch,
smoked and fed fuel to the fire. According to Inca law, elderly persons unfit
for work should still serve as scarecrows to frighten birds and rodents from
the fields.[48]

Tunstall, however, is doubtful about the contribution of the
elderly in the past.[49] Shanas *et al.* also question the view that
intergenerational contact and mutual exchange of services is less
today, even though the standard living pattern now is one of separate
households. They say:

The traditional assumptions about the changes in the family and the
disintegration of relations between the generations in modern societies have
never been supported by empirical evidence. On the contrary, a number of
studies have demonstrated that the generations, although preferring to live

apart, maintain contact and exchange mutual services. What is found between the generations is 'intimacy' at a distance rather than isolation.[50]

The British studies of the 1950s and 1960s came to very similar conclusions about help given by the elderly, i.e. that it is still given, though more in areas where the families are housed near the elderly. Young and Willmott in *Family and Kinship in East London* showed the amount of help given, especially by mothers to their daughters.[51] But migration of the families impedes this flow of services between the generations. They said: 'If they [the elderly] have children and grandchildren round them, they cannot only be of some value to youth, they can also enjoy the rewards of being appreciated.'[52] Townsend and Wedderburn also found in their sample of the elderly that there was an exchange of services.[53]

A study by Brockington and Lempert of the over 80s in Stockport observed their 'importance and active contribution to family life'.[54] Bracey's comparative study of pensioners in Great Britain and the United States notes the types of help the elderly gave.[55] They included those observed in the granny annexes sample[56] – helping with children, keeping the house key and so on. Help also included gifts of money and help with housekeeping services. The study of Woodford by Willmott and Young emphasised the care grandparents gave to children.[57] And the Shanas *et al.* study showed that in Great Britain 44 per cent of the elderly gave help to their children and 33 per cent to their grandchildren.[58] This compares with 59 per cent who received help from children and other relatives. But Harris points out that the giving and receiving may blur into one: 'Whereas the daughter sees her visits as "keeping an eye on Mum", Mum may see the visits as the daughter turning to her for help and advice.'[59] He points out that to be on the receiving end of help in old age amounts to an abrupt reversal of the parental role.

Evidence from studies in the 1970s confirm the extent of help given to families.[60] Hunt found that nearly one-third of her sample of elderly people were able to give help when they visited relatives, but that this declined sharply with age.[61]

Bell has pointed out that there may be class differences.[62] More financial help may be given by the older generation to the younger family in the middle classes. Fletcher says: 'The kinds and degrees of mutual aid, and the reasons for it, may differ between social classes also. For example, young middle-class parents may desire, and obtain, help from elder relations in order to send their children to public school.'[63]

One matter which has concerned a number of people has been the lack of legal rights and obligations that grandparents have in relation to their grandchildren. Until recently grandparents could find after death, divorce or separation had ended the marriage of their son or daughter that there was no way, short of going to the High Court for a wardship order, by which they were legally entitled even to see their grandchildren. However, clauses relating to the right of grandparents to apply for access to their grandchildren in certain circumstances were put into effect in 1979 following the Domestic Proceedings and Magistrates' Courts Act 1978.

To neighbours

Many elderly people give help to their neighbours. Sometimes the people helped are other old people. For example in the survey of old people in granny annexes the elderly often gave help to other old people and it was found that the design of the dwellings was an important factor in bringing this about.[64] There was a good deal of keeping keys for one another, letting in meter readers and so on. This was particularly noticeable in flats where the elderly lived in a row (if, for example, they were in a block under family flats) or in a square or corridor (above the family flats). It was less common in bungalows linked to the family house. Age Concern have also noted the extent of help elderly people give one another. They found that the help the elderly most liked giving was to other elderly people: 30 per cent visited someone sick or disabled and 24 per cent helped with shopping or errands.[65] And the reliance of old people in seaside resorts on their neighbours (usually also elderly) has already been mentioned in Chapter 10.

Voluntary work

The Aves Committee on volunteers thought that 'there may be considerable resources among the over 60s of both sexes'.[66] It was particularly poignant that this should have been one of their conclusions since they had started by paying tribute to their own honorary secretary who had 'devoted the greater part of her first year of retirement, in which she had planned to enjoy some leisure, to the gruelling task of helping us to formulate this report. We find it difficult to convey our gratitude in adequate terms.'

The view that there are untapped resources among the elderly to help the community is now widely held. Some also believe that if a sense of purpose and of belonging to the community can be given, mental health can be considerably improved.[67]

The Aves Committee in 1969 analysed the ages of volunteers in two research studies and concluded that retired people provided numerically only a minor source of voluntary service – less than 20 per cent in each case.[68] However, Hunt found that over one-third (36.2%) of her sample belonged to voluntary organisations.[69] She concluded: 'Membership of voluntary organisations may be of value to elderly people, particularly in enabling them to meet other people and to make a contribution to the life of the community.'[70] And in the *GHS 1977* the percentage of those over 60 years participating in social and voluntary work was 28 per cent, which was a higher figure than 10 years earlier.

Apart from voluntary work for any group, elderly or otherwise, that may need it, some writers and organisations consider that new schemes are in prospect. For example at a neighbourhood care workshop run by Age Concern it was suggested that elderly people could run self-help groups or provide a mutual service such as a food co-operative. The active elderly might provide a warden-type neighbourhood care scheme.

ROLE IN SOCIAL POLICY

The challenge to society over the elderly comes not only through the outward pressure of events such as the rise in numbers of the very old and frail or the increased cost of services. It comes also from within through the growth of an increasingly articulate group of people speaking for themselves. In some cases they may be speaking about their own needs but in others about other aspects of society.

Social policy for the elderly

Organisations and individuals concerned about the elderly are becoming more forceful in putting forward their views, as Age Concern's *Manifesto* stated:

Those who frame public policies, who set up systems of transportation and communication, and who plan social environments often fail to pay due regard to the special needs of the elderly when they differ from the needs of those who are more active and mobile. Those who administer medical and welfare services or who allocate resources of accommodation, recreation and education often fail to take their preferences and priorities fully into account.[71]

The acceptance of the elderly speaking for themselves was acknowledged in DHSS, *A Happier Old Age*, which declared that its policies so far had had two main aims but, 'Now we must add a third vital aim. Old people must be able to take their own decisions about their own lives. They must have the fullest possible choice and a major say in decisions that affect them.'[72]

Social policy in general

The elderly participate to a reasonable extent in elected bodies. They are well represented both among MPs and among local councillors, though there are fewer MPs over 60 than local councillors.

Of those elected to the House of Commons in 1977 10 per cent (and in 1974 13%) were over the age of 60 compared with about 20 per cent of that age in the total population in both years.

Hobman has declared that the elderly ought to be a more powerful and potent political force because of their sheer numbers. He has said that the politics of ageing should have their place within the mainstream of political decision making, and offered as a debating point the suggestion that: 'Pensioner organisations and those which serve the elderly should create an alliance which would have about it a force and permanence to define its own priorities: to test politicians' reactions to its proposals, and then to enlist support for its achievable objectives in the short-term so that it could then monitor progress in various ways including individual voting performances.'[73]

Figures are not available for the ages of all elected councillors, but two large surveys have been carried out. One was of 3,970 councillors for the Maud Committee on *Management of Local Government* in 1964. The second was for the Robinson Committee of Inquiry into the *Remuneration of Councillors*. This covered 4,643 councillors. As Table 9 shows, councillors are much older than the general population. For example in 1964 over half (52%) the male councillors were over 55 but only 31 per cent of the general male population were at that time over this age. In 1976 50 per cent of male councillors were over 55 but only 33 per cent of the general male population were over this age. If the equivalent figures for those over 65 were taken there were 14 per cent in the male population in 1964 and 17 per cent in 1976, while 22 per cent of councillors were of this age in 1964 and 21 per cent in 1976.

The Maud Committee saw value in a fairly high proportion of older councillors since they might bring wisdom and experience to

Table 9. Comparison of councillors in 1964 and 1976 with general population* – by age and sex (percentages in each age group)

| | *Men* | | | | *Women* | | | |
| | *Councillors* | | *Population* | | *Councillors* | | *Population* | |
	1964	*1976*	*1961*	*1976*	*1964*	*1976*	*1961*	*1976*
55–64	30	29	17	16	37	32	17	16
65–69	11	12	6	7	11	10	7	8
70–74	7	7	4	5	8	5	6	7
75 and over	4	2	4	5	5	1	7	10
Numbers	3,480	3,848†			490	795†		

* Census 1961 and Registrar-General's home population estimates, 1976.
† Excludes those who did not answer.

Sources:
1965 MHLG, *Committee on the Management of Local Government* (the Maud Committee). Vol. 2, *The Local Government Councillor*, Louis Moss and S. R. Parker, HMSO, 1967, Table 1.1, p. 15.
1976 DOE, *Committee of Inquiry into the System of Remuneration of Members of Local Authorities* (the Robinson Committee). Vol. 11, *The Surveys of Councillors and Local Authorities*, HMSO, 1977, Table 1, p. 8.

Note: The Maud survey covered England and Wales, whereas the Robinson survey included Scotland.

local affairs. On the other hand, they declared that they were anxious about the high average age of members and thought that no one aged 70 or over should be allowed to stand for election [doc 45].

CONCLUSION

The elderly, then, can and do give service in various ways, particularly to their families and as elected representatives. The opportunities in the future may be even greater. For example, the increasing number of mothers who work may lead to a demand for extra child care facilities. Grandparents, especially grandmothers, already play a major role in the care of their grandchildren as many surveys have shown. For example in one study by Bone for OPCS, *Pre-school Children and the Need for Day Care*, it was found that 25 per cent of children under five whose mother worked outside the home were looked after for at least part of the time by a grandmother. The increased emphasis on the value of voluntary help in many spheres may also lead to an expansion of help by the elderly.

On the other hand, there are other factors which should not be ignored. The numbers of young elderly, who might be expected to contribute through part-time employment or voluntary work, will decline at least in the short term (see Ch. 2). And society has also to be convinced of the value and usefulness of their contribution. For what everyone is able to contribute to society is determined in part by the social and psychological conditioning to which they are subjected. Those who feel wanted usually find it easier to give help than those who accept a public estimate of their own worthlessness.

REFERENCES

1. PINKER, R., *Social Theory and Social Policy*, Heinemann, 1971.
2. TITMUSS, R., *Commitment to Welfare*, Unwin, 1968.
3. TITMUSS, R., *The Gift Relationship*, Allen and Unwin, 1970.
4. PINKER, *op. cit.*
5. *Ibid.*, p. 142.
6. FORDER, A., *Concepts in Social Administration*, Routledge and Kegan Paul, 1974, p. 68.
7. TITMUSS, *The Gift Relationship*, pp. 210–24.
8. JONES, S. (ed.), *The Liberation of the Elders*, Beth Foundation Publications and Department of Adult Education, University of Keele, 1976, p. 93.
9. AGE CONCERN, *Easing the Restrictions on Ageing*, Age Concern, 1972, p. 49.
10. PINKER, *op. cit.*, p. 151.
11. HUNT, see Ch. 2 note 3, p. 130.
12. TINKER, see Ch. 7 note 27.
13. AGE CONCERN, *The Attitudes of the Retired*, see Ch. 3 note 48, p. 80.
14. NCSS, *Living Longer*, NCSS, 1954, p. 10.
15. *Ibid.*, pp. 12–13.
16. FORDER, *op. cit.*, pp. 142–3.
17. PINKER, *op. cit.*, p. 138.
18. *Ibid.*, p. 160.
19. AGE CONCERN, *Manifesto*, see Ch. 9 note 48, p. 3.
20. TITMUSS, *The Gift Relationship*.
21. GILHOLME, K., *The Emotional Needs of the Retired and the Elderly*, Age Concern, 1973, p. 6.
22. JONES, *op. cit.*, p. 27.
23. *Ibid.*, p. 28.

24. CSO, *Social Trends* (No. 9), see Ch. 2 note 12, p. 177.
25. HUNT, see Ch. 2 note 3.
26. JONES, *op. cit.*, p. 68.
27. STEWART, M., *Social Rehabilitation of the Elderly*, Age Concern, 1974, p. 8.
28. AGE CONCERN, *Manifesto*, see Ch. 9 note 48, p. 4.
29. PILCH, M., *The Retirement Book*, Hamish Hamilton, 1974, p. vii.
30. AGE CONCERN, *The Place of the Retired and Elderly in Modern Society*, Age Concern, 1974, p. 12.
31. *Ibid.*, p. 32.
32. AGE CONCERN, *The Attitudes of the Retired*, see Ch. 3 note 48, p. 74.
33. HUNT, see Ch. 2 note 3, p. 106.
34. SHANAS, *et al.*, see Ch. 3 note 7, Ch. 9.
35. *Ibid.*, p. 260.
36. TOWNSEND, see Ch. 4 note 1.
37. TUNSTALL, see Ch. 3 note 8.
38. SHANAS *et al.*, see Ch. 3 note 7.
39. ABRAMS, see Ch. 2 note 4, pp. 35–6.
40. SHANAS *et al.*, see Ch. 3 note 7, Ch. 9.
41. TUNSTALL, see Ch. 3 note 8.
42. PAGE and MUIR, see Ch. 4 note 13.
43. HADLEY, R. and WEBB, A., *Social Isolation and Old People – some implications for social policy*, Age Concern, 1974.
44. AGE CONCERN, *The Place of the Retired*, pp. 44–5.
45. SHANAS *et al.*, see Ch. 3 note 7, p. 271.
46. SAINSBURY, S., *Registered as Disabled*, G. Bell and Sons, 1970, p. 182.
47. ABRAMS, see Ch. 2 note 4, p. 38.
48. SIMMONS, L. W., 'Ageing in primitive society', *Law and Contemporary Problems*, Winter, 1962, p. 42.
49. TUNSTALL, see Ch. 3 note 8.
50. SHANAS *et al.*, see Ch. 3 note 7, p. 180.
51. YOUNG and WILLMOTT, see Ch. 9 note 8, pp. 196–7.
52. *Ibid.*, p. 192.
53. TOWNSEND and WEDDERBURN, see Ch. 3 note 6, pp. 66–7.
54. BROCKINGTON and LEMPERT, see Ch. 3 note 12, p. 2.
55. BRACEY, see Ch. 3 note 3.
56. TINKER, see Ch. 7 note 27, p. 26.
57. WILLMOTT and YOUNG, see Ch. 3 note 5, pp. 66–7.
58. SHANAS *et al.*, see Ch. 3 note 7, p. 205.
59. HARRIS, C. H., *The Family*, Allen and Unwin, 1969, p. 204.

60. AGE CONCERN, *The Attitudes of the Retired*, see Ch. 3 note 48, p. 80.
61. HUNT, see Ch. 2 note 3, p. 101.
62. BELL, C. R., *Middle Class Families*, Routledge and Kegan Paul, 1969.
63. FLETCHER, see Ch. 9 note 2, p. 169.
64. TINKER, see Ch. 7 note 27.
65. AGE CONCERN, *The Attitudes of the Retired*, see Ch. 3 note 48, p. 78.
66. NCSS, Aves Committee, see Ch. 10 note 15, p. 120.
67. JONES, *op. cit.*, p. 68.
68. NCSS, Aves Committee, see Ch. 10, note 15, p. 36.
69. HUNT, see Ch. 2 note 3, p. 126.
70. *Ibid.*, p. 125.
71. AGE CONCERN, *Manifesto*, see Ch. 9 note 48, p. 3.
72. DHSS, *A Happier Old Age*, see Ch. 3 note 61, p. 5.
73. JONES, *op. cit.*, p. 117.

Chapter twelve
SOME GENERAL PROBLEMS

Many of the problems encountered in providing for the elderly are the same as, or similar to, those for other groups. Many old people are disabled, and some who are housebound share some of the problems of mothers with small children. Those who are deaf, blind or socially isolated present difficulties of communication similar to those experienced by ethnic minorities.

Some of these problems, which will now be discussed, are: differing perspectives of need; variations in services; take-up of benefits and lack of knowledge of services; the evaluation of services; the meaning of community care.

DIFFERING PERSPECTIVES OF NEED

While theorists of social administration have become increasingly concerned with measuring needs there is a danger that those actually providing the service may become less so. If resources continue to be severely limited it is possible that agencies may deal solely with the obvious needs of which they are immediately aware. For example a local authority with a lengthy waiting list for housing can perhaps be forgiven if it does not go out of its way to uncover any fresh needs. Yet it might be possible for some people on the list to have their needs met in a more appropriate way. An elderly person on a council list for sheltered housing, for example, may not have considered (or been offered) ways of improving or adapting their home. Similarly, there may be many in need who, for one reason or another, are not on the list. It might, for example, be more economic (and make for greater individual happiness) if some old people in residential homes had their needs examined more closely and, if it were found appropriate, offered an alternative form of housing. One of the most interesting ways of distinguishing types of need is that developed by

The elderly in modern society

Bradshaw (*New Society*, 3.3.72, pp. 640–3). He divided needs into four types: normative, felt, expressed and comparative, and these will be discussed in turn.

Normative

This is need as defined by the experts. Examples of this concept of need, as used for the elderly, are the incapacity scale developed by Townsend[1] and the measures of social isolation used by Tunstall.[2] A number of subsequent researchers such as Shanas *et al*.[3] have constructed similar scales of disability to Townsend's by asking questions of the elderly about their capacity to perform certain tasks. In this way their dependency rates can be measured, so that they can be assessed as needing varying degrees of help, from slight to continuous, if they are to be able to remain in their own homes. Some of these different approaches are summarised in Isaacs and Neville [doc 46].

A variation of the idea of consulting 'experts' was that used by Harris who asked the appropriate officers in a sample of local authorities what criteria they used for assessing the needs of the elderly. But the expert may sometimes conceal needs. For example, a community physician has suggested that some old people are not put on a waiting list for accommodation by their professional advisers – health visitors and social workers – who wish to spare them from disappointment. Another disadvantage of this approach is pointed out by Forder. He said that the views of experts are likely to be strongly influenced by their own perspectives.[4] One of the dangers of leaving definitions of need to the experts, he declared, is that it appears an attractive and simple approach. On the other hand there is evidence from Goldberg that social workers with training identify more needs of elderly people than do those without training.[5]

Felt

Bradshaw's second category is felt need. This equates needs with wants. Many services are based wholly or partly on this notion of self-referral. The problem here is that what people feel they want is governed very much by their previous experience and their knowledge of what is available. What one elderly person may feel he or she needs may be very different from what another feels. Rising expectations will mean that felt needs will keep on growing. Some elderly people today do not expect central heating in their homes, but it is likely that their children will.

Felt need is probably one of the least satisfactory ways of measuring need. A number of studies have shown that the less people have and the more deprived they are the less likely they are to feel the need for a service. Forder discusses the view that 'a policy of provision based on felt need would require a wide dissemination of knowledge, and indeed a much greater openness about the criteria for decisions than most of those concerned with the provision of social service, professionals, administrators and representatives are generally prepared to show'.[6]

Expressed

Bradshaw's third category is expressed need. This is when felt needs are turned into action. Need then becomes equated with demand, for it is those who express their need who are said to be 'in need'. Some local authorities see the needs of their area through the expressed needs of a waiting list. But there may be many reasons why people do not demand a service. The following are just some examples:

1. They may not know that the service exists, especially if it attracts little publicity.
2. They may feel that they do not qualify. For example in a study of granny annexes one or two owner-occupiers expressed surprise that they had been offered a council house tenancy.[7] Not all local authorities do rehouse owner-occupiers.
3. They may feel that the service is overloaded and they have no possibility of obtaining it. As Harris commented in *Social Welfare for the Elderly* '. . . they decide, rightly or wrongly, that there is little point in asking for a home help or rehousing, as they "know they haven't got a chance"'.[8] Sumner and Smith in *Planning Local Authority Services for the Elderly* make the same comment about housing: 'Clearly there was a tendency for demands not to be expressed by the public unless there was some hope of their being met.'[9]
4. The service may be very poor.
5. There may be stigma attached to the service.
6. The person may feel it beneath his dignity to apply.

On the other hand the provision of a service – especially if it is of a high standard – will actually create a demand. This is as true in the

1970s as it was in the 1930s, as the following two examples show. Olive Matthews who was an early campaigner to obtain better provision for the elderly wrote in the *Sunday Graphic* (16.2.36):

I have had specimen blocks of one room flats designed and have submitted them to councils all over the country. At first there was an outcry against them – Ridiculous! What do single women want with flats? We never have any demand for them. Exactly. There has been no demand because there has been no supply. Yet when a certain mining town built ten cottages for old people over a thousand applications were received. Whenever the experiment is made the response shows how great the need has been.

And as recently as the early 1970s the James Butcher Housing Association in Reading, when planning to build a block of flats beside a prosperous 1930s estate of owner-occupiers, was told 'there was no demand, the owners were adequately housed'. But in the first two weeks after the flats were opened they had 48 applications from these 'satisfied owners'.

The conclusion must be that any assessment of demands is hypothetical until a service is actually provided. When it is provided then demand may rocket. Demand, therefore, is not by itself a simple and reliable guide to need. This distinction between demand and need was made by the DHSS in their evidence to a House of Commons Public Expenditure Committee in 1972 [doc 47].

Comparative

The fourth definition Bradshaw used is comparative need. 'A measure of need is found by studying the characteristics of those in receipt of a service. If people with similar characteristics are not in receipt of a service, then they are in need.' This is the same basis used by Harris in *Social Welfare for the Elderly*.[10] She examined the records of those getting a service or on live waiting lists. She then asked the elderly for details of the circumstances which led to their being given a particular service. From this she was able to make some assessment of need.

These four methods of assessing need (normative, felt, expressed and comparative) all have a place in the overall concept. But, as has been seen, each has advantages and disadvantages and none gives a complete picture. To achieve a comprehensive definition of need all four have to be taken into account. From a practical point of view Harris in case studies of some local authorities has shown how they interpreted need [doc 48].

VARIATIONS IN SERVICES

There may be variations in services between individuals, between different groups of people and between areas. Good reasons may well account for this variation. The personal circumstances of people are rarely identical, nor are local conditions.

Between individuals

In some services, such as provision of the basic pension, the standards are laid down with great precision. But for other services, such as supplementary pensions, there may be need for individual discretion so that any different factors (such as the need for a special diet or extra heating) can be taken into account. The only way to achieve some sort of standardisation is to have detailed codes issued to officers so that like cases are treated in a similar way. But while policies are different there can never be a guarantee that elderly people will get the same service. An example quoted by Harris is of an authority that did not give home help if a daughter was living there [doc 48]. What is helpful for the elderly is that the criteria on which services are provided should be known. It can help prevent the 'Mrs Smith next door has it why haven't I?' syndrome so well known to social workers.

Between groups

The second sort of variation is that which occurs between different client groups. In the case of the elderly it is held that not only is there need to improve care but provision must be made for the continuing increase in the elderly population. These points are developed further in Chapter 13 under Priorities.

Between areas and local authorities

Variations between areas occur largely because local authorities are elected bodies with considerable freedom of choice about what they do. One reason for local government is the variation in local conditions, and it is right that councils should be able to take this into account. Another powerful argument for a lack of uniformity is that there should be freedom to experiment and pioneer. If successful these services can then be copied by other authorities. Services that have started in this way include meals on wheels and sheltered housing. But local authorities also work under considerable constraints, not least the fact that about two-thirds of their income comes from central government. The controls exercised by central government include loan sanctions, subsidies, confirmation of plans, the right to vet certain key appointments and a whole range of informal advisory roles. Some ministries lay down standards in great detail, as the DOE has done over housing for the elderly (Ch. 7). In the case of the DHSS, departmental guidelines are laid down for many services as was seen in Chapter 8.

There are many reasons why there are differences between services provided by local authorities. Some of these were analysed by Davies *et al.* in *Variations in Services for the Aged*. These included the political composition of the council, the demand for the service and the extent of provision in the past. Research has pinpointed other reasons. Wealth came out as important in two studies done for the Royal Commission on Local Government in 1968. The Maud Committee on Management (1967) showed that the impact of personalities, both elected members and officers, was considerable. As the Royal Commission on Local Government (1969) discovered, it has been more difficult, however, to prove that the size of a local authority has any important effect on performance. What a large authority does have is the potential to provide better services. Variations may also be caused when services fail to catch up with a movement in population. For example Hunt found that retirement areas, which by definition included high percentages of people aged 65 and over, were badly off in respect of visits by nearly all the social services.[11]

Variations may also occur between non-elected bodies and this is acknowledged in health. The DHSS (1976) Report of the Resource Allocation Working Party stated: 'This report confirms the existence of large disparities between the way in which resources have traditionally been allocated to different parts of the country, and the way in which they would be allocated on our recommended criteria of relative need. Disparities of the order demonstrated could not be redressed at a stroke.'[12]

Following this the DHSS stated that 'there is also to be a shift of resources towards those regions and localities which, historically have received less funds per head of population than others, and where standards of service have suffered accordingly'.[13]

TAKE-UP OF BENEFITS AND LACK OF KNOWLEDGE OF SERVICES

Access to benefits in the welfare state is one of the most interesting and relevant subjects.

One consistent theme running through social surveys of the elderly is their reluctance to take up benefits which are theirs by right and their lack of knowledge of services. Townsend and Wedderburn made particular reference to the numbers not claiming state financial help to which they were entitled.[14] This has subsequently been borne out by the work of the SBC (see Ch. 5).

In the medical field Isaacs, Livingstone and Neville claimed that there were many old people who 'failed to seek help because of apathy, reluctance or fear' who had disabilities such as foot troubles, anaemia, visual impairment or depression which are amenable to treatment.[15]

Interesting evidence is presented in Hunt's study that elderly people in touch with one service seemed more likely to receive others. She found that those living in rented accommodation, particularly council tenants, were more likely than others to receive visits (from social services and similar bodies). This seems to be another indication that being in touch with one service increased the likelihood of contact with others.

In a useful discussion on rights to benefit, Hill in *The State, Administration and the Individual* gave some of the evidence about under-claiming by pensioners [doc 49]. One reason he put forward is the link between ignorance and stigma. 'Individuals who feel that they are likely to be stigmatised for claiming certain benefits, or even for simply revealing their needs, are likely to fail to take steps to overcome their ignorance of their rights.'[16] But stigma is not the only reason why people may fail to claim. They may, for example, be put off by whoever is the first person they approach. In *The Point of Entry* Hall makes a comment about the former children's departments which could apply to other social service departments: 'One of the many elements which may affect decisions about who received what is the person who looks after the telephone or sits behind the reception desk.'[17] These people are often referred to as 'gatekeepers'.

In addition to the points made here it is relevant to consider the expectations of the elderly. Many have lived through the privations of two world wars and a Depression and are grateful for what they now have. Whether the future elderly will take the same attitude is questionable. Generations used to a higher standard of living and used to questioning and a general awareness of 'rights' are less likely to be unaware of their entitlements. 'The rising level of education in the population is giving rise to a society which is less inclined to accept submissively the services provided by professionals' claimed speakers from the DHSS in a seminar.[18]

The need for more advice and information services has been made by a long line of government and other committees which have been summarised by Brooke in *Information and Advice Centres* (1972). Other suggestions for improving take-up are given in Burgess, *Selected or Neglected?* (Age Concern, 1974). If more advice is provided the problem of take-up of benefits and lack of knowledge of services may diminish.

THE EVALUATION OF SERVICES

One of the most difficult tasks in social policy is to measure the effectiveness of services. There is no simple way in which this can be done, but some key questions must be asked.

Some questions

What is the total *amount* of provision? It is possible to measure total provision in a number of ways – amount spent, units provided, numbers of staff or man-hours allocated – and all these give some indication of the service. But even these figures may mask a poor or unequal service. A large amount of money may be spent but be wastefully used. There may be better, possibly cheaper, ways of providing the service. The amount may not be distributed evenly, either between individuals or between areas, so again the amount spent does not tell the whole story.

What is the *range* of provision? A wide range gives choice. For example there are many ways in which food can be provided for the elderly, but unless all the options, which include meals on wheels, clubs, day centres, allowing home helps to cook the meal and paying a neighbour, are provided the service is not necessarily an effective one as it may not meet the needs of all the elderly. A range of provision may mean that specialist services and workers are provided.

What is the *quality* of the service? Quality is one of the most difficult things to measure. Some would argue that staff who are trained provide a better-quality service and this was borne out by

Goldberg's study where trained social workers uncovered more of the needs of elderly people.[19]

Does the service reach the people for whom it is intended? An elaborate, expensive service may be provided but be totally ineffective if it does not reach planned recipients. If this is because the elderly persons do not know about it, the remedy is to find ways of ensuring that they do know. If, however, the elderly person does not in fact want it, that is a different matter. The elderly, as other groups, have the right not to accept a service.

Some problems

There are also a number of problems in how a service is to be evaluated:

The subjective nature of evaluation The process of evaluation necessarily entails, as the word suggests, the placing of goods, services or actions in an order of values. What these values are and what level of importance is given to them ought always to be openly stated and not, as so often happens, be left as a hidden assumption, since not everyone will necessarily accept the same scale of values. In some research, for example, the assumption is made that to keep the elderly in their own homes is to some extent a mark of 'success'. But this assumption needs to be questioned as Malcolm Brown pointed out in *The Observer* (25.3.73):

The problem is that, of itself, keeping an elderly person at home can be both a measure of effectiveness and ineffectiveness. The true measure of effectiveness could be either keeping the old person at home or encouraging him to enter a hospital or residential home – depending on which course of action was appropriate to his own need and circumstances. Once the term 'appropriateness' enters in – and it must do if measures are to be meaningful – subjective judgement becomes an important factor. It brings with it the problems of whose judgement should be accepted and whether that judgement is valid and reliable.

Statistical measurement Another method of evaluation which is not open to subjective bias, is to assess a service in terms of the amount spent or the number of units provided, or in some other way which is easily quantifiable. The 'cost–benefit' approach is one which has become increasingly popular among researchers in social administration. But this method also has disadvantages in that it does not give room for an assessment of quality or the matching of need. For example, one agency may spend a great deal more than its neighbour on a service but may not necessarily provide a better service. It may not spend the money appropriately or it may spend wastefully.

Nevertheless, the quantitative method can be a valuable one and can be used, for example, in measuring sources of help for the elderly.

The views of the present consumers being used as a basis for provision for future generations Even when it is possible to find out people's views and feelings one has to assess what weight should be given to the views of the present generation when planning for the next, whose expectations may well be different. It would therefore be unwise to plan solely on the basis of what today's elderly think. It cannot, for example, be assumed that bedsitters and open fires, which find some favour today, will do so in the future.

Comparison between groups of elderly Another method of evaluation is to compare the information about the elderly given in various studies. Comparisons are an important form of evaluation, but again there are problems which have to be faced (see Ch. 2). For example, the definition of the elderly varies greatly. Some researchers take 'elderly' to mean those of retirement age, i.e. over 60 for women and 65 for men. Others take the same age for both. In the OPCS Social Survey study, *Handicapped and Impaired in Great Britain*, Harris divided the elderly (men and women together) into age groups of 50–64, 65–74 and 75 and over.[20]

A similar problem arises over the concept of social isolation (see Ch. 11). The method of scoring used by Tunstall in *Old and Alone*[21] was itself a modification of that used by Townsend in *Family Life of Old People*.[22] This again makes comparison difficult. Cross-national comparisons are even more complex because of the differing variables.

THE MEANING OF COMMUNITY CARE

The evidence of the previous chapters can now be brought together. The major findings are that some old people need some form of help and that this is substantial in the case of the frail elderly. This help comes mainly from the family, but the statutory services, voluntary organisations and friends and neighbours play an important role. They complement rather than compete. Many of the elderly give help to others and it is suggested that more of them could if given the opportunity. At the moment this help is mostly given to their families.

How do these findings contribute to a theory of community care? If we return to the definition of community care in Chapter 4 it was seen that the meaning is usually polarised between the provision of domiciliary services and a vague idea of caring by the community or society. Caring in this context is usually taken to mean the provision of help, support and protection. But as Titmuss pointed out: 'Unless we are prepared to examine at this level of concrete reality what we mean by community care we are simply indulging in wishful thinking.'[23] Or as a speaker to the Royal Society of Health in 1972 said: 'Community care is a treacherous, seductive· phrase which creates a warm glow like roses round the cottage door catching the rays of the setting sun.' The reality of care for elderly people is neither of the two extremes just mentioned but a synthesis of them. If anything it is nearer to the second description. Domiciliary services are important and provide that care which a family is not able to give. But the support of the family is of crucial importance. Apart from those who are severely incapacitated, some of whom are in residential care, it is often the combination of services which is important.

The concept of social policy based on community care thus contains a number of different elements. Firstly, there is the public recognition of the importance of the family. An example of this is the payment of a constant attendance allowance. If the family still plays the major role in meeting the needs of the elderly (physical, social and emotional) the aim of statutory services ought to be to enable them to discharge their task more effectively rather than the other way round. The community can care. It is up to the professional helpers and helping services to help it to do so. Policies that allow elderly people to move close to relatives who wish to care for them is an example of practical help.

At the same time there may be families who cannot or will not give help. It is not always possible for them to do so, nor is it always the right solution for all families. It may well be that a family is not suited to helping an old person. It would be as foolish to ignore the limitations of the family as to undervalue its potential. Nor is it sensible to ignore the fact that family care has up to now usually been provided by women and that equal opportunities may now mean that the men will have to take a larger share in the family caring. There are also elderly people without any relatives and for them family support is obviously impossible.

Secondly, it is foolish and shortsighted to see the elderly (and probably any other group) as being always recipients of services. Bracey says: 'For generations it has been the custom to speak, and equally important, to think of the "poor old pensioners". It is unfortunately true that many pensioners see themselves in this light.'[24] But the 80-year-old running her son's household after the death of his wife and the 76-year-old disabled man doing his 89-year-old uncle's shopping found in the granny annexe sample[25] are as much a part of the caring pattern as the family looking after a bedridden granny. Lack of economic status accentuates this feeling of being a taker rather than a giver. Pinker claims: 'The most profound humiliation of all, however, may be experienced in hearing that only money can preserve self-respect in conditions of dependency.'[26] This is why Age Concern's Link Scheme for exchange of services is so interesting because no money changes hands. All services are assessed on a time basis so that a professional task can be exchanged for a manual one.

Unless the elderly are seen in the role of contributors as well as takers they are not equal members of society. Or as Pinker puts it: 'Concepts like "the caring society" and the "welfare state" are subjectively meaningless to those who have not achieved citizenship in an authentic form. It may be that effecting changes in the social consciousness of ordinary people is now becoming more important than further changes in the statute book.'[27]

This is relevant to the discussion (in Ch. 11) of the isolation and loneliness of some old people. It has been noted that the problem of loneliness was particularly acute for those who felt that no one relied on them. Townsend had earlier suggested that it was time to look critically at the assumed 'burden' of old age. He said: 'We may be attaching too little weight to the contribution to society made by the aged and too much to their claims on it.'[28] Bayley suggested (in relation to families with a mentally handicapped member) that the fact that the families were not always on the receiving end, but had something to give, made a big difference to the family's morale.

The third element in a social policy based on community care must be the role of neighbours and friends. It was therefore disquieting to find that some of the most vulnerable old people in Hunt's sample felt that they could not ask for help from this source. Little is known about how this commitment can be fostered. Perhaps what is needed is a more structured framework for this form of care and it has been suggested that this could be done in conjunction with a voluntary organisation or a volunteer (who could come from either a statutory or voluntary body). One of the most interesting examples where this had been tried was in Nottingham (see Ch. 10 and document 50). An assessment of this scheme found that certain inputs were necessary in terms of manpower, administrative machinery and finance. One of those involved in the project concluded:

'Caring' is something which happens all the time: it will be to the advantage of both the community and the social services that this should be recognised and that, without losing existing warmth and spontaneity, a greater degree of rationality and effectiveness should be introduced in order to create a coherent policy which meets the actual needs of those to whom formal and informal care are directed (*Social Work Today*, 5.4.73).

It was held by the Seebohm Committee that one of the roles of voluntary bodies is the mobilisation of community resources and it may be that this will prove to be the case. At the end of the 1970s the key role of the informal sector was beginning to be better appreciated and in 1978 the Consultative Document on voluntary organisations stated: 'The time has now come to look systematically at the Government's relationships with this great and diverse field of activity which continues to attract the support of so many people in all walks of life.'[29]

But it must not be thought that the stimulation and organisation of the informal network is necessarily exclusively the role of voluntary bodies. It can be done through statutory bodies such as organisers of volunteers in hospitals and social service departments, good neighbour schemes and the Kent Community Care Project (see Ch. 8).

Finally, a fourth element in community care is the proposition that institutional care can be looked on as a form (and a very necessary form) of community care. Lapping argues that a hospital is an example 'of the community's decision that certain individuals' problems should be dealt with by pooling community resources'. If the two types of care were more fluid and there was an easy exchange between them it is probable that more families would take on the care of the elderly.

In conclusion the approaches outlined above are complementary and ought to dovetail into one another. It is the interleaving of informal care with statutory services that is so necessary but so difficult to achieve. Whether this can come about of its own accord or whether it needs the 'new long-term strategy' called for by the Wolfenden Committee in the form of a 'collaborative social plan'[30] is an open question.

The elderly in modern society

REFERENCES

1. TOWNSEND, see Ch. 4 note 1.
2. TUNSTALL, see Ch. 3 note 8.
3. SHANAS *et al.*, see Ch. 3 note 7.
4. FORDER, see Ch. 11 note 6, pp. 53–4.
5. GOLDBERG, see Ch. 3 note 28.
6. FORDER, see Ch. 11 note 6, p. 52.
7. TINKER, see Ch. 7 note 27.
8. HARRIS, see Ch. 3 note 9, p. 65.
9. SUMNER and SMITH, see Ch. 3 note 52, p. 157.
10. HARRIS, see Ch. 3 note 9.
11. HUNT, A., *The Elderly at Home. Supplementary Report*, 1979 (unpublished).
12. DHSS, *Sharing Resources*, see Ch. 6 note 40, p. 12.
13. DHSS, *Priorities for Health*, see Ch. 6 note 41, p. 13.
14. TOWNSEND and WEDDERBURN, see Ch. 3 note 6, pp. 125–33.
15. ISAACS, LIVINGSTONE and NEVILLE, see Ch. 3 note 13, p. 98.
16. HILL, M., *The State, Administration and the Individual*, Fontana, 1976, p. 70.
17. HALL, A. S., *The Point of Entry*, Allen and Unwin, 1974, p. 139.
18. BARNES, J. and CONNELLY, N. (eds), *Social Care Research*, Policy Studies Institute, Bedford Square Press, 1978, p. 13.
19. GOLDBERG, see Ch. 3 note 28.
20. HARRIS, see Ch. 4 note 18.
21. TUNSTALL, see Ch. 3 note 8.
22. TOWNSEND, *The Family Life*, see Ch. 3 note 4.
23. TITMUSS, see Ch. 11 note 2, p. 106.
24. BRACEY, see Ch. 3 note 3.
25. TINKER, see Ch. 7 note 27, p. 21.
26. PINKER, see Ch. 11 note 1, p. 175.
27. *Ibid.*, p. 174.
28. TOWNSEND, see Ch. 3 note 4, p. 63.
29. HOME OFFICE, *The Government and the Voluntary Sector*, see Ch. 10 note 51, p. 43.
30. WOLFENDEN, see Ch. 10 note 3, pp. 74 and 193.

Chapter thirteen
THE TOPIC IN PERSPECTIVE

In these chapters we have looked at the position of the elderly at the present time and at possible future developments. We have considered their needs and who might meet them. It is now possible to draw together some of the threads and to come to some conclusions. But before doing so we must relate the elderly to other groups. This is important because a group should not be singled out for special policies without taking into consideration its position in relation to the rest of society.

It is easy to be aware that the elderly is a group which is increasing in size, while other groups such as children, are at present declining in numbers. But it is not just this demographic fact alone that has caused an upsurge of interest in the elderly (as witnessed by official pronouncements, academic books and so on). Although it is difficult to know exactly why this has happened, pressure groups and an increasingly articulate and educated group of elderly must have had some impact. Some would argue, however, that this growing interest and public concern is not matched by increased provision of services. Nor is there any noticeable queue of people waiting to become geriatricians or to work in establishments that care for the elderly.

THE ELDERLY AND OTHER GROUPS

The majority of elderly people continue to live their lives with only marginal state intervention. While nearly all will receive a state pension and some form of state health care it is only the minority who receive the many other services available.

For those who do need help many of their problems such as ignorance of benefits and the feeling of stigma, will be the same as for those in other disadvantaged groups. The need for more information about benefits presented in a more lucid form is not peculiar to the elderly. Similarly, when sources of help are examined a pattern akin to that for other groups is found. This is particularly noticeable in the extent of family care. For the mentally handicapped for example, Bayley describes self-help by families as 'staggering'.[1] The bulk of the caring for this group is done by kin and so is care for the disabled. Sainsbury in *Registered as Disabled*[2] showed this conclusively, and later in *Measuring Disability*[3] emphasised again how the social services took second place to family care.

The general approach to the delivery of services for the elderly is similar in many ways to that increasingly being recommended for other groups such as children, the disabled and the homeless. The legislation (such as the National Health Service Reorganisation Act 1973, Section 10), the circulars issued by government departments and the reports of advisory committees (such as the DHSS report from the Working Party on *Collaboration between the NHS and Local Government on its Activities to the end of 1972*) have stressed the importance of joint planning, particularly between services concerned with personal social services, health and housing. The main emphasis should be on collaboration between all those involved in provision from the moment of assessment of need to the delivery of the service and subsequent monitoring. This is helped if both professionals and informal carers are well informed about each other and their respectives roles. Agreed procedures such as over the admission of elderly people to residential care or about criteria for selection to sheltered housing can help ensure that what one group provides is in line with others. The CPRS in *Housing and Social Policies: some interactions* concluded that 'a common reaction at all levels was that, in spite of the great efforts that have been made, effective consultation and collaboration still had a long way to go'.[4] The object of their study was to identify issues affecting relations between housing and the other services and to examine the effect of one service on another. For the elderly they saw the need for co-ordination on such issues as location of housing, housing allocations and lettings, choice of heating systems and the role of caretakers and wardens.

The elderly also share with other groups many of the uncertainties in social policy. What changes, for example, will be required in social policy when there are more ethnic minorities among the elderly? As a report for Age Concern has pointed out these people may feel insecure in their new environment, when they are remote from friends and in a different culture.[5] They may compare the expectation of care that they would have received in their home country, possibly with an extended family system and with enhanced status, with the reality of care in Britain.

Nor is it at all certain what changes in law and/or public opinion over equal opportunities between men and women will mean. There is not only the obvious difference at the moment in the age at which men and women are entitled to draw a pension; women are also at an advantage in other spheres. For example over free prescriptions and National Savings Retirement Issue they have entitlement at 60 compared with 65 for men.

PRIORITY FOR RESOURCES

A question that will be increasingly asked, particularly if resources continue to be limited, is what priority the elderly should have compared with other groups. In part the question is answered by the demographic facts. The large increase in the numbers of the very elderly (see Ch. 2) means, if present trends continue, a greatly increased demand on health and personal social services. Paradoxically, policies of prevention and care are enabling more people to live longer and in better health, but probably in the end they become more dependent and therefore increase the calls on national resources. Those who argue for priority to go to the elderly also point to the extent of the unmet need.

Some views about priorities have already been expressed. Age Concern, for example, decided in 1978 to invite the official spokesmen of the Conservative, Labour and Liberal Parties to answer a series of questions about their priorities.[6] Sometimes government departments also express views about priorities between groups. When the SBC were deciding about unclaimed benefits in 1978 they concluded 'that families with children should be the top priority in efforts to improve the take-up of supplementary benefits and that pensioners should be the other main group on whom efforts should be concentrated'. Similarly, housing departments reflect their priorities when deciding, for example, who should be offered a transfer from flats to houses, when these become available. Is it to be the family with a child or an elderly person who finds difficulty with stairs or lift?

The assumption has been made in many studies that the welfare state will continue to expand and that the questions to be answered are largely about where priority for expansion should take place. But the change that has now taken place was foreseen by Klein in 1975 [doc 51]. In a time of financial restraint it is essential that those who argue for resources for the elderly should do so on sound evidence. As the Royal Commission on the NHS pointed out, without a greater shift of resources to the elderly the community will have to bear the responsibility of coping with the care of the elderly at home.[7] The two DHSS Priorities documents in 1976 and 1977 had previously stressed the need for priority to certain groups including the elderly.

INTEGRATION OR SEGREGATION?

Another basic issue to be faced in deciding social policies for the elderly is that of integration versus segregation. Should the elderly be (as the dictionary puts it) combined into the whole or should they be set apart? Should they be integrated into society through housing, new forms of employment and social activities or should they be moved, or encouraged to move, away from the mainstream of life? Shanas *et al.* considered that both theoretically and practically this was the most important question affecting the elderly.[8]

As they, and others, have pointed out there are a number of different theoretical approaches to integration and segregation. Firstly, there are those related to historical changes. These assume that while the elderly used at one time to be integrated into both society and the family they are now much more segregated. However, as was pointed out in Chapter 9 when the family was discussed, evidence is lacking to substantiate such theories. What evidence there is does not support the view that the close three-generation family was the norm, and anyway few people actually survived into the old age.

Secondly, there are theories about the advantages and disadvantages accruing to groups when they are singled out for special treatment. The advantages include the value of a co-ordinated approach to provision and the focusing on the needs of the group. This has been argued strongly in the case of children. So it was too for the disabled who have had a Minister since 1974 to look after their interests. The plea for a Minister for the Aged is sometimes put but has been strongly rejected by, among others, Hobman. He argues that such an appointment would be psychologically damaging and could further disadvantage the elderly by setting them as a race apart. As far as administration is concerned, and particularly over the monitoring of services, it has been suggested that there should be an inspectorate based on client groups rather than on services. On the other hand a service concerned solely with a client group risks the danger of being out of the mainstream of function-based services. There may also be the problem that when a group is chosen for special treatment this may bring stigma with it. Also, as has been pointed out many times, the elderly are not a homogeneous group and may not gain from being treated as if they were.

The third approach is concerned with ageing and theories of disengagement. It is held to be normal for the elderly to disengage and therefore bring about their own segregation from society. The theory is that the individual's activities form a curve during his lifetime and gradually fall away. He 'prepares' for death by withdrawing from previous roles and limiting his social contacts. There is little evidence to back up these theories and some writers suggest that insufficient attention has been paid to forms of compensation, replacement and substitution. For example is there evidence of the elderly wanting to disengage and if they do, is it perhaps because it is forced on them rather than being something they wish to happen?

Perhaps the right basis for assessing the range of views is to note again the evidence presented earlier that the elderly are a varied group. Some want independence with privacy. Others want to live with other people. Some like quiet and to be able to associate mainly with people of their own generation. Others prefer the company of younger people.

Clearly, integration and segregation are two opposing principles, but that does not mean that one or other must be the right policy to pursue. It is more sensible to make varied provision, so that for example the elderly can choose to live either in mixed communities or in special schemes for their age group alone. The same course should be followed with other provision such as clubs, since some old people will want to belong to clubs for their own age group while others will prefer those without age restrictions.

THE ELDERLY IN MODERN SOCIETY: STRESSES AND COMPENSATIONS

Surveys of old people often concentrate on measurable needs and the extent of services provided. Many show up alleged deficiencies in services or focus on people in particular situations – found dead, suffering from cold, lacking income and so on. A good deal, therefore, is known about the stresses of growing old, but much less about the compensations. Nor is there a philosophy of retirement.

There is no doubt from recent evidence that for some old people life does present difficulties.[9] In their own judgement the greatest problems are caused by ill health closely followed by loneliness. It is interesting that these findings are the same in the surveys of Hunt and Abrams. Hunt found that financial difficulties were mentioned by comparatively few, but that when they were asked for suggestions for helping the elderly most of these were in fact related to finance.[10] However, even more old people wanted volunteers to chat or for company than any other single form of help. Abrams came to a very similar conclusion [doc 52].

But for the majority of old people life continues to have a great deal of satisfaction. Hunt comments 'looking at elderly people as a whole, it can be said that a great many appear to get a great deal out of life'.[11] Abrams found this too when he measured life satisfaction.[12] One of the things which enhances happiness is being able to help others and the feeling of being relied upon. Age Concern and others have commented that the elderly represent a large untapped source of help which could well be utilised to their own benefit and happiness in support of either other elderly people or of other groups in the community such as mothers with young children.

But to allow the elderly to achieve their potential and to be valued members of society there may need to be a change in the mental picture that people have of old age. Comfort has said that men of his generation knew that grandmothers dressed in black at 45, and looked like grandmothers, whereas today grandmothers often wear shorts and play tennis.[13] Twelve years later he stated that what was needed was a change of attitude.[14] He thought that social gerontology would only have made an impact when an older person came to be seen not as old first and provisionally a person second, but as a person who happens also to be old (plus experience and minus the consequences of certain physical accidents of time).

IMPLICATIONS FOR PROFESSIONALS

It is always important for professionals to remember that they are likely to be in contact with only a minority of the elderly. And just as one cannot generalise from a study based on the 5 per cent in residential care so groups such as social workers should not generalise from the elderly who present themselves to them. For they are bound to be those who have particular difficulties.

What it is hoped that this study has shown is that 95 per cent of old people live out their lives in their own homes supported in the main by their families. But this must not be taken to imply that there is no need to be concerned about them and about those services which they will all have recourse to, such as pensions and health care. There must be constant vigilance that these are adquate and, above all, provided in the most appropriate way with the elderly themselves having the maximum say in this. What is also crucial is that services for the growing number of frail elderly should be adequate. These are vital as back-up to what their families can do and particularly so for those old people who have no families to turn to.

Professionals, whether administrators, doctors, social workers, health visitors, nurses or others in the caring professions must aim to provide the sort of service they would wish for themselves when they reach retirement. But the welfare of society is not exclusively the concern of the professional. There are many skills and resources available to help in the community, and some indeed are to be found among the users of services. It is the dovetailing of professionals with others that is of importance so that each may contribute to the maximum advantage of society.

REFERENCES

1. BAYLEY, M., *Mental Handicap and Community Care*, Routledge and Kegan Paul, 1973.
2. SAINSBURY, see Ch. 11 note 46.
3. SAINSBURY, see Ch. 8 note 6.
4. CPRS, *Housing and Social Policies: Some Interactions*, HMSO, 1978, p. 6.
5. PYKE-LEES, S. and GARDINER, S., *Elderly Ethnic Minorities*, Age Concern, 1974.
6. AGE CONCERN, *Political Party Priorities for the Elderly*. Report of a discussion between the spokesmen for the Conservative, Labour and Liberal Parties, Age Concern, 1978.
7. ROYAL COMMISSION ON THE NHS, see Ch. 6 note 33, p. 358.
8. SHANAS *et al.*, see Ch. 3 note 7.
9. HUNT, see Ch. 2 note 3, p. 131.
10. *Ibid.*, p. 10.
11. *Ibid.*, p. 31.
12. ABRAMS, see Ch. 2 note 4, Ch. 6.
13. COMFORT, see Ch. 3 note 22, p. 119.
14. COMFORT, A., *A Good Age*, Mitchell Beazley, 1977, p. 27.

Chapter fourteen

DEVELOPMENTS SINCE 1980

INTRODUCTION

When this book was completed in 1980 it was clear that a watershed in social policy had been reached. Since then a new Conservative administration and continuing economic constraints have been the backdrop against which policies for elderly people have been pursued in the last four years. It was significant that the Labour Government's Discussion Paper *A Happier Old Age* in 1978 was followed by the new administration's White Paper *Growing Older* in 1981, which was noticeably less optimistic.[1] Few major changes in policy were outlined but the emphasis was rather on what could be achieved within existing resources. There was stress on the contribution of the private and voluntary sectors – an important theme of the last few years. *The Guardian* in a leader (6.3.81) criticised the White Paper, saying it 'makes no attempt even to identify the nature and scale of the problem. Its message is plain: the Government has no intention of spending any more money at all to cope with the extra demand. It is all up to "the community".'

Similar criticisms came from organisations representing elderly people. Most of the disappointment centred on the absence of many concrete proposals. A leader in *New Age* (Spring 1981) said that readers of the White Paper would look in vain for the usual outlining of proposed government measures. However, David Hobman, Director of Age Concern, welcomed the commitment of the government to four policy initiatives. These were a proposal to sponsor a number of experimental NHS nursing homes; a long-term commitment to flexible retirement; the equalisation of retirement ages between men and women; and a tax credit system.

The main aim of government policy in relation to elderly people as expressed in *Ageing in the United Kingdom*, produced in 1982 for the World Assembly on Ageing, was 'to enable them to lead full and independent lives in the community to the greatest possible extent'.[2] This is almost identical to the words of the 1981 White Paper, which said policies were 'to enable elderly people to live independent lives in their own homes wherever possible – which reflects what the majority themselves want'.[3] Similar policies are likely to continue with the Conservative victory in the 1983 election although it is doubtful if the other parties would have adopted a different stance.

Interest in the elderly, for whatever reasons, has developed rapidly. One illustration of this is the increase in the number of books (by authors from many different disciplines) published during this time. The period has also seen the completion of some major pieces of research which were brought together for discussion in an important seminar organised by DHSS in 1982.[4] This research is drawn on during this chapter. While no new major general survey of elderly people has been carried out the *General Household Survey 1980* contained questions, some repeated in 1981, to elderly people which enabled some of the Hunt data to be updated.[5] In fact, very few changes were shown in levels of disability [doc 503] or of services received (Table 10). The 1981 *Census* will in time yield more information and some results are already available and are referred to.

The pattern of this chapter follows that of the book and the later developments are noted under the headings used for the previous chapters. In some cases it has been possible to substitute more up-to-date material in the original chapters. Chapter 3 'General review of the literature' and Chapter 4 'A critical narrative of the main developments in social services' are unaltered. Additions have been made under the specific topic (e.g. the many official reports on community care are referred to in the health and personal social services sections).

THE FINANCIAL AND EMPLOYMENT POSITION

Pensions and benefits

Legislation on pensions has come thick and fast. The Social Security Act 1979 amended statutory provisions relating to the new earnings-related pension scheme. In 1980 a further Social Security Act amended the Social Security Act 1975 so that in future benefit

Table 10. Use of some services by elderly people aged 65 and over

	1981* G.B.	1980† G.B.	1976‡ England
Doctor at surgery	24	27	not given
Doctor at home	10	11	33
District nurse or health visitor	6	6	12
Chiropodist§	8	11	not given
Home help	9	9	9
Attendance at day centre	5	5	17 } (social centre
Lunch at lunch club or day centre	3	3	for the elderly)
Meals on wheels	3	2	3

★ In the month before interview. *Source*: *GHS, 1981*, HMSO, 1983, p. 151 and p. 153.
† In the month before interview. *Source*: *GHS, 1980*, HMSO, 1982, p. 211 and p. 213.
‡ Visits received during the past six months. *Source*: Hunt, *The Elderly at Home*, HMSO, 1978, p. 87 and p. 103.
§ Excluding private treatment.

increases were to be related to the movement of prices, and not of earnings. The Social Security Advisory Committee, which replaced the Supplementary Benefits Commission, commented in their first report in 1982 that they regretted the decision to break the link between the growth of earnings and pensions.[6] Pensioners, therefore, no longer had a guarantee that their living standards would rise in step with those of wage and salary earners. While the Advisory Committee did not single out benefits for retired people as a priority topic they emphasised their concern that the benefits for this group should be protected and improved as resources permit. The 1980 Act was followed by the Social Security Act 1981 which enabled the government to take account, at the next up-rating, of the fact that the previous up-rating had been higher than intended. The Social Security and Housing Benefits Act 1982 provided for a change in the way in which pension increases were calculated.

Expenditure on pensions continued to rise. Total expenditure on retirement pensions in Great Britain rose from £6.6 million in 1977/78 to a planned £13.5 million in 1982/83 and supplementary pensions from £0.7 million to £1.6 million in the same period.[7] Judge in the *Journal of Social Policy* (October 1981) identifies three factors which have accounted for the growth in pensions expenditure since 1951. One is the increase in numbers of elderly people which will not happen again in the next 20 years. The second is the decline of economic activity of elderly people. This is unlikely to fall further. It is the third, improvements in the real rate, which is the unknown quantity and he discusses what factors are involved.

The dependence of elderly people on supplementary pensions has already been shown (p. 50) and in Chapter 5 the growing number of discretionary payments was mentioned. These reached a peak in 1978 but have now dropped steadily for all claimants. In 1980 under the Social Security Act, a change, foreshadowed by the SBC, took place. This was a new structure for supplementary benefits which had as its major objective putting rights and clear entitlements in place of official discretion. Firm and clear rules were introduced and made public. While the new system has brought advantages a number of problems have occurred including the way the scheme is administered in local social security offices, rules relating to the beneficiaries capital and information given to claimants on their entitlements and how these are worked out.[8]

Other forms of financial help have become available. The Social Security Act 1979 extended the upper age limit for mobility allowance which can be claimed by people who cannot walk. When the scheme was introduced in 1976 it was progressively phased in by age. The last group, those aged 61–65, were included from 1979. Once a person receives this allowance it can be continued up to the age of 75.

A further change was the switch for help with housing costs to a Unified Housing Benefit following the Social Security and Housing Benefits Act 1982. The Act made provision for housing benefit to replace the two previous schemes of supplementary benefit for rent and rates and local authority rent and rate rebates and rent allowances. The scheme is administered by local authorities and guidance was given in 1982 in *DHSS Circular HB (82) (12) The Housing Benefits Scheme*. A major advantage of this scheme is that 70,000 people, the majority pensioners, were taken off supplementary benefit and no longer had to calculate whether this or rent and rate rebates and allowances were a 'better buy'.[9]

Retirement

Although little fresh evidence has been produced on poverty a powerful article on dependency in *Ageing and Society* (March 1981) by Walker illuminated some on the issues, especially those relating to retirement policies. His theme is that poverty is a result of low economic and social status prior to retirement which restricts access to a wide range of resources. He argues for flexible retirement, coupled with the pursuit of full employment and radical changes in the structures and organisation of work, to prevent flexible retirement being used to force earlier retirement. He also advocates policies aimed at increasing the value of retirement pensions relative to earnings.

A comprehensive review of the issues relating to the age of retirement was part of the House of Commons *Third Report from the Social Services Committee* in October 1982. They undertook their inquiry because of demands for changes in the male pension age and the trend towards early retirement. They concluded that the recent trend towards early retirement has in many cases been involuntary but if the pension was sufficient most people would 'happily retire earlier than at present'.[10] They warned however of the drawbacks to early retirement and concluded that premature and involuntary retirement may well have unfavourable mental and physical side-effects. To reach their objectives of flexibility and equal treatment between the sexes they recommended a common pension age of 63 (lowering male pension age to 60 would cost around £2.5 billion) but a flexible retirement policy. The Equal Opportunities Commission welcomed the report but was concerned that any proposals should take into account the views not only of expert witnesses and institutional interests, but also of the men and women who would be affected by any change. They therefore undertook a study of people's attitudes towards the principle of equalisation and their views on a common pension age, taking into account both general consequences and personal costs. The results were presented in *Paying for Equalisation* in 1983.[11] There was a high level of agreement that the male pension age should be lowered and that the pension age should be equalised (with a favoured common age of 60). There was also sufficient commitment towards equalisation on the part of most people for at least some of the cost to be borne through increased national insurance contributions.

Parker poses the question: 'Is it possible to find a selection of policies which will meet aspirations for flexible and earlier retirement, combined with a socially acceptable level of income for older people, yet at the same time minimise the potentially very large addition to pension costs?'[12] He suggests that giving opportunities for gradual early retirement on part pension, selective reduction of standard or normal retirement ages and positive inducements to continue in employment beyond standard retirement age would help. These issues are also explored and costed by Fogarty.[13]

Employment

The 1981 *GHS* showed that economic activity declined for most people aged over 65 between 1971 and 1980 (from 17 per cent to 11 per cent for men, from 7 per cent to 4 per cent for non-married women but remained constant at 5 per cent for married women).[14]

The rise and fall in the number of elderly people in paid employment is to some extent related to the state of the economy. Changes in government policy have been described thus 'twenty five years ago the labour shortage led to official encouragement of older people remaining at work, *inter alia* by promoting research to show that their capabilities were on a par with others; now the situation is different. The point has been made that official interest in the elderly employed has tended to be influenced by the state of the economy so that voluntary early departure from the labour force is now regarded as worth encouraging'.[15]

Phillipson argues that the treatment of the elderly as a reserve work force has led to confusion about the value of retirement. He makes a useful distinction between the experiences of men and women in retirement. He also argues that the experience of growing old is heavily influenced by class. He says that to view growing old 'as a period where the biological process of age assumes a primary role is to ignore the cumulative power and significance of life in a class society'.[16] However, class, while important, is only one element in a person's history.

Preparation for retirement has attracted a growing amount of attention particularly with the increase in early retirement. But the subject tends to be seen now in the wider context of education and opportunities for older people.

HEALTH

Policy development

A positive flood of official documents has come from the DHSS in the last three years most with community or care in the title and all concerned with two issues. One is the need to give priority to increasing and improving provision for elderly people and the other to promoting care at home rather than in institutions. These documents continued the theme of the mid-1970s following the concentration in the 1960s and early 1970s on hospital provision.

In February 1981 *Care in Action* was published.[17] This was a handbook providing national guidance for health and personal social services. It stated that priority was to be given to four groups one of whom was 'elderly people, especially the most vulnerable and frail'.[18] Four objectives were given.[19] First, to 'strengthen the primary and community care services, together with neighbourhood and voluntary support, to enable elderly people to live at home'. Second, to 'encourage an active approach to treatment and rehabilitation to enable elderly people to return to the community from hospital wherever possible'. Third, to 'maintain capacity in the general acute sector to deal with the increasing number of elderly patients'. Fourth, to 'maintain an adequate provision for the minority of elderly people requiring long-term care in hospital or residential homes'. In December 1982 the government stated that these priorities had not changed.[20] *Care in Action* drew on material included in a *Report of a Study on Community Care* written by DHSS officials based on research and published in September 1981.[21] It concentrated on assessing whether there had been any shift away from long-term hospital or residential provision for those people whose needs put them on the boundary between institutional and non-institutional care and also the contribution of the voluntary sector to all forms of community care. Some interesting findings and expressions of doubt emerged. The authors found little shift from hospital and residential care for elderly people on the margins of institutional and community-based care and they noted that there may have been a tendency to underestimate the number of elderly people who will always require long-term residential care. There was an acknowledgement that 'community-based packages of care may not always be a less expensive or more effective alternative to hospital or residential provision, particularly for those living alone'.[22] They also made some salutary points about the voluntary sector, which they wanted strengthening, and included the warning that 'it is important not to assume that the amount of informal care can be limitlessly increased'.[23] Some of the general pointers to emerge from this study were that it may be necessary to shift NHS expenditure from hospital in-patient to community health services, that manpower constraints (e.g. a shortage of district nurses) may become as important as financial constraints, that social and demographic changes may reduce the number of those people who have traditionally provided the mainstay of informal care and finally that demand for all community-based services are likely to continue to increase over the next decade. Published simultaneously were two complementary studies on hospitals. *The respective roles of the general acute and geriatric sectors in the care of the elderly hospital patient* indicated that an important area of concern was the impact on the acute sector of the shortfall in provision for elderly patients in departments of geriatric medicine.[24] The *Report of a study of the acute hospital sector* also showed that between 1968 and 1978 most of the increase in activity rates throughout the acute sector were accounted for by services to elderly people.[25] In between *Care in Action* and the three reports came (March 1981) the White Paper *Growing Older* (see p. 194) with its firm commitment to community care but again with the warning that community services and families 'cannot be expected to provide a solution to every problem, and should not normally be used to support people who can only properly be cared for elsewhere'.[26]

Then in July 1981 *Care in the Community* was published.[27] This was subtitled 'A consultative document on moving resources for care in England' and it was concerned with how patients 'together with resources for their care', may be transferred from the NHS to the personal social services in addition to existing joint finance arrangements. As a subsequent DHSS note explained (*Explanatory Notes on Care in the Community* 1983) the policy thrust was different from before. 'The joint finance arrangements have assisted the development of community care and in doing so have contributed to the important objective of enabling people to *remain* in the community instead of having to be taken into hospital. But the *Care in the Community* initiative has a different and quite specific aim: to help long-stay hospital patients unnecessarily kept in hospital to *return* to the community where this will be best for them and is what they and their families prefer'.[28] The section in *Care in the Community* on elderly people was as follows:

it is often not possible to make a once and for all assessment of the long-term needs of an elderly person. Some of those discharged from hospital will return later, sometimes for good. While there are differences of opinion about the scope for discharging long-stay patients from hospitals to the care of social services, there are elderly people in hospitals who do not need to be there. The objective of enabling elderly people to live as far as possible in the community requires the development not only of personal social services but also of primary health care services and of acute geriatric services. The patterns of health and social services provision and the interactions between the different forms vary greatly according to local conditions and these variations make it impossible to provide overall figures for the numbers of elderly people who might suitably move one way or the other'.[29]

While no estimate could be given of numbers of elderly people who might be more suitably cared for by the personal social services it was stated that each patient cost the NHS on average about £8,000 in 1979/80.

A number of suggestions were put forward including transfer of hospital buildings, lump sum or annual payment, central transfer of funds and extending joint finance arrangements. Comments on the suggestions were sought and received by DHSS and a circular was issued in March 1983. This was DHSS (HC (83)6 and LAC(83)5) *Health Service development. Care in the Community and Joint Finance*. One of the main decisions was that District Health Authorities could offer lump-sum payments or continuing grants to local authorities or voluntary organisations for people moving from hospital into community care. Another was the extension of joint financing from 7 to 13 years. A further decision was that joint financing could now be given to housing departments and housing associations. This needed legislation and was part of the Health and Social Services and Social Security Adjudications Act 1983. A programme of pilot projects was proposed and these are to be monitored.

It is clear that joint financing has provided a welcome additional source of funds for elderly people. Money earmarked for joint finance rose to £68.5 million in 1981/82 and was planned to rise to £96 million in 1983/84.[30] About 40 per cent of this money has been spent on services for the elderly.[31] While attempts have been made to change policies and to direct resources away from hospitals to health services in the community an analysis of costings shows that there has actually been little variation in percentages spent.[32] In England in 1974/75 hospital services absorbed 63.1 per cent of health service expenditure and in 1981/82 62.8 per cent. In 1974/75 family practitioner services took 23.3 per cent and in 1981/82 22.8 per cent. In 1974/75 community health services took 6.5 per cent and in 1981/82 6.7 per cent.

But a simple switch of resources away from hospital care may not always be in the best interests of elderly people. *Health Care and its Costs* showed that more advanced and safer anaesthetic procedures, together with more refined surgical techniques, have enabled surgical treatment to be given to patients who would previously have been considered too frail for major surgery.[33] Between 1971 and 1979 the number of operations per elderly population rose by 21 per cent for the 65–74 age group and 29 per cent for the over-75s.

Health and special groups

The danger of generalising about elderly people is well illustrated in the DHSS Black report *Inequalities in Health* subsequently reproduced with comments by Townsend and Davidson.[34] The report points to inequalities in health as being a direct reflection of inequalities in the social division of labour. Not only do some workers' bodies wear out first but material fortunes or misfortunes of old age are closely linked with occupational class during working life.

The 1981 *GHS* confirmed the extent of ill-health of elderly people (p. 58) and their use of health services (Table 10). When personal mobility, self-care and ability to perform certain domestic tasks were compared almost identical percentages unable to manage on their own were found [doc 53]. Particular attention is drawn in the 1980 *GHS* to the 'considerable proportion of the elderly living alone'[35] who were unable to manage particular activities involving personal mobility. For example, as many as a fifth of those aged 75 and over who were living alone were unable to walk down the road on their own. Furthermore, small proportions of elderly people living alone, mainly women aged 75 and over, were unable to get around the house, to the lavatory or in and out of bed on their own.

The mentally disordered   The implications of the growing number of mentally disordered elderly people over 75 were taken much more seriously and the medical profession in particular stressed that problems of mental illness such as dementia would rise dramatically. *The Rising Tide* was an aptly named title of a report by the NHS Health Advisory Service (HAS) in 1982 which claimed that unless the challenges are met 'the flood is likely to overwhelm the entire health care system'.[36] In a briskly written report a very positive approach is taken with particular emphasis given to underlining that the problem is not just one for specialist psychiatric services. The difficulties of people attempting to care for elderly people at home, in private nursing homes or residential homes are acknowledged. Unlike many reports which meekly accept that solutions must be within existing resources this one has no such compunction. It is argued that 'until a lot more money is put into the care of the elderly mentally ill, it will in fact be impossible to provide what we already know can and should be done'.[37] Nevertheless HAS also put the case for a truly comprehensive service (involving as they put it 'style') which is well led and has high morale. The report was followed by an announcement (4.1.83) that an extra £6 million was to be given by the government to finance about 14 demonstration projects. A useful complement to this report is Norman's *Mental illness in Old Age: Meeting the Challenge* with its careful description of the types of mental illness and its account of the various forms of service in both residential and community settings.[38] Enlivened with local examples, Norman pleads for these innovative services to be a part of a strategy for shared caring which looks first at need and then at ways in which resources can be moved round or mobilised to meet that need.

Much that has been written has focused on dementia. Work done by Levin has shown that there is a heavy burden upon the families supporting the demented elderly at home.[39] Over one third of the supported were so stressed as to be in probable need of psychiatric help themselves. Bergmann and Jacoby say that until scientific research provides a means of altering the prognosis of dementia fundamentally, the main focus has to be on maintaining the autonomy and viability of the elderly person for as long as possible.[40] In the absence of the family, or when it collapses, homelike institutional settings in the community can substitute. Arie has argued in *The Health Services* (14.1.83) that there are some patients, and he includes some with senile dementia, for whom institutional care is the only humane and proper answer.

The dying   Another group who have received more attention have been the dying. In *The Hospice Movement in Britain: its role and its future* Taylor has charted the development and aims of one particular solution. He details the current pattern of services, location, organisation and funding and on balance favours independent organisations outside the NHS.[41] But others argue that the development of hospices within the NHS will enable a different attitude to develop within hospitals where death is not seen as a defeat. Both hospices and hospitals are developing services to support the dying and their families at home, offering where necessary spells in hospital to control pain or relieve relatives.

The need to support relatives is brought out clearly by Bowling and Cartwright in *Life after a Death: A Study of the Elderly Widowed*.[42] Some require emotional support, others practical help and advice, while many probably need both.

It is interesting that euthanasia, about which there has been much debate in the media, was thought to justify a paragraph in *Growing Older* and repeated in the UK contribution to the World Assembly on Ageing. 'There is a small body of opinion which believes euthanasia should be legalised. Most people believe that legalised euthanasia could expose very vulnerable people to undesirable pressures, and would not wish to see it made possible. The Government considers euthanasia unacceptable, and is firmly opposed to changing the law to allow it.'[43]

Granny battering   A group who have received increasing attention are elderly people who are assaulted by families and other carers. 'Granny battering' has taken its place in the matters of concern taken up by journals (for example, *Geriatric Medicine*, November 1982) and especially the media. Non-accidental injury to children has long been a subject researched and written about, but the identification of elderly people as objects of battering is relatively new. Its discovery owes much to Mervyn Eastman, a social worker (*Community Care*, 27.5.82). But there is still a lack of research in this country on the whole subject and also a lack of agreement about how to define abuse, which can range from screaming and threats to actual violence.

Health care

The growing interest by doctors from many different disciplines in the treatment of elderly people is illustrated by Arie's *Health Care of the Elderly* which is a collection of essays written from different points of view. Arie admits that 'very aged people get a poor deal from services; and not all the services which we disburse, often enthusiastically and almost always expensively, have been shown to be effective'.[44] On the other hand, he points to the great advances made in treatment in some areas; for example, the growing clinical and epidemiological understanding of functional mental disorder which is often treatable.

The pioneering work of Gray in his writing about the importance of prevention of handicap and attention to the old person's ability to function has been refreshingly practical (for example, *BMJ* 21.8.82). Measures to prevent unfitness (e.g. encourage exercise:

the motto is 'use it or lose it') and social problems are outlined. To get over these messages he favours using the potential offered by a normal primary care consultation (because most elderly patients will contact the practice at some time during the year) rather than full-scale screening.

The Royal Commission on the NHS had already reported on the physical problems of access which elderly people have to their GPs[45] and fresh evidence came to light about primary health care in inner cities (where many elderly people live).[46,47]

Another issue which has received much publicity is the power of compulsory removal by doctors usually referred to as 'section 47' (after section 47 of the National Assistance Act 1948). Little is known about how often the powers are invoked and whether they are abused, but, as Gray reveals, opinion is divided over whether section 47 should be repealed (*Health Trends*, 1980, Vol 12).

A further problem of health care arises when frail elderly people are kept at home or sent out of hospital in unsatisfactory circumstances. A number of schemes are being tried out in various parts of the country. For example, in Cleveland an augmented home nursing service for chronic elderly invalids provided a cost effective alternative to providing additional long-stay beds (*BMJ* 30.1.82). In other areas Continuing Care Projects (*Social Work Today* 9.6.81) and intensive domiciliary care schemes (*Health and Social Services Journal* 29.4.82) have proved successful. Another option now is a place in a NHS nursing home. A pilot programme of three homes was announced in 1982 and is described in *Geriatric Medicine* (May 1982).

Nutrition

A study of the nutrition and wellbeing of elderly people at *Three Score Years . . . and then?* by Davies in 1981 rejected the simple approach to nutrition needs.[48] She pointed out for instance that the provision of meals on wheels, or extra meals on wheels, will not automatically increase the food intake in those who are ill or neglecting their diet. In her survey she found that the majority of elderly people were taking several types of drug either on doctor's orders or self-prescribed. She pointed to some of the possible effects of this including confusion, depression and apathy or impairment of food flavours. Runcie states (*The Practitioner*, December 1981) that elderly people are liable to nutritional deficiency, a particular problem being the maintenance of their water-soluble vitamin status and says that the development of nutritional monitoring programmes should become a major objective.

HOUSING

Policy developments

Of major importance has been the Housing Act 1980 which may potentially affect elderly people in all tenures. The right to buy clauses enable council (and some housing association) tenants to buy their homes (at a discount) from the local authority or housing association. Although purpose-built or adapted accommodation for the elderly is specifically excluded (Housing Act 1980 Schedule 1, Part 1. Circumstances in which right to buy does not arise), this covers only a small proportion of the stock. Many elderly people are therefore free to buy their own local authority homes. While the Act is controversial (opponents believe it will lead to council housing becoming a residual service and there are suspicions that some families may lend or give parents the money so that they may eventually sell the home at a profit or use it as a second home) it may result in more elderly people becoming owner occupiers.

Elderly people in the council sector have gained from some of the other provisions of the Act such as security of tenure, greater freedom over conditions (e.g. the right to take in lodgers) and the statutory duty of authorities to give information about allocations and to consult tenants.

The 1980 Act also widened the grant system so that more owner occupiers became eligible for improvement and repairs grants. Grants were also made more flexible (e.g. an inside lavatory can be provided without all the other three standard amenities being insisted on). In cases of hardship, grants of up to 90 per cent of costs became available as they also were for elderly people on low incomes under the *Homes Insulation scheme* (*DOE Circular 60/78* amended by the Housing Act 1980).

The poor state of housing of some elderly people makes any attempt to give greater flexibility in the grants system or encourage higher take-up a worthwhile objective. Research continued to confirm the inadequacy of the housing occupied by some elderly people. The 1981 *English House Condition Survey* found that defects were heavily concentrated in pre-1919 stock (where a disproportionately large number of elderly people are housed). However, there has been a significant reduction in the number of dwellings lacking amenities (from 2.8 million in 1971 to 0.9 million in 1981).[49] However, the *GHS 1980* revealed that elderly households continue to have worse housing conditions than households containing no elderly people as Table 11 reveals.

It is difficult to tell what effect another change will have. This is the abolition of building standards (Parker Morris) and the withdrawal of Circular 82/69 (which technically still lies on the table but is no longer a standard to be adhered to). These are all part of the move to give local authorities more freedom to choose what they provide and how to do so. But advice on good practice and new developments has still been given sometimes; for example, DOE made a film on housing elderly people which was first shown in June 1983.

Another factor which has affected elderly people has been the decline in housebuilding. Houses and flats completed in the UK were 159,800 in 1981 compared with 358,600 in 1971.[50] There was a drop in every sector except housing associations. But numbers of small units have increased which must help elderly people who want to move. The percentage of one-bedroom accommodation increased from 13.5 per cent in 1969 to 18.5 per cent in 1979.

Sheltered housing

Sheltered housing has been the subject of two major pieces of research–one in England and Wales and one in Scotland. The former was undertaken at Leeds University and the conclusions of the four-year research study were published in 1981[51] and subsequently in 1983 in a book.[52] The authors estimated that there were 400,000 elderly people in England and Wales in sheltered housing in 1981 compared with 10,000 in 1951.[51] Based on a study of the literature, case studies in 12 areas and interviews with 608 tenants and 237 wardens, the authors concluded that most tenants were satisfied with their housing but that this satisfaction was generally linked to the wish for small, warm, easy-to-run accommodation rather than the provision of an alarm and warden. Tenants were found to be of similar dependency as old people in the community and yet received much more help from the domiciliary services. The Scottish study came to similar conclusions.[53] The authors of the Leeds study queried the lack of clarity about the purpose of sheltered housing and disproved some of the benefits claimed (e.g.

Table 11. Amenities of households in Great Britain (%), 1980

| | Households containing at least one elderly person | | | | Households containing no elderly persons |
	Elderly person living with spouse only	Elderly person living alone	Elderly person in household of miscellaneous type	Total	
WC outside the accommodation, but inside the building	1	2	1	2	2
WC outside the building	4	5	4	4	1
No WC	0	0	1	0	0
Has no bath/shower	3	4	3	4	1
Has no central heating	49	55	54	53	39

Taken from OPCS, *GHS, 1980*, HMSO, 1982, Table 10.4(a), p. 184.

that it increased longevity and broke down isolation of elderly people).

A notable feature of the last four years has been the development of very sheltered housing (pp. 87–88) by both local authorities and housing associations. Little is known about the kind of tenants being accepted, extent of extra help given and cost of such schemes. On the one hand it can be a useful way of joint provision by housing and social service departments but on the other hand some social service departments are encouraging housing departments to build sheltered housing purely in the absence of their own Part III accommodation. Question marks over very sheltered housing have been raised by Butler *et al.* [54]

Alternatives to sheltered housing

The last four years have seen more attention paid in policy and research to alternatives to sheltered housing.[55] Butler has identified some of the reasons which include danger to health and psychological wellbeing by the need to relocate, creation of geriatric ghettoes, cost, over-provision of support, schemes beginning to resemble the institutions they were intended to replace and dependence undermined rather than fostered among tenants.[56] Not all the criticisms are proved, as he points out, but they are nevertheless some of the reasons for a changed view of sheltered housing.

Two major pieces of research in DOE were due for completion in 1983. Tinker, in *Housing the Elderly in the Community*, has looked at initiatives by housing and social service authorities to enable elderly people to remain in their own homes.[57] Methods include surveillance and alarm systems and intensive domiciliary care schemes. Fleiss has examined the growing number of initiatives in the private sector, namely private sheltered housing and schemes to enable elderly owner-occupiers to use some of the capital they have locked up in their homes (e.g. through Home Income Plans).[58] Home income plans enable an elderly owner-occupier to buy an annuity by remortgaging his home. He or she pays the mortgage interest, less income tax relief if eligible, from the annuity but capital is not repayable until the death of the elderly person.

Other initiatives are particularly related to improving the homes of elderly owner-occupiers. In one of these Anchor Housing Trust set up a team to help elderly owner-occupiers in seven areas with property repairs, improvements, adaptations and heating alterations. Abbey National have provided interest-only mortgages either to supplement a grant or to provide the full amount. Capital does not have to be repaid until the house is sold. Many elderly people have not proceeded after initial interest. Wheeler writing in *Housing Review* (Sept./Oct. 1982) and *Ageing and Society* (Nov. 1982) has shown that among the reasons for failure to proceed with the work appear to be a dislike of borrowing, anxiety over its effect on eventual legacies, worry over the ability to repay the interest and unwillingness to face the disruption of building work.

Another interesting initiative was developed by Help the Aged Housing Trust in conjunction with Shelter in South Wales. Here the Ferndale Home Improvement Scheme employed an architect and had its own building team which did the repairs. It was intended to assist owners who seemed to have no other means of help (i.e. by filtering out those who could afford a builder or who were eligible for a council grant). A small charge was made but this could be waived. The key concepts were: a maximum cost, a client responsive approach, automatic follow-up and repairs for 'lifetime use'. Research has concluded that the work was inexpensive and gave good value for money.[59]

Special groups

The housing needs of special groups have been the subject of recent research. The working of the 1978 Circular *Adaptations of housing for people who are physically handicapped (DOE Circular 59/78)* was investigated. The subsequent report, *Organising house adaptations for disabled people*, showed that the majority of authorities had adopted the recommendations which were thought to have provided a good basic framework.[60] However, there were some problems and the report suggested ways of overcoming them.

Research has continued to highlight the problems of elderly people who are homeless. A survey published in 1982, *Single and Homeless*, found that 8 per cent of the sample were over retirement age.[61] In a survey of rehoused hostel residents, *A Home of their Own*, 39 per cent of the sample were 60 or over.[62] The authors found that choice was limited for ex-residents and, while some hostel residents were not realistic in their views of the type of accommodation best suited to their needs, 'it may well be that given a wider choice, a proportion of the sample would have chosen and lived more successfully in housing where some support was provided'.[63]

Elderly people in the public sector who wish to move may, as

previously indicated, have particular problems. Two new schemes
have been started. The National Mobility Scheme began in 1981
to enable public sector tenants to be nominated for a move to
another council's area. One criterion for nomination is the need to
be nearer relatives or friends. The other scheme, the Tenants
Exchange Scheme, started in 1982, is a computerised service to help
people exchange homes with someone in another council's area.

Another group who have been the subject of recent research are
those who fail to take up benefits. Take up of benefits often seems
low for elderly people but one of the things that research on rent
allowances showed was that elderly people fared better in this case
than other groups. This seemed to be because they were given extra
help by staff or, as the researchers put it, there is 'greater likelihood
of encountering intervention from other people'.[64] Maybe there is
a message there for local government. It remains to be seen whether
the new Unified Housing Benefit which replaced rent allowances
will have more impact on elderly people (see p. 197).

PERSONAL AND OTHER SOCIAL SERVICES

Recent trends and community care policies

The growing emphasis on community care policies (see pp. 199–
203) has inevitably meant that attention has been focussed on the
two elements necessary to make these policies a reality. One is informal care, especially that provided by the family (see pp. 119–32 and
pp. 225–29) and the other is personal social services.

The practicalities of both moving elderly people out of institutional care and of keeping frail elderly people in homes of their
own depend on a combination of statutory and voluntary help.
What evidence is there of a change of direction away from residential care and towards an expansion of community care services? One
measure is to look at the proportions of elderly people in various
forms of care. The proportion in long-stay hospitals has remained
constant.[65] In part III numbers of elderly people have gone up
(from 163,500 in 1976 in Great Britain to 183,400 in 1981)[66] but
as a proportion of people aged over 65 the figure remains unchanged
at 2 per cent. What has happened though is that many more in
residential care are older and frailer than previously.

Have community care services expanded? This question has to

be answered with careful attention to the evidence about recent trends. For example, claims and counter claims have been made about whether cuts have taken place. A mere scrutiny of expenditure yields only part of the picture: *The Government's Expenditure Plans 1983–84 to 1985–86* (Cmnd 8789–1983) show that local authority public expenditure on health and personal social services doubled between 1977/78 and 1981/82 (from £983 millions to £1,862 millions) with a further forecast increase to £2,128 millions in 1983/84.[67] It is likely that wage settlements for people working in the health and social services accounted for some of the increase and inflation for a good deal of the rest. In *Public Administration* (Spring 1983) Wistow and Webb have shown how necessary it is to look behind figures and their expertise was drawn on by the House of Commons Select Committee on Social Services. They argue that crude public expenditure figures may conceal what is actually happening to a service. They favour using a constant level of service output as the benchmark against which standards can be assessed. They instance total personal social services expenditure which grew by rather more than 2 per cent per annum in the years 1976/77 to 1980/81 but services did not necessarily expand to that extent. For example, expenditure on residential care, meals, home helps and day care increased but only day care grew in real terms. Changes in unit costs are identified as the major source of deviation between expenditure and output trends (Table 12).

The Association of Directors of Social Services have carried out their own monitoring of personal social services in a series of surveys. In December 1982 they found that the 1982/83 budgets of social service departments indicated an overall increase in expenditure in real terms of 1.1 per cent.[68] This compared with a cut of just under one half of 1 per cent in the 1981/82 budgets. However, this marked a varied pattern with 31 of the 81 departments planning reductions. The Association also point out that the small rise is unlikely to cover the extra services they will be expected to provide; for example, for more very elderly people, let alone to improve the quality of services.

This point about the over-75s is one made by the House of Commons Social Services Committee (based on evidence from Webb and Wistow) examining the 1982 Public Expenditure White Paper:

Evidence suggests that most services for the elderly have not been maintained at a constant level of service over the past four years. Meals and

Table 12. A comparison of trends in services, expenditure and unit costs for elderly people – England and Wales

Activity	Services per 1,000 population 65+ ★		Expenditure trends (November 1980 prices)		Unit cost trends (November 1980 prices)	
	1975/6	1980/1 on 1975/6	Expenditure in 1975/6 (£m.)	1980/81 on 1975/76	Unit costs in 1975/6 (£000s)	1980/1 on 1975/6
Residential	17.7 = 100	94.4	260.3 = 100	119	2,261 = 100	117
Day Care†	2.9 = 100	127.6	20.5 = 100	155	1,029 = 100	113
Home Helps‡ (WTE)	7.4 = 100	93.2	177.3 = 100	109	4,172 = 100	100
Meals‡	6,060 = 100	92.9	25.5 = 100	102	629 = 100	100

★ Numbers of elderly people aged 65+ were 6,811,200 in 1975/76 (index 100) and 7,325,480 in 1980/81 (index 107.6) (+7.6%)
† England only.
‡ These figures give the total provision of services not just for the elderly. WTE = Whole time equivalent.
Source: Evidence of A. Webb and G. Wistow to House of Commons Social Services Committee 1982. Reprinted in Public Administration, Spring 1983, Vol. 61, No. 1, p. 33 and p. 35.

home help services have scarcely grown in volume terms, and almost certainly insufficiently to meet the growing demands. There is some evidence that the shift from residential to day care provision has begun in terms of the number of day care places available; but even day care places have fallen in proportion to the population over 75 since 1979/80 as have the number of hours of home help contact for that population. Between 1975/76 and 1980/81, home help hours of service to those over 75 failed by 8 per cent to keep pace with the growing numbers of elderly, and meals served to these over 75 failed by 11.6 per cent.[69]

DHSS in *Community Care* also showed that the growth of numbers of every elderly people has presented difficulties. They found little evidence of a shift towards community care of people who might be regarded as on the margin of community and institutional care.

There are some small glimmers of light on the scene especially over the innovatory schemes being adopted by both housing and social service departments. These include schemes being monitored by DOE (p. 210) and the Kent Community Care Project which is specifically concerned with cost effective ways of keeping frail elderly people out of residential care. Clients referred are those assessed by the area team to be sufficiently at risk as to make them eligible for admission to residential care. A feature of the scheme is that the social worker, in agreement with the elderly person, can buy in services from any source (private, statutory or voluntary). Challis and Davies in *British Journal of Social Work* (Spring 1980) describe the scheme as a new approach to community care for the elderly and the monitoring team at the Personal Social Services Research Unit, University of Kent have produced numerous papers and articles on many aspects of the Project. However, Davies has pointed out some of his reservations about these innovatory services. These include the fact that most are geographically very localised and do not form part of a coherent strategy by the local authority.[70]

Another problem in trying to monitor what has happened to the personal social services, as Booth has pointed out (*Policy and Politics*, April 1983), is the difficulty in discovering patterns of provision since the suspension after 1979 of the system of three-year planning known as LAPS (Local Authority Planning Statements).

Standards and effectiveness

Another development has been the move away from standards of provision laid down by DHSS. Although these have not been explicitly dropped much more recognition is given to local conditions. In *Care in Action* it was stated that for personal social services 'The Government indicates broad national policies, issues guidance where necessary and has a general concern for standards. There are only a small number of direct controls and these are being reduced as a matter of general government policy towards local government'.[71]

The view of the Association of Metropolitan Authorities on this was that all priorities seemed to be given equal weight.[72] How could priorities be monitored without any financial or other yardstick?

In December 1982 the position was made even clearer when DHSS were asked by the House of Commons Committee on Social Services (Cmnd 8775) whether some indication could be given of the informal minimum personal social services standards which they used. They replied that they did not have any formalised or precisely quantified minimum standards. 'Written evidence from the Department and oral evidence from the Association of Directors of Social Services argued against such standards, and the Committee accepted that it would not be helpful to lay these down. For similar reasons, we do not have a set of private and informal minimum standards which it would be possible to codify and publish in the way that the Committee has implied.[73]

A recent example of attitudes was given by a DHSS Minister in May 1983 when he was asked about local authority policies for charging for domiciliary services. He said: 'We feel that the local authority associations are the most appropriate bodies to provide general guidance for their members on charging for day and domiciliary services and they have been invited to do so' (*Hansard* 12.5.83).

With concern about the most effective use of resources to the fore and the fruition of much research on elderly people the two have been linked in Goldberg and Connelly's *The Effectiveness of Social Care for the Elderly*.[74] In this book they have attempted to draw together much of the research (mainly on personal social services) and consider what evaluation has taken place in the various fields. Based on research evidence they then draw out the general issues for the development of policy and practice.

Social service departments and social work support

The debate about the purpose and organisation of local social service departments has continued with the *Barclay report* favouring a community, locally based approach.[75] However, Pinker, in a powerfully argued note of dissent, points out the dangers of this with the possibility of conflict between social workers as 'advocates' of 'community needs' and their employers. He also argues for the continuation of the trend towards specialised social workers rather than community workers.

Additional evidence has been provided in the last three years of the low priority which elderly people appear to occupy with social workers. The Barclay committee set up to review the role and tasks of social workers reported in 1982. They discussed the sort of problems which require social work support and comment. 'If an elderly person has problems of these kinds, we consider they are as much in need of social work help as a child might be. We cannot accept what in effect is rationing by age.'[76] Rowlings, in *Social Work with Elderly People*, discusses some of the reasons for the reluctance of social workers to work with elderly people. She also examines the problem of assessing and managing dependence and risk while preserving individuality for elderly people living on their own, those living with their families and those in residential care.[77] Marshall, in *Social Work with Old People*, distinguishes between work with the young old and the old old and concludes with a useful section on new ideas.[78]

Special groups

The disabled Turning to particular groups of elderly people attention was focused on the disabled in 1981 which was the International Year of Disabled People. Some have argued that although attitudes may have changed, little was achieved in practical terms (*Social Work Today*, 20.10.81). In Parliamentary debates Ministers claimed that advances had been made but that economic circumstances prevented more being done. In the House of Lords (17.11.82) Lord Trefgarne said that disabled people could not be isolated from the effects of the recession, and in the House of Commons (22.11.82) the Minister, Mr. Hugh Rossi, said that until the economy was back on its feet the government would not be able to make the improvements which they would all like to see.

There were a number of attempts in 1981 and 1982 to enforce the Chronically Sick and Disabled Persons Act 1970. Voluntary organisations tried to persuade the Minister to use default powers after it had been shown that a particular service was not being

The elderly in modern society

provided for specific disabled people. In some cases the Minister wrote to the local authority and the service was provided. Alf Morris, who helped draw up the Act, asked (*The Times*, 26.5.82) whether departmental procedures could be speeded up and made more effective for enforcing the law, whether the Minister would accept that it was his duty to intervene where local authorities were breaching their duties on a wide scale and whether the Minister 'will ensure that they have adequate resources fully to discharge their statutory duties under the Act?'

In 1983 the Royal Association for Disability and Rehabilitation (RADAR) published, on behalf of a number of charities, a Code of Practice on the provision of services by social service departments under Section 2 of the 1970 Act.[79] They felt that national criteria for assessing needs were required and drew up a code to provide guidelines. Bristow, in *The Housing and Care Needs of Disabled People and their Families*, concluded that greater priority should be given to services for disabled people and their families.[80] She also wanted a further development of the Crossroads Care Attendant schemes.

Ethnic groups   The needs of another group, ethnic minorities, have come more into prominence. CPA in *Out of Sight – out of mind*, a study of the interface between social service departments and ethnic elderly people, found that social service departments were beginning to recognise the specialised needs of older Afro Caribbean and Asian people but felt relatively helpless. 'Housing came up again and again as a key component in social wellbeing, and similarly education, health care, income and the take-up of welfare benefits arose again and again as basic issues in wellbeing'.[81] It was felt that the main problem was over Asians, who for various reasons (e.g. their complex religious and dietary customs and the language barriers) 'were seen as presenting almost insuperable difficulties in identifying need and offering appropriate services'. A picture of lack of knowledge by ethnic elderly groups of statutory services and vice versa is painted in *Elders of the Minority Ethnic Groups*.[82] Further evidence about ethnic groups has come in an Age Concern report by Barker.[83]

Domiciliary services

Home helps   The home help service illustrates how different conclusions can be drawn from varied statistics (Table 12). The total number of home helps went up in the 1970s and there was also a steady rise in the number of elderly people *served* by home helps. In 1971/72 67.1 per thousand elderly people aged 65 and over had a home help whereas in 1979/80 the number had risen to 95.5.[84] But there is difficulty in interpreting information on home helps as the CIPFA figures do not distinguish between elderly and other clients and DHSS have not collected statistics on cases attended since 1979/80.

Research has illuminated some of the issues. Hedley and Norman in *Home Help: key issues in service provision* concluded that the service was being spread more thinly 'so that more clients are receiving less service and that, even so, a significant number of those in need are not getting any help at all'.[85] They also plead for allocation according to clearer priorities and raise queries about a changing role. The rise of intensive domiciliary care schemes causes them to question whether home helps should be domestic cleaners or personal carers. Should the service be of an intensity that it can be seen as an alternative to residential care? They also point out:

> residential care offers a different range of services to intensive care. If the old person wants or needs surveillance, comprehensive medical and personal care, removal of the majority of domestic and financial worries, and some sort of social intercourse and therapeutic treatment, at the cost of some independence – then residential care can offer it. If the client wants to stay at home and is prepared to accept physical and social isolation, then intensive care can offer it.[86]

A matter of concern has been the growing practice of charging for the home help service. Charging is a discretionary matter for local authorities. Some provide the service free of charge, some make a standard charge to all recipients, while others use a 'means test'. An account of charging concluded: 'in recent years the pressure to reduce local government expenditure has resulted in many authorities reviewing their policies on charges for the home help service. Decisions have been made on political, administrative and pragmatic grounds, and many social services departments have introduced increased charges in order to avoid what they see as ever more damaging reductions in service'.[87] Under the Health and Social Services and Social Security Adjudications Act 1983 anyone who satisfies a local authority that they cannot reasonably pay the standard charge for any service shall not be asked for more than is 'reasonably practicable'.

Meals The provision of meals shows a pattern of rising provision in the 1970s and then a fall. In 1969 total meals (at home or elsewhere) served per 100 people aged over 65 in England were 335 but in 1980/81 this had risen to 592. The numbers peaked in 1976/77 (619) and have since declined to the present figure[88] (Table 13). In 1981 the *GHS* showed that 3 per cent of elderly people had received meals on wheels and 3 per cent lunch elsewhere in the previous month. Question marks have been raised about the purpose of meals on wheels by Johnson *et al* in *Ageing, Needs and Nutrition*.[89]

Table 13. Provision of meals 1969–82★ and residential care 1976–82† – England

	1969	Peak year	1981/82
Total meals★ served per 100 pop. aged 65+	335	1976/77 = 619	565
Meals served★ at *home* per 100 pop. aged 65+	224	1979/80 = 391	380
Meals served★ *elsewhere* per 100 pop aged 65+	111	1976/77 = 249	185
	1976	Peak year	1981/82
Residents 65+† supported by local authorities			
in local authority homes	99,027	1981/82 = 103,668	103,668
in voluntary homes	13,988	1976 = 13,988	10,999
in private homes	2,096	1980/81 = 3,267	2,178
Total	115,111 peak	1980 = 118,813	116,845

Sources: ★ *DHSS Personal Social Services. Local Authority Statistics.* A/F/82/18 – Domiciliary services, meals, aids and adaptations year ending March 1982, England, March 1983, p. iii.

† *DHSS Personal Social Services. Local Authority Statistics.* RA/82/1 – Residential accommodation for the elderly and for younger physically handicapped people, year ending 31.3.82, England, January 1983, p.v.

They show that few are either acutely in need of a nutritional supplement or properly identified as being at nutritional risk. Is the purpose nutrition or social support? They make a plea for allocation according to need which may vary at particular times. They also argue that an extension of luncheon club provision might be a better use of resources given that few meals on wheels recipients are house-bound. The researchers conclude by asking whether the service is a symbolic one. 'For many old people it represents the local community's willingness to do something, even if it cannot give what they really need.'[90]

Day Care   Day care services are among those which have recently been researched in a more systematic way than in the past. The main national study was done by Carter in *Day Services for Adults: somewhere to go*[91] but a number of local studies were carried out to complement this. Goldberg and Connelly in Chapter 7 of *The Effectiveness of Social Care for the Elderly* summarise all recent research and say that possibly the most important issue is how to integrate day care into a continuum of community services.[92] The second main issue they identify concerns the effective organisation of day care and the third relates to staffing.

Other services   Confirmation that provision of some other services in 1981/82 was dropping is shown elsewhere. DHSS Statistics for England for 1982 show that compared with 1980/81 assistance with holidays, telephone rentals, television installations and licence fees fell but there were increases for installation of communication equipment and for personal aids. With adaptations to property the number of cases rose for non local authority dwellings.[93]

Boarding out

As interest has grown in alternatives to residential care there was a particular welcome in 1980 for the findings of a research study funded by DHSS on elderly people who were boarded out. Thornton and Moore found 23 schemes operating in England and Wales. Some were long term and some short term with a wide range of objectives from providing a cheap form of care, to enhancing the quality of life of elderly people.[94] They report satisfaction by both the elderly people and their carers with many elderly people needing constant attention. They emphasise the importance of selecting and matching elderly people and carers. The working of a number of local authority schemes were described in a workshop (*New Age*, Autumn 1982).

Residential care

While the overall proportion of elderly people in residential care has remained constant at about 2 per cent for some years there has been a shift towards voluntary and private provision. Between 1976 and 1981 in England numbers of residents over 65 in local authority homes rose from 97,719 to 103,295, in voluntary homes from 23,788 to 26,037 and in private homes from 21,320 to 31,838.[95] In 1981 36 per cent of residents aged 65 and over in homes were in voluntary or private homes compared with 32 per cent in 1976.[96] But the percentage of elderly residents *supported* by local authorities in voluntary and private homes declined from 14 per cent in 1976 to 11 per cent in 1982[97] (Table 12). The cost of supporting some residents in private homes by DHSS, including Attendance Allowance, was as high as £100 per week in 1983. The average gross cost per week for an elderly person in a local authority home in 1982/3 was estimated by CIPFA to be £84.05, excluding capital costs, and the average income from charges per resident was £32.15.[98] Under the Health and Social Services and Social Security Adjudications Act 1983 local authorities were given power to recover fees when a person has deliberately disposed of their assets before entering a home.

The average age of admission to local authority homes in 1981 was 82.[99] In 1981 36 per cent of admissions were people over 85 and 45 per cent were between 75 and 84 and the average age of permanent residents was 82 years 6 months.[100] Some argue that an expansion of residential care is needed bearing in mind the expected growth in numbers of very elderly people. Using the old DHSS guidelines of 25 places per 100 population over 65, Grundy and Arie estimate (*BMJ*, 13.3.82) that over 32,500 additional Part III places will be needed simply to ensure provision at the same rate as in 1976. Grundy and Arie feel that community care cannot provide a real alternative to residential care for those who need round-the-clock support and live alone. This view is not shared by the Association of Directors of Social Services who welcome the tendency to reduce the number of residential places which should be for those who are totally dependent (*The Times Health Supplement*, 19.3.82). They say that what is needed is good community services and sheltered accommodation. Others pin their faith in very sheltered housing (p. 210). In an attempt to produce guidance on the need to go into institutional care, Rodgers and Gray suggest (*BMJ*, 11.9.82) that a starting point should be that it is demonstrably shown that they cannot manage at home with the full range of domiciliary services and a comprehensive social and medical assessment has shown that nothing further can be done to reduce the level of disability.

Concern about standards in private and voluntary homes is considerable. In 1980 the Residential Homes Act consolidated certain legislation relating to the registration, conduct and inspection of homes but made no changes in powers. In 1982 DHSS issued a consulative document, *A Good Home*, which proposed a code of practice. Under the Health and Social Services and Social Security Adjudications Act 1983 a new classification of residential care homes, as distinct from nursing homes, was set up for establishments which provide residential accommodation with both board and personal care by reason of old age, disablement and certain other categories. Each home looking after four or more residents has to be registered with the local authority who may impose conditions.

An unknown number of elderly people live permanently in boarding houses which at their best provide homely care but may also lack privacy, have low standards and exploit their residents. Particular problems relating to the suitability of the premises and relations between staff and residents occur when the latter are not able to lead a wholly independent life. The report of a Working Party, *At Home in a Boarding House*, in 1981 by Clarke and Stone proposed guidelines.[101] 'A boarding house charter rather than a landlady's lament', as the Chairman, David Hobman put it (*Community Care*, 1.10.81). It emphasised higher standards of care and raised issues such as the lack of clarity about which homes need to be registered before they can operate legally, the criteria for determining which providers of homes are suitable for registration and the period of registration. A working party was set up to establish a code of practice.

Concern is growing over the frailty and confusion of residents in homes. The trend for elderly people to be older on admission is adding to the problem. One research project directly concerned with this issue was a feasibility study for NHS nursing homes and has led to three experimental ones being set up (p. 206). *Different Care Provision for the Elderly* by Wade, Sawyer and Bell in 1982 showed that some elderly people were inappropriately placed in most forms of care.[102] They argued for nursing homes which would mainly take elderly people from long stay hospitals but could take others as well.

On the subject of mentally and physically impaired elderly people living alongside less dependent elderly people, Wilkin and Jolley's research has led them to argue for full integration of the two groups so long as no home has to cope with more than 30 per cent of the moderately or severely confused. Wilkin has misgivings about the increasing number of different specialised institutions. He feels that they expose elderly people to the risks of moving from one institution to another and alienate staff from the process of care by limiting their role to that of cogs in a production line. He feels that the long-term solution is provision of institutional care for the elderly by a single agency (PSI Seminar, 26.5.83).

A number of other important studies covering elderly people in residential care have recently been concluded. In *A Balanced Life* by Peace, Kellaher and Willcocks (a consumer study of residential life in 100 local authority old peoples homes) the authors concluded that a major problem is lack of privacy.[103] They recommended that the future design of homes should allow for more private and less communal space. They argued for residential flatlets which are more akin to sheltered housing. Inevitably this leads to questions about the role of old people's homes, the cost of such schemes and whether some of the elderly people currently in homes could not remain in ordinary accommodation with some support but without the constant presence of staff. There can, however, be little dissent from the view that ideally those elderly people who do have to live in an old people's homes should have more space and privacy and that design should take into account the growing number of elderly people who have walking aids. Peace *et al.* were also critical of staff attitudes. A positive role for social workers over admission to care and after admission is outlined by Rowlings.[104]

The purpose of old peoples homes is becoming less clear the more they become involved in a diversity of roles. One developing function is acting as a short stay home for elderly people. In 1981 numbers of short-stay residents were up 70 per cent on 1976.[105] Allen, in *Short-stay Residential Care for the Elderly*, found that these placements should not be accepted as necessarily a good thing, that the needs of short stay residents were often different from long stay and that the former seemed to be most successful when in a separate home or wing.[106] The main beneficiaries seemed to be the carers.

COMMUNITY CARE – THE FAMILY

Policy developments

The family came into even greater prominence in the period 1980/83. The White Paper *Growing Older* not only recognised that families were still the principal source of support but held that there was 'no evidence to suggest that the modern family has given up its caring functions or transferred its responsibilities to the State'.[107] The emphasis in policy was to be on providing support for families. The family became a major theme for political speeches. For example, the Secretary of State for Social Services described the family and community as 'front line providers of social care' (*Guardian*, 21.1.81) and other Ministers stressed the role of the family. A special committee called the Family Policy Group, which included eight Cabinet members and the Prime Minister, was set up. *The Guardian* published excerpts from a draft report which looked at a number of ideas. These included proposals to encourage mothers to stay at home and more family involvement in looking after groups such as the elderly, perhaps by adjusting tax and benefit allowances to see if families might be better rewarded (*Guardian*, 17.2.83). More encouragement to community-based services for the elderly like day, or short-term, care were also suggested.

The 1983 political party manifestos all had some mention of the family with obvious recognition of the position of women. The Conservatives, in a chapter entitled 'Responsibility and the family', declared under a heading 'Supporting family life' that 'it is not for the Government to try to dictate how men and women should organise their lives. Our approach is to help people and their families fulfil their own aspirations in a rapidly changing world' (*The Conservative manifesto*, 1983). The Labour manifesto had a section 'Helping families' but their main remarks came when they discussed personal social services and said 'the Tory cuts in its social services have hit women hardest. They have meant lost jobs for many women and a loss of support for the elderly and disabled, thus forcing women to stay at home as unpaid carers' (*The New Hope for Britain*, 1983). And the SDP/Liberal Alliance stated that 'we favour caring for people in the community – for example, helping the elderly to live among family, friends and neighbours. We will support and sustain the family, in particular by helping

225

those, especially women, who carry the burden of this care' (*Working together for Britain*, 1983). The same script writer could have written all three of these excerpts.

Grave doubts about the implications of family care unless backed up by appropriate financial and supportive arrangements are expressed by some bodies. The Equal Opportunities Commission (EOC), for example, 'noted with deep concern' the assumption in *Growing Older* of the increasing involvement of families in community care.[108] They felt that family care 'is too often a euphemism for "care by the nearest female relative"'.[109]

It is to be hoped that the new family study centre set up with joint DHSS and Social Science Research Council funding will be able to monitor the impact of family care. The Centre grew out of the Study Commission on the Family which concluded its investigation in 1983, having produced much useful work on many aspects of the family.

Policy developments have gone hand in hand with research which was concentrated on three areas. The extent of help given by families to elderly people, the need for care for the carers and an analysis of the limitations of family help. Before discussing these aspects it is worth looking at a useful distinction which Parker makes between 'care' and 'tending'. He says that the word care is used to convey the idea of concern about people. 'On the other hand "care" also describes the actual work of looking after those who, temporarily or permanently, cannot do so for themselves. It comprises such things as feeding, washing, lifting, cleaning up the incontinent, protecting and comforting.'[110] He prefers the word tending for these active manifestations of care. Much of what follows is concerned with tending.

Help given by families

Research reports continued to emphasise the important role of the family in providing help with personal and domestic tasks. For example, although attention is rightly given to factors such as geographical mobility, which mean that some families and elderly people no longer live close to each other, a specific question in the 1980 *GHS* directed to elderly people who lived alone showed that 30 per cent had relatives living nearby.[111] The *GHS* also revealed the extent of care by families for elderly people. An EOC report found that two thirds of their sample of carers were giving help to elderly people.[112] Only two fifths of the carers lived in the same home and the others often had awkward expensive journeys to contend with before they could give help.

An analysis of the physical care, emotional demands and time spent caring has also been given by the EOC together with the costs involved.[113] These included loss of employment opportunities. Similar information is given by Nissel and Bonnerjea in *Family Care of the Handicapped Elderly: who pays?*[114] Allen, in a paper summarising recent research on the elderly and their informal carers, stressed that carers do not constitute a homogenous group of people and failure to appreciate this can lead to inappropriate expectations of their role.[115] For instance, the duration and type of the relationship will affect what carers feel able to do. The nature of the caring role will have an effect too. A son or daughter may feel embarrassed at performing personal tasks for a parent which may be easier for a professional.

The extent of care by elderly spouses and the effect this subsequently had on their lives is documented by Bowling and Cartwright in *Life after a Death*.[116] Elderly people who have cared for a spouse who has died not only lose the person they cared for but may have to come to terms with anxiety, loneliness and adjustment to their lives.

Care for the carers

There was a growth of interest in the position of those who do the caring. Indeed the word carer was one increasingly used. It had not become familiar enough to be used in the 1981 White Paper *Growing Older* but it was in *Care in Action*. The formation of the Association of Carers in 1981 gave another boost towards recognition of this group of people, most of whom are family members. The media increasingly focussed on the problems of carers too and they featured prominently as a topic at conferences. These developments were helped by an upsurge of research reports which spelt out the implications for carers. The EOC spearheaded the research with *The Experience of Caring for Elderly and Handicapped Dependants* in 1980,[117] *Who Cares for the Carers*[118] in 1982, and *Caring for the Elderly and Handicapped*[119] in 1982. Their main findings, understandably, have been the impact on women because they are the main carers.

Practical suggestions about ways carers could be helped have been put forward and actual schemes started. These include self-help groups or opportunities to meet and discuss problems with fellow carers. The work of Levin and Siddell has shown that not only are more services needed but greater flexibility would help as would an explanation from a professional about what is happening to the person they are caring for.[120] Others simply want a recognition of what they are doing. The EOC are among those who argue for an extension of the invalid care allowance to married and cohabiting women.[121] Invalid Care Allowance (first payable in 1976) is a non-contributory benefit for men and single women under pension age who are in paid employment or in full-time education and who look after a severely disabled person for at least 35 hours a week. The severely disabled person must be receiving Attendance Allowance or a Constant Attendance Allowance. The EOC also put the case for a non-taxable, non-contributory carers benefit, for a more flexible approach to the working week and domestic responsiblities and extended leave.[122] Others argue for tax concessions for carers and/or higher benefits for elderly people who could then buy in help from carers. McKenzie believes one of the greatest needs is for relief for the carer by way of sitting-in services (*New Age*, Spring 1982).

Growth in the number of books aimed at those who are caring, or about to take care of a dependent elderly relative (e.g. Agate,[123] Gray and McKenzie[124]), are another acknowledgement of the need to support the supporters.

Limitations of family help

Some of the limitations on family help were given in Chapter 9. In addition the growing complexity of family life has to be taken into account. Divorce and re-marriage mean new sets of in-laws, stepparents and varying relationships. To which older people will the younger feel bound?

Recent research has also identified that there are some problems which may particularly lead to carers giving up their task.[125] These include aggression, disturbance at night and behavioural problems.

The sad fact is that the evidence points to families only reluctantly relinquishing the care of an elderly person while a little more support would have tipped the balance. But it is also only fair to recognise that other generations have rights too. Who can argue that a disturbed grandparent in a family should be cared for at the cost of a mother's breakdown in health with the consequent effect on her children? Hopefully women's role will be shared more by men but even so it is likely that the future will continue to see middle-aged women looking after other women a generation older. If present evidence is anything to go by they will also receive less statutory help than their masculine counterparts. The Crossroads study of 172 carers found that while 4 per cent of mothers, 20 per cent of wives and 24 per cent of daughters received home help support 75 per cent of caring sons and 68 per cent of husbands received this service.[126] Finch and Groves (*Journal of Social Policy*, October 1980) raised serious question marks over community care based so much on families (e.g. women), claiming that equal opportunities were not being given. They felt that the forces pulling women back into domestic caring roles were an inevitable consequence of community care policies. Unless there were a greater degree of financial and practical support for the carers and changes in employment patterns (e.g. the development of job-sharing, 'caring' leave, etc.) women will continue to be disadvantaged.

The dividing line between a family being able to cope or not is a narrow one. As Rapoport and Rapoport concluded in *Families in Britain*: 'if the State shifts too much of a burden on to families themselves, it may produce another kind of erosion of its vast store of popular care-givers-erosion through overloading'.[127] There is little disagreement that policies in the future must concentrate on a partnership between families and statutory services. How this is to be spelt out is far from clear.

COMMUNITY CARE – SUPPORT FROM THE WIDER
COMMUNITY

General policy developments and problems

Community care remained an attractive phrase yet an ethereal concept. But those who talk about community care are far more likely now to be asked to be specific than in the heady days when 'community care' was just a vague cosy description. Then there did not even seem to be a distinction between care in the community and care by the community.

The previous section has spelt out some of the recent developments in family care in the spectrum of community care but what of the role of the other participants in the informal caring network? Voluntary bodies, volunteers and friends and neighbours have all come into the limelight recently. As Michael Power said in a Policy Studies Institute Seminar (26.1.83), it is a 'don't call us – call each other' approach. The central role for the voluntary or informal network was argued by Patrick Jenkin, then Secretary of State for Social Services, when he responded to what he thought were criticisms of this policy. 'It is not caring on the cheap – it is a way of getting a great deal more for our money', he said (*The Guardian*, 21.1.81). But the danger of stressing this aspect of care was put by Nicholas Hinton later in the year when he feared that there would be antagonism 'if voluntarism is over-sold' (*The Times*, 7.9.81).

Perhaps one of the main dilemmas, apart from those mentioned in Chapter 10 and that of insufficient funding, is how to ensure that needs are met by the much vaunted statutory and voluntary twinning. To make this a certainty a central strategy and some kind of central co-ordination is needed. This was well put by Wicks in relation to care for the elderly. Discussing the evidence for neighbourhood care, he suggested that a strong role for central government and local authorities is needed if community care is to become a reality.[128] For instance, the role of a social services department as planner, initiator, enabler and co-ordinator may be as important as the role of provider in the future. But in many ways informal care would then have to develop, what Peter Westland calls, 'a coherence and unity which it lacks' (*Community Care*, 19.11.81). The strength of informal care is precisely because it is not an entity and does not have to reconcile its differences. Westland then goes on to pose the extreme question: 'if central government relinquishes its traditional planning role, abandons its attempt to monitor and assess social needs and rolls back the frontiers of the State in the guise of freedom, choice and familial duty – all of which it says it is attempting to do – then it is clear that we are in for a major revolution in social welfare policy'.

If a central strategy is to be possible, Walker holds that the objectives must be related to a plan intended to achieve them (e.g. changes in duties and allocation of staff).[129] However, Bayley believes that no one strategy will provide community care. Apart from the need for genuine commitment by formal agencies to work with kin and kith he considers that a number of approaches must be used. 'Some of these are community work techniques, some are special intervention techniques worked out for a particular group of people like the Kent Community Care Project, some are broader organizational approaches like the patch system.'[130] And the danger of generalising is shown by research which distinguishes between communities in urban and rural areas. Wenger's work on ageing in rural areas, for example, has shown that the rural elderly have higher levels of contact with neighbours and are more likely to be involved with activities involving social contacts than their urban counterparts. In rural areas, dependency on family appears to be lower (*Ageing and Society*, July 1982).

It is only fair to acknowledge that a great deal of the questioning about informal care has come, or been prompted by, government departments. For example, the detailed questions posed in the Consultative Document *The Government and the Voluntary Sector*[131] were followed up in 1981 with a very comprehensive analysis of the responses.[132] A thorough discussion of such issues as the possible need for a long-term strategy were examined and the relationships between volunteers and trade unions. Subsequently extra help was given for local voluntary initiatives.

Many of the recent examples of informal care have been evaluated and they are summarised by Goldberg and Connelly, who conclude that a great deal more thought and experimentation has to be devoted to working out patterns of fruitful relationships with the statutory sector.[133] They also point to the need for ways of monitoring voluntary activities not only for purposes of accountability but to provide voluntary bodies with some idea of how they are doing and where they are going.

Voluntary organisations

The growing number of voluntary organisations and the development of existing ones concerned with the elderly is illustrated by the increased activity by both voluntary residential homes (p. 222) and housing associations. Between 1971 and 1981 provision of homes by housing associations rose from 217,000 to 465,000. Provision for the elderly has always featured strongly in housing association programmes and it seemed likely that in 1982/83 as much as 50 per cent of additional homes to rent would be for this group (*Voluntary Housing*, August 1982).

The church too has played an important role, sometimes in housing associations, but especially in the rapid development of good neighbour schemes. A recent survey of 3,000 schemes found that two fifths of those studied owed their existence to the church (*Community Care*, 10.12.81). The report of the schemes *Action for Care: a Review of Good Neighbour Schemes* by Abrams *et al.* found that good neighbouring represents a major initiative.[134] They stressed, however, the need for effective discussion between voluntary and statutory organisations. Elsewhere (*Social Work Service*, No. 22, 1980) Abrams has concluded:

I would suggest that attempts to revive traditional local social networks are largely misguided if it is hoped thereby to secure patterns of neighbourliness which will provide care with anything like the measures of coverage and reliability possibly achieved by the most tightly-knit versions of such networks in the past. One cannot and should not want to recreate the conditions for that sort of neighbourliness. What *is* possible is to accept that the so-called 'informal' system of social care – except as a system of care between kin – is irretrievably lost, but that an adequate substitute for it can be found in the formal projects and schemes of the new neighbourhoodism. This means recognising that the networks generated by the new neighbourhoodism are essentially and necessarily political in nature; their energy and effectiveness tied to the fact that they are making *demands*. This in turn means that instead of patronising or colonising the local community, as envisaged by the original conception of neighbourhood care, the existing statutory and voluntary agencies are going to have to learn to live with it as an equal.

Another feature has been the growing partnership between statutory and voluntary agencies. An illustration of this is the extension of joint financing to the latter and the push by DHSS to involve the latter. The Health and Social Services and Social Security Adjudications Act 1983 provides for additional members of joint consultative committees (see p. 76) to be appointed by voluntary organisations. Voluntary organisations are also eligible under the new joint finance arrangements for pilot projects enabling elderly people to move into the community (DHSS Circular HC (83) 6 March 1983. *Health Service Development. Care in the Community and Joint Finance*).

Another interesting development has been the co-operation between different voluntary bodies for very specific purposes. One of the values of this as outlined by David Hobman (*New Age*, Winter 1980) is that the alliance, as it is usually called, can be flexible, costs little to administer and can be wound up quickly when its purpose has been achieved. Age Concern, England for example belonged in 1983 to the Disability Alliance, Dignity in Death Alliance and the National Fuel Poverty Forum.

However, close links between statutory and non-statutory bodies are not without their dangers especially when public funding becomes of major importance. Grants from government departments inevitably mean that voluntary bodies have to tread a delicate line. As Alison Norman, Deputy Director of CPA, put it in an aptly named unpublished paper 'Pigs in the middle', whether they like it or not major voluntary agencies are involved in political issues and political decisions. If they then bite the hand which feeds them, continued sustenance cannot be taken for granted. She also cites examples of voluntary agencies being pressed to take on a task such as running a day centre which would otherwise be the local authority's responsibility and to do it more cheaply and with lower standards.

Volunteers

One of the few recent pieces of empirical research on the use of volunteers to help elderly people has been done by Power in a study of volunteer support to elderly people living in residential homes.[135] In a study of six residential homes he found that there was a demand for volunteers; the latter could be organised but they were not found to make much difference to the quality of life of the elderly people. From his research, which he suggests needs replicating, Power found that a small number of people are willing to volunteer to work with elderly people, but they need a good deal of support and overall have a role of modest dimensions which should not be inflated (Policy Studies Institute Seminar, 26.1.83).

In another study based on the Kent Community Care project, Bleddyn Davies would like to see greater use made of volunteers in caring for vulnerable old people living in their own homes.[136] It is clear that far more evaluation has to take place on the quality and acceptability of community care and also on the interchangeability between informal and formal care. For example, in what circumstances is help to elderly people of a personal and intimate nature better coming from a professional, such as a nurse rather than a volunteer? Or is it the timing and delivery of statutory services which calls them into question? The research on the Crossroads Care scheme seems to indicate that volunteers, albeit paid, are able to work how and when those they care for wish and deliver an acceptable service.

Friends and neighbours

The 1980 *GHS* asked questions about contact between elderly people and friends and relatives. The overwhelming majority, about six out of seven elderly people, said that they saw relatives or friends at least once a week, and almost a third did so every day or nearly.[137] Only 3 per cent said that they did not see relatives or friends at all. It is interesting that elderly people living alone were more likely than those living in other types of household to see relatives or friends daily or nearly every day.[138]

THE CONTRIBUTION OF THE ELDERLY

Growth of participation?

Perhaps one of the most encouraging developments over the last three years has been the growing and belated recognition that elderly people have as much, and sometimes more, to contribute to society than many younger people. This recognition was acknowledged by the UK government which nominated as their topic to the United Nations World Assembly on Ageing in 1982, 'The Contribution Elderly People can make to Society'. In the paper sent to the Assembly, *Ageing in the United Kingdom*,[139] two aspects were highlighted. One was the value to elderly people themselves of their distinctive and valuable contribution and the other was the help that can be given. 'The failure of a community to draw on that contribution can greatly diminish the lives of its older members, as well as depriving the community itself of a major source of talent and energy'.[140] It was thought that greater participation would substantially help not only the very old and frail but also, for example, single parents and families coping with handicap.[141]

As has been seen (pp. 154–172) the contribution of elderly people is already considerable. Fresh evidence was provided in the *1981 GHS* when questions about voluntary work were included.[142] It was found that 23 per cent of respondents had participated in voluntary work in the year before the interview.[143] For those aged 65–74 it was 21 per cent and for those over 75, 11 per cent. It is interesting that the recently retired participated less than any group except those under 24 and the over 75s. One reason could be that help to families and friends was not included in the survey and it is well known that elderly people do give a great deal of help here. But it could be that some things could be done to expand help from this group. One enterprising initiative was started by Age Concern in 1982. Called 'lifeskills', it is a programme of community involvement for older people. Funded by the Carnegie United Kingdom Trust schemes are being set up involving direct partnership with other appropriate organisations. Schemes include using retired people as volunteers in day and residential centres with children, a gardening co-operative in conjunction with a Youth Opportunities Scheme and a project to care for pets when owners have to go into hospital. Marshall in *Social Work with Old People* has a section on selling the skills of the newly retired. She points out that many newly retired people lack confidence and also that they can be very short of money. Not only may there be problems organising them but the temptation to exploit them must be avoided.[144] Although many of the constraints on older people participating are those of attitudes some of the more practical ones are becoming less pronounced. For instance, in 1981 the number of elderly households with a telephone had risen to 66 per cent (the average for all households was 75 per cent), and to 32 per cent for a car (the average for all households was 59 per cent).[145] This represents an increase on the 1976 figures (p. 161).

Another interesting development has been along self-help lines. An example of this is the University of the Third Age. Started in France, it now has branches in this country and aims to provide educational opportunities for the retired as a group. Some of the tutors are retired and some groups are managed by the retired too. One reason for the movement is that education is seen as a right for every age group yet at present benefits mostly the under 25s. It is also considered that education will help create a fulfilling lifestyle and postpone dependence.

In a summary of research on older people as volunteers, Goldberg and Connelly found that a common thread was for them to feel useful, to meet and relate to other elderly people and to support each other, rather than to take up issues with outside bodies on general problems.[146] Voluntary work was seen as a therapeutic measure enhancing self-esteem and life satisfaction.

There are also indications of a growing unwillingness to be passive receivers of services (e.g. an article by Rosalind Chambers, an octogenarian and resident in a home in *New Age*, Spring 1981). She argued for a radical change in the running of such homes, giving much more consumer participation.

Political involvement

The growing importance of elderly people in the political context also seems clear. Age Concern, for example, produced a leaflet, *Campaign Priorities*, for the 1983 General Election with questions about specific policies for people to put to all their local candidates. In *Political Attitudes and Ageing in Britain* Abrams and O'Brien concluded from a National Opinion Poll survey that elderly people were as likely as younger people to have voted in a general or local election, stood for public office, paid individual membership to a political party and taken an active part in a political campaign.[147] They also found that in every general election since 1964, irrespective of which party had an overall victory, support for the Conservatives was highest in the 65 or more age group. The Conservatives acknowledge that Britain's pensioners represent a major slice of the electorate. They say that they draw almost 30 per cent of their voting strength from this group.[148] Abrams and O'Brien speculate on why elderly people have not become a powerful political pressure group. Among possible explanations are differences between elderly people (e.g. car owners may oppose free public transport on buses), dislike of being labelled old and an awareness of lack of power (e.g. at being unable to withdraw their labour).

In the United States elderly people are becoming increasingly involved in lobbying and advocacy and Oriel has speculated about the effect that this growing citizen participation will have on programmes.[149] Phillipson argues that older people in this country have been slower to become a political force but claims that there is a gradual emergence of more radical groups of pensioners. Some militant groups of pensioners have developed links with trade unions.[150]

The Future

But what could be the greatest boost for the contribution of elderly people would be a re-thinking of what people do when they do not work and the whole concept of retirement. If a large proportion of people are going to spend long periods not in paid employment, because they are retired or unemployed, then what they do has to be seen as valuable. Contributing in some way to society could give the self-esteem, status and role that many sadly only find now in paid employment. Parker has said that at least some of the present generation of elderly people are seeing retirement as offering a new lease of life, a liberation and an incentive to live actively and positively.[151] He believes that we should not talk about retirement *from* but retirement *to*.

When Geoffrey Finsberg, then Parliamentary Secretary for

Health, spoke at the World Assembly on Ageing in July 1982, he said that 'a conscious and informed effort by the whole community is needed if elderly people are to make the full contribution of which they are capable to the life of the society in which they live'. A more aggressive attitude by a new generation of elderly people who refuse to be treated as second-class citizens may make this hope a reality.

SOME GENERAL PROBLEMS

Introduction

The theoretical framework of the chapter on general problems is still valid but changing factors have inevitably led to less emphasis being placed on some of them and more on others. For example, much less has been heard about need and its measurement. But the combination of scarce resources and discussions about what are the right policies for the change in the balance of numbers of elderly people especially the growth in the likely number of frail elderly have led to fierce debates about value for money and how services are to be evaluated. Perhaps in less dire times research will again turn to the measurement of need. But it has to be said that the development of research into value for money and a more stringent approach to evaluation, though still in their infancy, are long overdue. Similarly, the research of the last few years which has explored more fully the issues and implications of one of the other policies previously mentioned (community care) has given a more realistic basis for discussion than some of the much woolier thinking that went before.

The questions which now take precedence in most discussions of policy are those relating to finance and who does what, state or private sector, and especially the balance between the two. It is proposed to discuss these two problems (finance and the role of the private sector) first and then turn to developments in the debate over variations in services and evaluation.

Finance

Economic constraints and spending Economic constraints have dominated social policy in recent years. On the positive side closer scrutiny of budgets can lead to a radical and valuable reappraisal

237

The elderly in modern society

of policies which might not otherwise have happened. Knapp, for example, argues that shortage of resources does not necessarily mean that the well-being of clients must take a back seat. Discussing residential care for the elderly he says, 'rather, the sensible analysis, interpretation and employment of cost information can ensure that unnecessary inefficiencies are avoided. This could mean that more and better care is provided from a fixed, or even contracting, budget' (*Ageing and Society*, July 1981).

More than anything else it has been the continued growth in the number of very elderly people which has concentrated people's minds on finance, since it is normally the care of the very elderly which is the most costly. But there have been a number of other factors which have contributed to the current interest in costs, such as variations in costs of apparently similar services, the growing interest generally in value for money studies, and the increasing number of economists and accountants becoming involved in matters of social policy.

Costings studies In government departments, in the Audit Commission and in bodies connected with local government costings studies are mushrooming. But the problems should not be minimised. As DHSS said in evidence to the House of Commons Social Services Committee in 1980:

the methodological problems associated with assessing both the total costs and the effectiveness of different methods of caring for people have made it particularly difficult to draw firm conclusions from much of the research work completed so far. Moreover, it is important to recognise that each of the hospital, residential and community options represents a particular mode of care which needs to be judged on its appropriateness for the individual concerned (e.g. in terms of relative dependency and domestic circumstances). To some extent, therefore, attempts to compare the relative costs of differing modes of care run the risk of not comparing like with like. There are, nevertheless, a number of continuing research projects, some of them funded in part or in whole by the DHSS, which will, it is hoped, build on past research findings to increase our understanding of the trade-offs between different forms of care.[152]

The Committee recommended that 'high priority' should be given to research on the cost-effectiveness of different packages of care.

Wright's work has contributed much to laying the foundations of a methodology of costings; but he has admitted that the actual measurement of costs and benefits is 'fiendishly difficult'.[153] His

238

explanation of the methods of costing is one of the clearest expositions on the subject. In particular he describes the two major ways of measuring costs. The simplest is the public expenditure approach in which costs are measured in terms of the cash expenditures falling on public authorities. The other approach is the opportunity cost which arises from the premise that, as resources are limited, using them in one way means that a benefit is foregone for use for an alternative. Therefore cost is a measure of sacrifice or opportunity lost. The latter approach includes all the resources used in the provision of care, whether or not they belong to public authorities. Wright, Cairns and Snell have undertaken one costings study involving four geographical areas. In their report *Costing Care* they discussed the measurement of dependency and how to estimate and allocate costs of alternative patterns of care.[154] They found that considerable daily help has to be given to higher dependency groups. 'This means that a good system of familiar and friendly help must be available if people in these dependency categories are to be kept at home. At the higher levels of the scale it may even be difficult to keep people in residential care'.[155] They found that generally residential care was much cheaper than hospital care but problems arise when the former cannot cope with the demands placed upon it. The differences between hospital and community care were considerable and had implications for giving financial help to informal carers.

While caution should be exercised in any discussion of costs (for example, capital costs are often left out of calculations) some comparative running costs are significant. In 1981/82 the average cost per week per patient[156] in an acute hospital of over 300 beds was £555.38, in a long stay hospital £232.89, in a geriatric hospital £215.53 and in a Part III home £83.82 (average income received from charges was £31.71 in Part III).[157] Some comparative costings on elderly people living in the community were expected in the DOE study (p. 210).

Other issues A prerequisite to any understanding about patterns of expenditure is adequate information. Some of the most interesting evidence on finance in the last few years has come from the House of Commons Social Services Committee. For example, in 1980 they examined the government's White Paper on Public Expenditure relating to the social services and asked fundamental questions on spending plans and the impact of these policies.[158] They also asked whether the information provided enabled Parliament to form judgements about the government's priorities and policies. In 1982, the Association of Metropolitan Authorities also pointed out difficulties over the availability of reliable information to the House of Commons Social Services Committee.[159] They said that better monitoring of information is required and it is considered that this is not at odds with local government's need to maintain local discretion to spend. Indeed better information will enable local government to discuss more effectively with central government the allocation of resources for new and improved services. Local government expenditure decisions can be better defended if accurate information relevant to comparative analysis can be made available. They also held that the present arguments about overspending and under-spending are sterile rhetoric in the absence of any worthwhile information about needs and the relative significance of the different ways of meeting these.[160]

Another problem is how to achieve any desired shift in resources. Research may show that it is possible and cheaper to keep an elderly person at home rather than in residential care but it may not be possible to switch buildings and staff at the drop of a hat. How to achieve a shift to domiciliary care when there is a shortage of resources is not easy. The carrot of joint finance has been one way of attempting to bring about this switch.

The role of the private sector

In most of the services discussed the impact of the private sector has been seen to be becoming more important. For sheltered housing, pensions and residential care the trend has been particularly pronounced. There seems no reason why other areas should not open up; for instance, private domiciliary care of a more intensive kind than that provided by the traditional domestic 'help' of the middle classes.

But while the development of private sector provision has gone forward it has not been without criticism and questioning. Perhaps the most important of these relate to standards of care, for what little research there is on private residential homes reveals that there are dramatic differences between the standards of the best and the worst. And in private sheltered housing elderly people or their advisers need to look closely at leases to see what the service charges are likely to be and whether the full capital amount on the investment will be returned when the property is sold. The question of standards becomes more acute where public money is involved, as it is for instance when social security payments are used for private residential care. The different financial help an elderly person gets on the one hand and the different charges to be paid on the other show up clearly the difference in value for money of the different provisions. But it has to be said that these anomalies are also to be found within the state sector. The only free (to the old person) form of provision is the hospital; whereas in sheltered housing rent must be paid or the home bought, and for Part III accommodation a person may have to sell their home or realise any other capital to pay for their stay.

The dilemma of the respective role of state and non-state sectors of public welfare is put by Challis when she asks 'how can any government of whatever political colour, whether central or local, influence the level and type of activity in those sectors of care for which it is not itself directly responsible?' (*Political Quarterly*, July-September 1982). Citing residential care for old people as an example, she says that the most obvious way of exerting control is through registration of rest homes by local authorities and of nursing homes by the District Health Authorities. Although registration is contingent upon standards such as space and, in the case of nursing homes, a certain level of qualified nursing staff, she claims this measure of control does not amount to a system of regulation of the private and voluntary sector. But she says that regulation of standards of care leaves untouched such issues as 'the extent of non-State provision, the kinds of people non-State care should be providing for, the price charged for care and so on'. Challis maintains that few mechanisms have been developed to assist the non-state sectors of care to respond to new (and old) problems. She believes that the reluctance on the part of the public authorities to get too closely involved with private care in particular is fuelled by two different streams of thought. At one extreme, there is the view that the state should leave well alone because there is no need for intervention; that the hidden hand of the market economy of care will do what is necessary. At the other, there is mistrust of the private sector and a belief that it is exploitative because of the profit motive, that it is aimed at the well-off and therefore not the concern of government which should concentrate its activities on the most needy. These stereotypes are at the two extremes and Challis hopes that evidence will accumulate which will break the mould of purely public/private/voluntary/informal care.

The blurring of the respective roles of public and private sectors can be seen in a number of ways; for example, the large number of state-supported elderly people in private old people's homes, and equity sharing housing schemes where a person owns part of the home and pays rent for the rest. A coherent social policy becomes more difficult to establish when there is mixed public and private provision.

Variations in services

Research on services continued to find varied provision. For example, Johnson looking at a local meals service was surprised to find the variation 'far in excess of differences in circumstances which exist in local areas'.[161] Variations were found between individuals, between groups and between areas and the search for reasons was pursued. Bebbington and Davies have shown the considerable differences in levels of provision and spending on local social services for elderly people.[162] Examining trends closely, they found that although there was considerable responsiveness to the pattern of need, other factors intervened. For example, political factors were clear (i.e. spending was relatively high in areas of high Labour Party representation). They also comment that 'it is noteworthy that not only are those authorities which face above average costs spending disproportionately more on the elderly, but that this trend is continuing to advance'.[163] Uneven provision can also result from demographic changes where, for instance, large numbers of elderly people move into an area. Allon-Smith believes that, economic and planning factors permitting, there will be continued pressure for the development of certain coastal regions and retirement towns and villages.[164] If this is not matched by increased provision, especially of health and social services, discrepancies over provision will widen. Nor is it just a simple case of assessing the amount of provision. Performance, intensity, quality of care and charges may all vary and cause there to be wide differences between areas.

Variations in services seem to be a considerable source of irritation to elderly people. In a BBC television programme 'Are we being served?' (2.9.82) a member of the National Executive Council of the Old Age Pensioners Association raised three issues, two concerned with anomalies. Why, she wanted to know, were some old people only paying 5p for their television licence, while others just as needy pay the full fee, and why is there discrepancy in areas in travel concessions? The latter is a matter for local authorities but the former is an interesting example where it is laid down under the Wireless Telegraphy (Broadcasting Licence Charges and Examption) Regulations 1970 that elderly people in residential homes and sheltered housing may have a concessionary licence (5p per year each). Some local authorities have been trying to circumvent this by providing a warden service so that more elderly people may benefit. In December 1979 an Opposition motion was moved to abolish the licence fee for all pensioners but it was defeated. The Home Secretary said that the licensing system could not afford to lose revenue from a third of all households (*The Times*, 7.12.79). The question of equity between elderly people was also raised by the Leeds sheltered housing survey which found that the elderly people there in sheltered housing, while very little different from those in the community, were however receiving more help from domiciliary services.[165]

Findings about variations have led some to press for more central direction. For example, Hedley and Norman on home helps argue for 'an official directive that local authorities are not expected or indeed permitted to make savings by cutting back on home help or by charging those who by definition cannot afford to pay'.[166] Johnson also asks for more guidance. 'At national level there should be an attempt to specify the purposes of the different forms of meals service which currently exist and to indicate the usefulness and applications of others which are at the developmental stage'.[167] An increase in central control of this kind would mean a shift away from the prevailing political attitude of central government in the 1980s which is to encourage local authorities to make their own decisions. Though some may argue that central control is a reality through the overall power of the purse strings, it is the Conservative government's view that within these financial constraints, it is for local authorities to make their own assessment of local needs and provide accordingly. Research has an important role to play in providing factual information and in particular finding out about and publicising good practice. Whether more could be done in the way of a clearing house for evaluative studies is another question. This could easily become a role for local authority associations but few have the resources, and perhaps the interest, to undertake this function.

The evaluation of services

Some of the problems involved in evaluating services for elderly people were outlined in Chapter 12. Recently however there have been some useful contributions to methodology. Foremost among these is the work of Goldberg and Connelly at the Policy Studies Institute and that of members of the Personal Social Services Research Unit (PSSRU) at the University of Kent.

In the *Effectiveness of Social Care for the Elderly* Goldberg and Connelly claim that evaluation must incorporate consideration of aims and outcome.[168] They suggest that evaluation is important to get public accountability, to ensure that resources are deployed to obtain a measure of territorial and social justice, to determine what impact the service has on the well-being on its users, to assess cost effectiveness and as a 'safeguard against the new' (i.e. to assess the usefulness of new schemes which are being pushed but are not tested). They then describe how to evaluate, from description to field experiment, and finally go on to look at some evaluative pieces of research which have been done in the various areas of care in the community (e.g. social work and day care services) and in special accommodation. Some of the studies discussed are small-scale, some are sophisticated experiments and others are large scale comparisons.

Much of the work done at the PSSRU at the University of Kent has been of an evaluative nature particularly that in the Kent Community Care Project. An example of the latter is Challis's article 'The Measurement of Outcome in Social Care of the Elderly' in the *Journal of Social Policy* (April 1981) which concentrates on one aspect of evaluation, the effectiveness of services in attaining their objective. The objective is described as the quality of life, in relation to which seven dimensions (nurturance, compensation for disability, independence, morale, social integration, family relationships and community development) are identified and the evidence weighed.

Evaluative studies have travelled a long way since it was thought sufficient to ask recipients of services simple questions about satisfaction. More searching questions are now being asked about what the aim of the service is and how this had been achieved. What effect has it had on the elderly person? On other services provided? On carers? What is the cost? Other interesting aspects are developing too such as the replicating of research projects (e.g. the Kent Community Care Scheme) in other areas.

But evaluation still has a long way to go and often seems a relatively esoteric exercise to practitioners. Unless practitioners can become more involved and evaluation is built in as part of their normal work, there is a danger of them ignoring findings. Certainly better dissemination of evaluative studies could go a long way to spread the good news, but nothing brings home the value of research more than a small taste of it at first hand. Greater field involvement and peer reviews would enhance evaluation. It also has to be said that a number of other things are needed as well. Long-term follow-up studies are needed when the impact of social intervention cannot be assessed in the short terms of a normal research project. More work is needed on positive aspects of ageing. Why and how do some people appear to cope against all the odds? What is a normal old age? And much better measures are needed to make evaluation a reality. I have argued elsewhere for more work on measures for assessing dependency, for without this it is impossible to compare like with like.[169] Measures also need to be developed to indicate both the number and intensity of services people receive and/or need. What combination or packages of care are essential for what sort of elderly people? Can measures be developed which take account of both formal and informal care?

Finally, when evaluations have taken place it is essential for policy makers and practitioners to be aware of them. Whether it is good practice resulting in successful outcomes or the reverse, people need to know. They, professionals and elderly people alike, also have to be prepared to accept changes.

THE TOPIC IN PERSPECTIVE

The elderly and other groups

If one of the most distinctive features of old age for most people is the absence of paid employment then this is now an experience which they share with millions of unemployed people. Is it too much to hope that this could bring about a change in the way in which leisure is seen? If more people could find status and satisfaction in their lives through activities other than paid work then this would be bound to have repercussions on the way in which people see ageing. Instead of old age being the end of 'real' life, it could be a more natural continuation of the life that has gone before.

Even if unemployment diminishes it is almost inevitable that other factors are going to affect the strict division between being in work and not. More equality between the sexes will hopefully mean that job sharing and more flexible working patterns will become more normal than at the present. If caring roles are shared by men and women, not only for children but for older and disabled people as well, then the blurring between work and other activities could become even greater.

Early retirement is yet another influence which needs to be considered. Those who come into this category could provide a bridge between those in work and those of pensionable age. On the other hand who is to say what would be the results of any future Age Discrimination Act? A Bill was introduced in 1983 but fell on the dissolution of Parliament. The purpose of the Bill was to make discrimination against people on the basis of age illegal. Any future Act could mean more older people keeping their jobs and this could cause ill feeling among younger age groups. Inevitably decisions have sometimes to be taken about priorities between social groups. It says much for the pressure groups acting for children, the disabled, the elderly and others that there has so far been little attempt to win resources for one against the other. However, it still seems true that children are the centre of interest of many professionals (and possibly many elderly people too).

But the fact is that elderly people will be the client group to whom a great many professionals will have to devote a good deal of attention. The growth in numbers of very elderly people have inevitable consequences for the caring professions. In 1981 40 per cent of all health and personal social services resources was spent on elderly people.[170] Demographic pressures seem to make it inevitable that a greater priority will have to be given in social policy to elderly people. The immediate effect of the bulge of much older people in the population will be that their visibility will be more pronounced. But it will be unfortunate if undue attention is given to frailty rather than accepting that although more services will have to be provided for this group they are in a minority. Society tends to think mainly in terms of frailty and, despite evidence to the contrary, the public image of the elderly is often of hypothermia, dementia and loneliness, though these effect only a small minority. Even an article full of evidence of enjoyment of old age was entitled 'Too happy to be old – Joy Melville finds there is life after retirement' (*New Society*, 10.6.82).

The quality of life of elderly people

Growing attention has been focused recently on the quality of life of elderly people and this was one of the subjects chosen for the DHSS Seminar in 1982.[171] *How* you measure quality of life is

difficult to decide. Some research studies are based on the perceptions of professionals with questions asked of them rather than of
the elderly people themselves as, for example, in some studies of
sheltered housing tenants where wardens rather than the elderly
tenants have been questioned. This may save time and achieve
answers in a more standard form but it may be dangerously
misleading as a way of finding out how elderly people themselves
really feel. Power, in his study of support to very elderly people
living in residential homes, showed how easy it is to be misled by
appearances. Professionals in homes might see elderly people sitting
passively and apparently apathetically; but when they were interviewed it was found that 'nothing could be further from the truth
. . . although they were still able to find an edge to life, group
living, in near total care, presented a major challenge to their
continued sense of worth and identity'.[172] When attempts are made
to measure quality of life by asking the elderly themselves directly
there is no agreement among researchers about how this should be
done. In some cases direct questions, albeit open-ended ones, are
put but others prefer a less structured biographical approach.
Certainly there are some aspects of life which do not always come
out clearly in a questionnaire yet do so in the latter approach. No
one who reads Ronald Blythe's *View in Winter* can fail to be moved
by his chapter on prayer and the importance of a spiritual life to
many elderly people.[173] Would this have come out in a general
questionnaire so vividly? Ideally each approach contributes a
different dimension to measuring quality of life so that the two can
be interleaved.

What is strikingly apparent in all recent studies is the variety in
the conditions and responses of the elderly which certainly gives the
lie to any attempt to generalise about them. As Brearley has said,
each person's attitudes and life are unique and satisfaction for each
of us is a highly personal experience.[174] Differences between elderly
people of different ages, between men and women and between
social classes are but three examples.

Of growing interest – and concern – is the first of these and in
particular differences between the quality of life of what have been
termed the young elderly and the old elderly. The dividing line
between the two is usually taken as 75. Nearly all of Hunt's data
in *The Elderly at Home* is analysed on this basis and she found that
one of the most interesting aspects of her findings is the extent to
which many of the disadvantages are strongly age-related (*Population Trends*, Spring 1978). More recently Taylor, Ford and Barber

drew up a profile of 11 risk groups.[175] They found that the most disadvantaged risk groups were the very old, those who had recently moved or been discharged from hospital and the divorced or separated. On the other hand some over-75s were doing very well. In Power's study of volunteers in residential homes one fifth of the residents in this age group were still healthy, fully mobile, could look after themselves and seldom felt lonely.[176]

Hunt also made much of the differences between men and women in the quality of life as measured by health and access to services. In most cases women came off worse though one can speculate that some of the disadvantages, such as lower income, were the result of fewer having been in paid employment or employment with equality of pay. This position may improve. But Abrams shows in his second report that there were striking differences between women who lived alone and women who lived with others.[177] Not only were women living alone worse off economically and in their likelihood of having family links but feelings of loneliness, depression and alienation were much more widespread among elderly women living alone than among those who lived with others.

Abrams also considered whether there were differences relevant to the quality of life between social classes. The overall picture that emerged in the life-styles of *very* elderly people from different social classes was that in both indoor and outdoor behaviour 'those from a professional background or managerial background lead more active lives than did those with a manual working class background'.[178] But he found no evidence that as a result 'middle class old people found their lives more satisfying than did working class old people. The replies to the various statements contained in the Life Satisfaction Index showed broadly similar feelings for all four groups about their circumstances'.[179] Where there *were* differences they were in looking back and regretting what they did not do. 'Working class elderly people are more prone than middle class elderly people to look back on a life of frustrated aspirations and disappointed expectations.'[180] Isaacs has also commented on class difference. He said 'what makes elderly people happy has been the opportunity to acquire sufficient culture, the raw material to enable one to enjoy life – like knowledge of gardening, books, the arts. Happiness in old age is class-related. The well-to-do are happy. If you go to people who have an adequate income and adequate health; you will find happiness' (*New Society*, 10.6.82).

Another distinction in quality of life is over those who live alone.

Concern about the quality of life of elderly people living alone is often expressed, but the evidence is mixed. On the one hand common sense suggests that elderly people living alone will have no one to share domestic tasks with and less chance of contacting someone else in an emergency; and Karn's research showed up clearly the problems and dissatisfaction of those living alone.[181] But it is perhaps salutary to remember that Abrams found, when he asked his sample of elderly people about satisfaction with particular aspects of their lives (e.g. health, financial position, income), that on all these matters those living alone were consistently more satisfied than those living with others. And, in a follow-up study of his sample, he noted that more of those living alone had survived.[182] Power too found that those living alone were healthier than those living with children (this could of course be that the least healthy go to live with their children).[183] He also observed that the higher rates of acute loneliness were to found amongst those in the late 80s living with their children – a finding similar to Abrams.

The three dominant themes in all recent studies are the importance to elderly people of social relationships, health and income.[184] Although fears are often expressed about other aspects of life it is salutary to remember these three. Some aspects of elderly people's lives assume much more publicity at certain times. To take one example, the government noted in *Ageing in the United Kingdom* 'the stress caused by such crimes as burglary and vandalism can have severe effects on the health and well-being of elderly people. Although evidence suggests that elderly people are not the main victims, the Government is concerned that many of them are alarmed by the increasing number of violent crimes'.[185] In fact, the *GHS 1980* showed that the burglary rate is less for elderly people than for the population as a whole[186] and *The British Crime Survey* showed that elderly people were the least likely to be victims of violent crime.[187] Nevertheless, fear of crime has to be taken into account too. Age Concern and the National Westminster Bank's 'Action against Crime' campaign was a direct result of anxieties expressed by elderly people.[188]

Implications for professionals

One of the most encouraging developments concerned with the care of elderly people who need help is a growing awareness of their needs by the professionals. Part of this is an increase in a multi-disciplinary approach (already evident in books such as Hobman's

Impact of Ageing[189]) and part is an attempt by professionals to define what it is they are trying to do. For example, Rowlings considers that three aspects of social work have a particular contribution to make.[190] These are the management of care systems in the community, life in residential establishments and caring for the carers. There seems to be more awareness in the medical press too of the positive contribution which professionals can make to the lives of elderly people.

And yet evidence continues to be produced about poor standards and a lack of understanding of the needs of elderly people. One of the most consistent themes running through the conclusions of recently completed research for DHSS has been the importance of attitudes of staff. Studies such as *Risk and Ageing* by Brearley, Jennings, Jeffreys and Pritchard[191] and Norman's *Rights and Risk*[192] have proved a useful focus for such issues. In the latter, Norman argues that what is needed above all is for a shift in underlying attitudes 'away from a patronising and paternalistic over-protection from risk and towards acknowledgement of their right to as much self-determination as is possible for each individual within the limits of the resources available'.[193] She asks, 'should old people be allowed to live in squalor or danger if they refuse help? Should residential homes and longstay hospitals protect old people from physical risk at the cost of depriving them of independence? How can old people prevent medical treatment from being forced upon them?'[194].

The issues of rights and risk seem most acute in residential settings and as Clough remarks, 'the more services staff provide, or the more they do for residents, the more power they have over their lives'.[195] It is a problem not only in institutions specifically for old people, such as geriatric hospitals but for acute hospitals too, since an increasing proportion of elderly patients are using beds in the acute sector.[196] This leads on to another point, that while professionals may not consciously opt for working with the elderly (e.g. medical students who declare adamantly that they wish to work with other age groups), most of them will do so. For example, 40 per cent of acute beds are occupied by elderly people at any one time, and elderly people occupy nearly half NHS beds in hospitals.[197] Livesley started a perceptive article in *The Health Services* (28.5.82) 'Like Peter Pan, British medicine wishes to stay with the young, dreaming of transplanting this and pioneering that – while avoiding the *real* health-care needs of our ageing population'. And Grimley Evans, discussing the case for absorbing geriatric medicine as a speciality into general medicine asks, in view of demographic trends, whether there is a future for general medicine that is not geriatric.[198]

Some would argue that a fundamental shift in society is needed for elderly people to have more rights and to be taken more seriously by professionals. Townsend argues that the dependency of the elderly is being manufactured socially. The major influences he believes are the imposition, and acceptance, of earlier retirement; the legitimation of low income; the denial of rights to self-determination in institutions; and the construction of community services for recipients assumed to be predominantly passive (*Ageing and Society*, March 1981). Wilding is more radical and suggests in *Professional Power and Social Welfare* that the professions trample on people's rights, help some but disable others, have been guilty of serious failures of responsibilities and are an example of power without accountability.[199]

The dilemma of those who write about elderly people is acute. On the one hand there is need to describe their social problems and try to activate society's conscience. There is no room for complacency while the problems of dementia, unreported health needs, poor housing, the burden on carers and the unattractiveness of elderly people to many professionals are still prevalent. On the other hand, as Midwinter had said, 'we are as urgently yelling "ghettoism" at those who try to shepherd the elderly into a corral separate from the rest of humanity'.[200] Hobman agrees that it is fashionable to argue that if elderly people are to be treated as first-class citizens, there should be no form of discrimination which sets them apart from the rest of society in any way. But he cites (*Community Care*, 10.12.81) examples from commerce, travel, education, health care, technology and access to show how positive discrimination would increase the options open to elderly people. By helping them to shop, to travel, to learn to keep fit and to function their need for care is reduced and their capacity for pleasure increased.

After all the discussion on research and the views of others perhaps the last word is best left to Mary Stott. In a passionately written book as she entered her eighth decade, *Ageing for Beginners*, she declared that ageing is not a 'condition' to be treated by doctors or social workers but a process that brings with it possibilities of new experience and achievement.[201] Her book is full of such examples. The next few years will bring problems, there is no doubt about that, but the most encouraging thing is that elderly people are more and more taking an active role in saying what sort of society *they* want. Long may it continue.

REFERENCES

1. DHSS, *Growing Older*, Cmnd 8173, HMSO, 1981.
2. DHSS, *Ageing in the United Kingdom*, DHSS, 1982.
3. DHSS, *Growing Older*, *op. cit.*, p. 6.
4. DHSS, *Elderly People in the Community: their service needs. Research contributions to the development of policy and practice*, HMSO, 1983.
5. OPCS, *General Household Survey, 1980*, HMSO, 1982.
6. SOCIAL SECURITY ADVISORY COMMITTEE, *First report of the Social Security Advisory Committee, 1981*, HMSO, 1982, p. 2.
7. CSO, *Social Trends* (No. 13), see Ch. 2, note 12, p. 69.
8. SOCIAL SECURITY ADVISORY COMMITTEE, *op. cit.*, pp. 41–2.
9. *Ibid.* p. 20.
10. HOUSE OF COMMONS, *Third Report from the Social Services Committee, Session 1981–82, Age of Retirement*, HMSO, 1982, p. LXXXI.
11. RITCHIE, J. and BARROWCLOUGH, R., *Paying for Equalisation*, EOC, 1983.
12. PARKER, S., *Work and Retirement*, Allen and Unwin, 1982, p. 177.
13. FOGARTY, M., *Retirement Age and Retirement Costs*, Policy Studies Institute, 1980.
14. OPCS, *GHS, 1981*, HMSO, 1983, p. 90.
15. JOLLY, J., CREIGH, S. and MINGAY, A., *Age as a Factor in Employment*, Department of Employment, 1980, p. 8.
16. PHILLIPSON, C., *Capitalism and the Construction of Old Age*, Macmillan, 1982, p. 167.
17. DHSS, *Care in Action*, HMSO, 1981.
18. *Ibid.*, p. 20.
19. *Ibid.*, p. 32.
20. DHSS, *Public Expenditure on the Social Services. Reply by the Government to the Second Report from the Select Committee on Social Services, Session 1981–82*, Cmnd 8775, HMSO, 1982.
21. DHSS, *Report of a Study on Community Care*, DHSS, 1981.
22. *Ibid.*, p. 3.
23. *Ibid.*, p. 5.
24. DHSS, *The respective roles of the general acute and geriatric sectors in the care of the elderly hospital patient*, DHSS, 1981.
25. DHSS, *Report of a study of the acute hospital sector*, DHSS, 1981.
26. DHSS, *Growing Older*, *op. cit.*, p. 43.
27. DHSS, *Care in the Community*, DHSS, 1981.

28. DHSS, *Explanatory Notes on Care in the Community*, DHSS, 1983, p. 1.
29. DHSS, *Care in the Community*, *op. cit.*, pp. 2–3.
30. DHSS, *Health Care and its Costs*, HMSO, p. 25.
31. DHSS, *Care in the Community*, *op. cit.*, p. 5.
32. DHSS and WO, *Health Services Costings Returns, Year ended 31.3.82*, NHS, 1983, p. 7.
33. DHSS, *Health and its Costs*, *op. cit.*, p. 17.
34. TOWNSEND, P. and DAVIDSON, N., *Inequalities in Health*, Penguin, 1982.
35. OPCS, *GHS, 1980*, *op. cit.*, p. 172.
36. HEALTH ADVISORY SERVICE, *The Rising Tide*. Developing Services for mental illness in old age, NHS, Health Advisory Service, 1982, p. 1.
37. *Ibid.*, p. 44.
38. NORMAN, A., *Mental Illness in Old Age: Meeting the Challenge*, CPA, 1982.
39. DHSS, *Elderly People in the Community*, *op. cit.*, paper by ALLEN, I.
40. DHSS, *Elderly People in the Community*, *op. cit.*, paper by BERGMANN, K. and JACOBY, R.
41. TAYLOR, H., *The Hospice Movement in Britain: Its role and its future*, CPA, 1983.
42. BOWLING, A., and CARTWRIGHT, A., *Life after a Death: A Study of the Elderly Widowed*, Tavistock, 1982.
43. DHSS, *Ageing in the United Kingdom*, *op. cit.*, p. 11.
44. ARIE, T., *Health Care of the Elderly*, Croom Helm, 1981, pp. 12–13.
45. SIMPSON, R., *Access to Primary Care*, Royal Commission on the NHS, Research Paper No. 6, HMSO, 1979, p. 56.
46. PRIMARY HEALTH CARE STUDY GROUP, *Primary Health Care in Inner London*, London Health Planning Consortium, 1981.
47. SNOW, T., *Services for old age: A growing crisis in London*, Age Concern, 1981.
48. DAVIES, L., *Three Score Years . . . . and then?*, Heinemann, 1981.
49. DOE, *English House Condition Survey*, 1981, Part 1, Report of the Physical Condition Survey, HMSO, 1982.
50. CSO, *Social Trends* (No. 13), see Ch. 2, note 12, p. 112.
51. GREVE, J., BUTLER, A., and OLDMAN, C., *Sheltered Housing for the Elderly*, report on study, Volumes 1, 2 and 3, Department of Social Policy and Administration, University of Leeds, 1981.

52. BUTLER, A., OLDMAN, C. and GREVE, J., *Sheltered Housing for the Elderly: Policy, Practice and the Consumer*, Allen and Unwin, 1983.
53. SCOTTISH OFFICE, *Sheltered Housing in Scotland*, Central Research Unit, Scottish Office, 1982.
54. BUTLER *et al, op. cit.*, Chapter 9.
55. BUTLER, A. and TINKER, A., Housing Alternatives for the Elderly, University of Leeds, 1983.
56. DHSS, *Elderly People in the Community, op. cit.*, paper by BUTLER, A.
57. TINKER, A., *Housing the Elderly in the Community*, forthcoming.
58. FLEISS, A., *Housing initiatives for the Elderly in the Private Sector*, forthcoming.
59. MORTON, J., *Ferndale: a caring repair service for elderly home owners*, Shelter, Help the Aged, 1982.
60. PRESCOTT-CLARKE, P., *Organising House Adaptations for Disabled People*, HMSO, 1982.
61. DRAKE, M., O'BRIEN, M. and BIEBUYCK, T., *Single and Homeless*, HMSO, 1982, p. 20.
62. DUNCAN, S., DOWNEY, P., and FINCH, H., *A Home of their Own*, DOE, 1983, p. 75.
63. *Ibid.*, p. 64.
64. RITCHIE, J. and MATTHEWS, A., *Take up of Rent Allowances: an in depth study*, Social and Community Planning Research, 1982, p. 75.
65. DHSS, *Community Care, op. cit.*, p. 27.
66. CSO, *Social Trends*, (No. 13), see Ch. 2, note 12, p. 108.
67. CHANCELLOR OF THE EXCHEQUER, *The Government's Expenditure Plans 1983–84, 1985–86*, Cmnd 8789, HMSO, 1983, p. 13.
68. ASSOCIATION OF DIRECTORS OF SOCIAL SERVICES (ADSS), *Fourth Survey of Personal Social Services Expenditure, Staffing and Activities*, ADSS, 1983.
69. HOUSE OF COMMONS, *Second Report from the Social Services Committee, Session 1981–82, 1982 White Paper: Public Expenditure on the Social Services*, Volume 1, Report, HMSO, 1982, pp. XLIV–XLV.
70. DAVIES, B., 'Strategic goals and piecemeal innovations: adjusting to the new balance of needs and resources', in GOLDBERG E. M. and HATCH, S., *A New Look at the Personal Social Services*, Policy Studies Institute, 1981.
71. DHSS, *Care in Action, op. cit.*, p. 19.

72. HOUSE OF COMMONS, *Second Report from the Social Services Committee, session 1981–82, 1982 White Paper: Public Expenditure on the Social Services*, Volume II, 12.7.82, HMSO, p. 226.

73. DHSS, *Public Expenditure on the Social Services*, Cmnd 8775, HMSO, 1982, p. 17.

74. GOLDBERG, E. M. and CONNELLY, N., *The Effectiveness of Social Care for the Elderly*, Heinemenn, 1982.

75. NATIONAL INSTITUTE FOR SOCIAL WORK, *Social Workers: Their Role and Tasks*, (Barclay Report), Bedford Square Press, 1982.

76. *Ibid.*, p. 47.

77. ROWLINGS, C., *Social Work with Elderly People*, Allen and Unwin, 1981.

78. MARSHALL, M., *Social Work with Old People*, Macmillan, 1983.

79. Royal Association for Disability and Rehabilitation (RADAR), *Code of Practice on the provision of services by social services departments under Section 2 of the Chronically Sick and Disabled Persons Act*, 1970, RADAR, 1983.

80. BRISTOW, A., *The Housing and Care Needs of Disabled People and Their Families*, Crossroads, 1981.

81. CPA, *Out of sight – Out of mind*, CPA, 1982, p. 43.

82. BHALLA, A. and BLAKEMORE, K., *Elders of the Minority Ethnic Groups*, All Faiths for One Race, Birmingham, 1981.

83. BARKER, J., *Black and Asian Old People in Britain*, Age Concern, 1983.

84. DHSS, Personal Social Services, Local Authority Statistics, AF80/1, *Home Help Service 1979–80, England*, DHSS, 1980.

85. HEDLEY, R. and NORMAN, A., *Home Help: key issues in service provision*, CPA, 1982, p. 11.

86. *Ibid.*, p. 32.

87. JUDGE, K., FERLIE, E. and SMITH, J., *Charging for the Home Help Service*, Policy Studies Institute, 1982, p. 2.

88. DHSS, Personal Social Services, Local Authority Statistics, AF/81/18, *Personal Social Services, year ending 31.3.81, England*, DHSS, 1981.

89. JOHNSON, M., with DI GREGORIO, S. and HARRISON, B., *Ageing, Needs and Nutrition*, Policy Studies Institute, 1981.

90. *Ibid.*, p. 134.

91. CARTER, J., *Day Services for Adults: somewhere to go*, Allen and Unwin, 1981.

92. GOLDBERG and CONNELLY, *op. cit.*, Ch. 7.
93. DHSS, Personal Social Services, Local Authority Statistics, AF/82/18, *Domiciliary Services, Meals and Adaptations, year ending 31.3.82*, DHSS, 1982.
94. THORNTON, P. and MOORE, J., *The Placement of Elderly People in Private Households*, Department of Social Policy and Administration, University of Leeds, 1980.
95. DHSS, Personal Social Services, Local Authority Statistics, RA/81/2, *The Statistics of Residential Accommodation for the Elderly and Physically Handicapped at 31.3.81*, England, DHSS, 1981, p. v.
96. *Ibid.*
97. DHSS, Personal Social Services, Local Authority Statistics, RA/82/1, *Residential Accommodation for the Elderly and for Younger Physically Handicapped People, Local Authority Supported Residents, Year ending* 31.3.82, England, DHSS, 1983, p. v.
98. CIPFA, *Personal Social Services Statistics, 1982–83 Estimates*, CIPFA, 1982.
99. DHSS, RA/81/2, op. cit.
100. *Ibid.*
101. CLARKE, R. and STONE, M., *At Home in a Boarding House*, National Institute for Social Work, 1981.
102. WADE, B. , SAWYER, L. and BELL, J., *Dependency with Dignity – Different Care Provision for the Elderly*, Bedford Square Press, 1983.
103. PEACE, S., KELLAHER, L. and WILLCOCKS, D., *A Balanced Life*, Survey Research Unit, School of Applied Social Studies and Sociology, Polytechnic of North London, 1982.
104. ROWLINGS, *op. cit.*
105. DHSS, RA/81/2, op. cit.
106. ALLEN, I., *Short-Stay Residential Care for the Elderly*, Policy Studies Institute, 1983.
107. DHSS, *Growing Older, op. cit.*, p. 37.
108. EOC, *Who Cares for the Carers?*, EOC, 1982, p. 1.
109. *Ibid.*, p. 1.
110. PARKER, R., 'Tending and Social Policy', in GOLDBERG, E. M., and HATCH, S., *op. cit.*, p. 17.
111. OPCS, *GHS, 1980, op. cit.*, p. 169.
112. EOC, *The Experience of caring for Elderly and Handicapped Dependants*, EOC, 1980.
113. EOC, *Caring for the Elderly and Handicapped: Community Care*

Policies and Women's Lives, EOC, 1982.

114. NISSEL, M. and BONNERJEA, L., *Family Care of the Handi-capped Elderly: who pays?*, Policy Studies Institute, 1982, p. 51.

115. DHSS, *Elderly People in the Community, op. cit.*, paper by ALLEN, I.

116. BOWLING and CARTWRIGHT, *op. cit.*

117. EOC, 1980, *op. cit.*

118. EOC, *Who Cares for the Carers, op. cit.*

119. EOC, *Caring for the Elderly and Handicapped, op. cit.*

120. DHSS, *Elderly People in the Community, op. cit.*, paper by ALLEN, I.

121. EOC, *Caring for the Elderly and Handicapped, op. cit.*, p. 3.

122. EOC, *Who Cares for the Carers, op. cit.*, p. 29.

123. AGATE, J., *Taking care of Old People at Home*, Unwin, 1979.

124. GRAY, J. A., MUIR and MCKENZIE, H., *Take Care of Your Elderly Relative*, Allen and Unwin, 1980.

125. DHSS, *Elderly People in the Community, op. cit.*, paper by ALLEN, I.

126. EOC, *Caring for the Elderly and Handicapped, op. cit.*, p. 33.

127. RAPOPORT, R., and RAPOPORT, R., in RAPOPORT, R., RAPO-PORT, R., and FOGARTY, M., (eds) *Families in Britain*, Routlege and Kegan Paul, 1982, p. 491.

128. WICKS, M., in WALKER, A., (ed) *Community Care*, Blackwell and Robertson, 1982, pp. 97–117.

129. WALKER, A., *Ibid.*, p. 20.

130. BAYLEY, M., in *Ibid.*, p. 195.

131. HOME OFFICE, *The Government and the Voluntary Sector*, Home Office, 1978.

132. HOME OFFICE, *The Government and the Voluntary Sector*, Home Office, 1981.

133. GOLDBERG and CONNELLY, *op. cit.*, pp. 178–79.

134. ABRAMS, P., ABRAMS, S., HUMPHREY, R. and SNAITH, R., *Action for Care: a Review of Good Neighbour Schemes*; The Volunteer Centre, 1981.

135. CLOUGH, R., GIBSON, P. and KELLY, S., *Helping Lively Minds*, University of Bristol, 1983.

136. DAVIES, B., *The cost-effectiveness imperative, the social services and volunteers*, The Volunteer Centre, 1980.

137. OPCS, *GHS, 1980, op. cit.*, p. 174.

138. *Ibid.*, p. 175.

139. DHSS, *Ageing in the United Kingdom, op. cit.*

140. *Ibid.*, p. 1.
141. *Ibid.*, p. 6.
142. OPCS, *General Household Survey, 1981*, *op. cit.*, Ch. 8.
143. *Ibid.*, p. 166.
144. MARSHALL, *op. cit.*
145. CSO, *Social Trends*, (No. 13), see Ch. 2, note 12, p. 87.
146. GOLDBERG and CONNELLY, *op. cit.*, pp. 173–74.
147. ABRAMS, M. and O'BRIEN, J., *Political Attitudes and Ageing in Britain*, Age Concern, 1981.
148. CONSERVATIVE POLITICAL CENTRE (CPC), Contact Brief, *Pensions: the ways ahead*, CPC, 1981, p. 5.
149. ORIEL, W., in HOBMAN, D. (ed); *The Impact of Ageing*, Croom Helm, 1981.
150. PHILLIPSON, *op. cit.*, pp. 124–25.
151. PARKER, S., *op. cit.*, pp. 175–77.
152. HOUSE OF COMMONS, Social Services Committee, session 1979–80, *The Government's White Papers on Public Expenditure; the Social Services*, Volume II, Minutes of Evidence and Appendix, question 61(1), HMSO, 1980.
153. WRIGHT, K., 'The Economics of Community Care' in WALKER, A. (ed), *op. cit.*
154. WRIGHT, K., CAIRNS, J. and SNELL, M., *Costing Care*, University of Sheffield, Joint Unit for Social Services Research, 1981.
155. *Ibid.*, p. 43.
156. DHSS and WO, *Health Services Costings Returns*, *op. cit.*, p. 34.
157. CIPFA, *Social Services Statistics 1981–82 Actuals*, CIPFA, 1982, p. 20.
158. HOUSE OF COMMONS, Report from the Social Services Committee, *The Government's White Papers on Public Expenditure: The Social Services, Volume 1*, Report, 9.7.80, HMSO, 1980.
159. HOUSE OF COMMONS, *Second Report, 1982 White Paper*, *op. cit.*
160. *Ibid.*, p. 228.
161. JOHNSON *et al*, *op. cit.*, p. 127.
162. BEBBINGTON, A. and DAVIES, B., 'Patterns of social service provision for the elderly in WARNES A. (ed), *Geographical Perspectives on the Elderly*, Wiley, 1982.
163. *Ibid.*, p. 373.
164. ALLON-SMITH, 'The evolving geography of the elderly in England and Wales', in WARNES, *op. cit.*, p. 51.

165. BUTLER, OLDMAN and GREVE, *op. cit.*, pp. 189–190.
166. HEDLEY and NORMAN, *op. cit.*, p. 36.
167. JOHNSON *et al.*, *op. cit*, p. 126.
168. GOLDBERG and CONNELLY, *op. cit.*
169. DHSS, *Elderly People in the Community*, *op. cit.* paper by TINKER, A.
170. DHSS, *On the State of the Public Health*, HMSO, 1981, p. 89.
171. DHSS, *Elderly People in the Community*, *op. cit.*, paper by TINKER, A.
172. POWER, M., *Volunteer Support for very elderly people living in residential homes*, Report to DHSS, 1981, p. 2.
173. BLYTHE, R., *The View in Winter*, Allen Lane, 1979.
174. BREARLEY, see Ch. 3, note 29, p. 21.
175. TAYLOR, R., FORD, G. and BARBER, H., *The Elderly at Risk*, Age Concern, 1983.
176. POWER, 1981, *op. cit.*
177. ABRAMS, M., *Beyond Three Score and Ten, Second Report*, Age Concern, 1980.
178. *Ibid.*, p. 29.
179. *Ibid.*, p. 29.
180. *Ibid.*, p. 30.
181. KARN, see Ch. 10, note 67, p. 179.
182. ABRAMS, M. , *People in their late Sixties: A Longitudinal Survey of Ageing, Part 1., Survivors and Non-Survivors*, Age Concern, 1983.
183. POWER, M., *The use of volunteers in the home care of the very old*, Report to DHSS, 1979, p. 69.
184. DHSS, *Elderly People in the Community*, *op. cit.*, paper by TINKER, A.
185. DHSS, *Ageing in the United Kingdom*, *op. cit.*, p. 11.
186. OPCS, *GHS, 1980*, *op. cit.*, p. 80.
187. HOME OFFICE, *The British Crime Survey*, HMSO, 1983.
188. AGE CONCERN AND NATIONAL WESTMINSTER BANK, *Crime against the elderly campaign report*, Age Concern, 1982.
189. HOBMAN, *op. cit.*, p. 165.
190. ROWLINGS, *op. cit.*
191. BREARLEY, C. P., JENNINGS, R., JEFFREYS, P. and PRITCHARD, S., *Risk and Ageing*, Routledge and Kegan Paul, 1982.
192. NORMAN, A., *Rights and Risk*, NCCOP, 1980.
193. *Ibid.*, p. 8.
194. *Ibid.*, back cover.

195. CLOUGH, R., *Old Age Homes*, Allen and Unwin, 1981, p. 162.
196. DHSS, *The respective roles of the general acute and geriatric sectors in the care of the elderly hospital patient, op. cit.*, p. 20.
197. DHSS, *Ageing in the United Kingdom, op. cit.*, p. 15.
198. EVANS, J. GRIMLEY 'Institutional Care' in ARIE, T. (ed.), op. cit.
199. WILDING, P., *Professional Power and Social Welfare*, Routledge and Kegan Paul, 1982.
200. MIDWINTER, E., *Ten Million People*, CPA, 1983.
201. STOTT, M., *Ageing for Beginners*, Blackwell, 1981.

Part four
DOCUMENTS

Document one
THE NEW ELDERLY

Dr Mark Abrams discusses important demographic trends relating to the elderly:

So far and currently, society has the relatively easy task of providing support and care for a population of elderly people who for the most part are comparatively young, mobile, and healthy. From now on the balance of concern will have to shift in favour of the very old, the immobile and the frail.

He goes on to say why he thinks the focus will change in the future:

Since the 1960s the fortunes of the teenager have been the focus of discussion and research by those interested in age-stratification. He has had his day; from now on the centre of the stage is likely to be occupied by the growing millions who will live well beyond the traditional allotment of three score years and ten.

From: Abrams, M., 'The new elderly', *New Society*, 26.6.75, p. 778.

Document two
MYTHS AND REALITIES OF AGEING

The Director of Age Concern describes some images of ageing:

The ageing process is deeply enshrined in a range of images leading to stereotypes based on notions of intense wisdom and even God-like proportions at one end of the spectrum, to uselessness and semi-idiocy at the other.

None of these extremes serve the elderly well. They are no more universally wise or nice or kind than they are stupid, but there are a range of half truths and fantasies about age, knowledge and experience which have become enshrined in the folk culture of ageing. Some of them stem from the professionals who practise in care. They also have their root in art and literature.

Perhaps the most important perception to be missing is that of the elderly themselves: People like a 60-year-old woman who wrote about her feelings on having reached the statutory retirement age. She said: 'Pensioners are being got at. We must prepare to do battle to maintain our independence and preserve our attractive personalities . . . now I am haunted by the fear that if I cannot dispel the assumption that I am a senior citizen, the following events may reasonably occur. (1) I shall have a gang of young thugs sent to my home to paint my kitchen instead of going to prison; (2) I shall have patients from the local mental hospital drafted to dig my garden; (3) I may be forced to go to suitable entertainments, drink tea and wear a paper hat; (4) I may receive vast boxes of assorted food to which I feel I am not entitled. We pensioners are in a terrifying position. We are *recipients* . . . hands off, please. I am in charge of my life.'

This person recognises, but does not accept, one widely held image of ageing full of assumptions and value judgements with its underlying theme of patronising attitudes, setting the elderly as a race apart to be pitied as people who are no longer capable of managing their own lives. It assumes that ageing is synonymous with a changing personality and that the retired adopt common characteristics with an incompetent level of social functioning. It also implies limited intellectual thresholds devoid of critical faculties.

Not only does this image suggest the old are incapable of exercising informed or rational choice and of maintaining a degree of control over their circumstances; but it also implies that they do not have sufficient resources to meet their own needs for recreation, or welfare when, in fact, the young retired now represent a very important resource which could well make a substantial contribution to the health and social well-being of the community as a whole.

From: Hobman, D., 'Myths and realities of ageing', *Social Work Today*, 3.1.78, p. 18.

Dr Alex Comfort argues that the concept of ageism is part of the prejudice against the elderly:

AGEISM is the notion that people cease to be people, cease to be the same people or become people of a distinct and inferior kind, by virtue of having lived a specified number of years. The eighteenth-century French naturalist Georges Buffon said, 'to the philosopher, old age must be considered a prejudice'. Ageism is that prejudice. Like racism, which it resembles, it is based on fear, folklore and the hang-ups of a few unlovable people who propagate these. Like racism, it needs to be met by information, contradiction and, when necessary, confrontation. And the people who are being victimised have to stand up for themselves in order to put it down.

From: Comfort, A., *A Good Age*, Mitchell Beazley, 1977, p. 35.

Document four
SEX AND AGE STRUCTURE OF THE POPULATION

The OPCS give census, estimated and projected numbers from 1901 to 2001.

Table 1.2 Sex and age structure of the population of the United Kingdom

Millions

	0–4	5–15	16–29	30–44	45–59	60–64	65–74	75–84	85+	All ages
Males										
Census enumerated										
1901	2.2	4.4	4.8	3.6	2.2	0.5	0.6		0.2	18.5
1911	2.3	4.6	5.0	4.3	2.7	0.6	0.7		0.2	20.4
1921	2.0	4.6	4.9	4.3	3.4	0.7	0.9		0.3	21.0
1931	1.8	4.2	5.4	4.5	3.8	0.9	1.1		0.4	22.1
Mid-year estimates										
1941	1.7	3.8	5.4	5.5	3.9	1.1	1.4		0.5	23.3
1951	2.2	3.9	4.9	5.5	4.5	1.1	1.6		0.7	24.4
1961	2.2	4.5	4.9	5.3	5.1	1.2	1.6	0.7	0.1	25.7
1971	2.3	5.0	5.6	4.9	5.0	1.5	2.0	0.7	0.1	27.1
1976	1.9	5.1	5.8	5.0	4.8	1.5	2.2	0.8	0.1	27.3
1980	1.8	4.8	6.0	5.4	4.8	1.3	2.2	0.9	0.1	27.3
1981[1]	1.8	4.7	6.0	5.5	4.8	1.4	2.3	0.9	0.1	27.4
Projections[2]										
1986	2.1	4.1	6.4	5.7	4.5	1.4	2.1	1.0	0.2	27.0
1991	2.3	4.1	6.2	6.0	4.6	1.3	2.2	1.0	0.2	28.0
1996	2.3	4.7	5.6	6.2	5.0	1.3	2.1	1.0	0.2	28.4
2001	2.1	4.9	5.3	6.5	5.2	1.3	2.0	1.0	0.2	28.6
Females										
Census enumerated										
1901	2.2	4.4	5.2	3.9	2.4	0.6	0.7	0.3		19.7
1911	2.2	4.6	5.4	4.6	2.9	0.6	0.9	0.4		21.7

Table 1.2 (cont'd)

Millions

	0–4	5–15	16–29	30–44	45–59	60–64	65–74	75–84	85+	All ages
Females										
1921	1.9	4.6	5.5	5.0	3.6	0.8	1.1	0.5		23.0
1931	1.7	4.2	5.7	5.2	4.2	1.0	1.4	0.6		24.0
Mid-year estimates										
1941	1.7	3.7	5.4	5.8	4.6	1.3	1.7	0.8		25.0
1951	2.1	3.8	4.9	5.7	5.1	1.4	2.1	1.1		26.1
1961	2.1	4.3	4.8	5.3	5.5	1.5	2.4	1.2	0.2	27.3
1971	2.2	4.7	5.4	4.8	5.2	1.7	2.7	1.4	0.4	28.6
1976	1.8	4.9	5.6	4.9	5.0	1.7	2.9	1.6	0.4	28.7
1980	1.7	4.6	5.7	5.3	4.9	1.5	2.9	1.7	0.4	28.7
1981[1]	1.7	4.4	5.8	5.4	4.9	1.6	2.9	1.7	0.5	28.9
Projections[2]										
1986	1.9	3.9	6.1	5.6	4.6	1.6	2.8	1.8	0.5	28.9
1991	2.2	3.9	5.9	5.9	4.7	1.5	2.7	1.8	0.6	29.2
1996	2.1	4.4	5.3	6.1	5.1	1.4	2.7	1.8	0.6	29.6
2001	2.0	4.7	5.0	6.4	5.4	1.4	2.5	1.8	0.6	29.7

[1] Great Britain figures for 1981 are on the new census base and definition of population, they include residents absent from Great Britain and exclude overseas visitors. The reverse was the case in earlier years. Northern Ireland figures included are 1980 mid-year estimates.

[2] Projections based on mid-1979 estimates of total population

From: CSO, *Social Trends* (No. 13), 1983, Table 1.2, p. 12.

Document five
THE DEMANDS WHICH DIFFERENT AGE GROUPS MAKE ON HEALTH AND PERSONAL SOCIAL SERVICES

Elderly people make higher demands on health and personal social services which increase with age.

Table 8.24. Estimated current expenditure per head on health and personal social services, 1975–76

| | *Great Britain* | | | *£ per head* |
	Hospital and community health	*Family practitioner services*	*Personal social services*	*Total expenditure per head*
All births★	455	30	10	495
Persons aged:				
0– 4	85	20	20	125
5–15	30	15	25	70
16–64	45	20	5	70
65–74	150	25	25	200
75+	350	50	125	525
All ages	75	20	20	115

★ Cost per delivery, including pre- and post-natal care; this is excluded from the costs by age group.
From: CSO, *Social Trends* (No. 9), 1979, Table 8.24, p. 143.

Estimated average hospital and community health current expenditure per head of population in 1980–81, and by age group.

| | | *England* | | | *£ per head* | | |
	Total Population	Births	0–4	5–15	16–64	65–74	75+
Expenditure per head	160	855	155	65	85	310	765

From: DHSS, *Health Care and its Costs*, HMSO, 1983 p. 11.

Document six
BRITAIN'S CHANGING AGE STRUCTURE 1931–2011

The balance between those who are primarily producers of resources and those who are primarily consumers is now more unfavourable than at any time since the early 1930s. But in the foreseeable future – to the turn of the century and beyond – the balance will improve.

The demographically determined dependency ratio (Figure 2b) has a similar shape to that of the index of ageing because, at least over the past forty or so years both curves have been dominated by the growth in the numbers of elderly people. This Figure shows that while in 1931 there were only 51 people under 15 or over retirement age for every 100 people in the so called working age-groups, by 1974 every 100 workers had to support 68 dependants. However, because the recent sharp decline in fertility more than

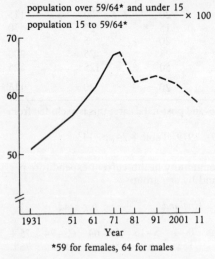

$$\frac{\text{population over } 59/64^* \text{ and under } 15}{\text{population } 15 \text{ to } 59/64^*} \times 100$$

Year

*59 for females, 64 for males

Fig. 2b Demographic dependency ratio, Great Britain

270

compensates for the further increase over the next few years in the number and proportion of elderly people in the population the dependency ratio will fall quite sharply during the remaining years of this decade and into the early 1980s. Thereafter it will increase slightly but remain fairly stable at a rate below the present level until the turn of the century when it will fall again.

From. Davis, N., 'Britain's changing age structure 1931–2011', OPCS *Population Trends* (No. 3), Spring 1976, p. 15.

GROWING INTEREST IN THE PROBLEMS OF OLD AGE

Two researchers comment on the lack of interest in the elderly in the first half of the twentieth century and a resurgence from the late 1940s.

Between 1901 and 1947 the numbers of persons in Britain who were aged 65 and over grew from under two to five millions. Yet in that period very little information on the problems of the aged living at home or receiving treatment and care in hospitals and other institutions was published. It is an extraordinary fact. At the turn of the century there had been a few studies on pensions and the effect of the Poor Law, three of them by Charles Booth.[1] In 1909 the reports of the Majority and Minority of the Royal Commission on the Poor Laws appeared, and they both contained sections on the aged.[2] In later years there were short passages on the problems of old age in various reports of general surveys.[3] Otherwise there was a dearth of published information and, apparently, of interest too.

Suddenly, in the late forties and fifties, or so it may seem to the historian of the written and spoken word, the problems of old age were discovered. The Nuffield Foundation pioneered the financing of a few studies, including the remarkable work of J. H. Sheldon.[4] The trickle of carefully documented studies became a modest stream, slightly preceding the floodwaters of interest and research in the subject which were released in the United States in the mid-1950s. Among some of the influential studies in Britain have been those of Dr Alex Comfort on the biology of senescence,[5] Dr Alan Welford and his colleagues on psychological adjustment in old age,[6] and Mr F. Le Gros Clark on ageing in industry.[7] There have been many sociological socio-medical and socio-economic surveys which have been based on interviews with samples of the elderly population.[8]

1. BOOTH, C., *Pauperism: A Picture; and the Endowment of Old Age: An Argument*, London, Macmillan, 1892; *The Aged Poor: Condition*, London, Macmillan, 1894; and *Old Age Pensions and the Aged Poor*, London, Macmillan, 1899.
2. *Report of the Royal Commission on the Poor Laws*, Cmnd 4499, London, HMSO, 1909.

3. See, for example, CARADOG-JONES, D., *The Social Survey of Merseyside*, London, Hodder & Stoughton, 1934; ROWNTREE, B. S., *Poverty and Progress*, London, Longmans, 1941.
4. SHELDON, J. H., *The Social Medicine of Old Age*, Oxford University Press for the Nuffield Foundation, 1948.
5. COMFORT, A., *Ageing: The Biology of Senescence*, London, Routledge & Kegan Paul (revised edition), 1964.
6. WELFORD, A, T., *Ageing and Human Skill*, London, Oxford University Press for the Nuffield Foundation, 1958.
7. For example, LE GROS CLARK, F. and DUNNE, A. C., *Ageing in Industry*, London, The Nuffield Foundation, 1955.
8. A selected list is given in Appendix I for readers who may wish to learn more about old people in particular localities or regions.

From: Townsend, P. and Wedderburn, D., *The Aged in the Welfare State*, G. Bell & Sons, p. 10.

Document eight
TERMS OF REFERENCE OF THE ROWNTREE COMMITTEE

One of the first large-scale social surveys was undertaken in 1944–46 for the Rowntree Committee on the problems of ageing and the care of old people. The terms of reference of the Rowntree Committee, which was appointed by the Nuffield Foundation, were:

TERMS OF REFERENCE
1. The terms of reference under which the Survey Committee were appointed by the trustees of the Nuffield Foundation were:

'To gather as complete information as possible with regard to (i) the various problems – individual, social, and medical – associated with ageing and old age; (ii) the work being done by public authorities and voluntary organisations, and the public and private resources that exist, for the care and comfort of old people in Great Britain; (iii) the provision made for old people in those countries that have given special thought to this matter; (iv) medical research on the causes and results of ageing; and (v) the lines on which action might usefully be taken in the future by public authorities and private organisations, including the Foundation.'

From: Rowntree, B., *Old People. Report of a Survey Committee on the Problems of Ageing and the Care of Old People*, The Nuffield Foundation, Oxford University Press, 1947, p. 1.

A selected list of social surveys 1945–64 was given by Professor P. Townsend and Professor D. Wedderburn.

Social surveys of old people 1945-64 (selected list)

Date of Survey	Area	Numbers interviewed	References
1945-46 (?)	Lutterworth, Midhurst, Mid-Rhondda, Wolverhampton, Oldham, Wandsworth and St Pancras	2,302 people of pensionable age	Nuffield Foundation, Survey Committee on the Problems of Ageing and the Care of Old People (1947), *Old People*, London, Oxford University Press
1945-47	Wolverhampton	477 people of pensionable age	Sheldon, J. H. (1948), *The Social Medicine of Old Age; Report of an Inquiry in Wolverhampton*, London, Oxford University Press
1948	Sheffield	1,596 people of pensionable age	Greenlees, A. and Adams, J. (1950), *Old People in Sheffield*, Sheffield
1948	Birmingham	2,230 people over 70	Shenfield, B. E. (1957), *Social Policies for Old Age*, London
1949-50	Plymouth	Chiefly 80 housebound on list of 350 kept by home help service	Plymouth Council of Social Service (1950), *Housebound*, Plymouth

Date of Survey	Area	Numbers interviewed	References
1949–51	Sheffield	476 living alone or with spouse (mainly health but also social)	Hobson, W. and Pemberton, J. (1955), *The Health of the Elderly at Home*, London; see also Bransby, E. R. and Osborne, B. (1953), *British Journal of Nutrition*, 7, 160. Osborne, B. (1951), *The Nutrition of Older People* (unpublished report of a government social survey)
1950	Northern Ireland	759 people aged 60 and over	Adams, C. F. and Cheeseman, E. A. (1951), *Old People in Northern Ireland. A Report to the Northern Ireland Hospitals Authority*, Belfast
1950	Great Britain	1,950 men and 482 women aged 55–74	Thomas, G. and Osborne, B. (1950), *Older People and Their Employment* (Social survey for Ministry of Labour and National Services. Report No. 150/1 – and unpublished). Summarised by Moss, L. (1955), A sample survey of older people and their employment in Great Britain in 1950. In: *Old Age in the Modern World* (Report of the Third Congress of the International Association of Gerontology, London, 1954), Edinburgh, Livingstone, p. 353

Date of Survey	Area	Numbers interviewed	References
1951	Lewisham and Camberwell	1,082 households with at least one person over 65 being helped by domestic help and/or district nursing service	Chalke, H. D. and Benjamin, B. (1953), *Lancet*, 1, 588
1951–52	Liverpool	500 people of pensionable age in 5 selected districts	Liverpool Personal Service Society and Liverpool University, Department of Social Science (1953), *Social Contacts in Old Age*, Liverpool
1953	Hammersmith	100 people over 70 living alone	Sir Halley Stewart Trust and National Old People's Welfare Committee (1954), *Over Seventy*, National Council of Social Service, London
1954	Edinburgh	2,768 people aged 60 and over	Gordon, C., Thompson, J. G. and Emerson, A. R. (1957), *Medical Officer*, 98, 19
1954	Great Britain	120,000 people receiving assistance aged 80 years and over and living alone	Great Britain, National Assistance Board (1955), *Report for the year ended 31 December, 1954*, London, H.M. Stationery Office
1954–55	Rutherglen	323 men aged 65 and over	Anderson, W. F. and Cowan, N. R. (1955), *Lancet*, 2, 239

Date of Survey	Area	Numbers interviewed	References
1954–55	Bethnal Green	203 people of pensionable age	Townsend, P. (1957), *The Family Life of Old People; an Inquiry in East London*, London, Routledge & Kegan Paul
1955	Aberdeen	244 retired men aged 65–74	Richardson, I. M. (1956), *Scottish Medical Journal*, 1, 381
1955	Nottinghamshire (two areas)	340 people aged 65 and over	Marsh, D. C. (1955), *Elderly People*, Nottingham
1955	Dundee	400 people aged 65 and over	Mair, A., Weir, I. B. L. and Wilson, W. A. (1955), *Public Health (London)*, 70, 97
1956–57	Stockport	2,073 people aged 80 and over	Lempert, S. (1958), *Report on the Survey of the Aged in Stockport*, Stockport, County Borough of Stockport
1957	Anglesey	160 persons aged 65 and over	Wynne Griffith, G., *The Needs of Old People in Rural Areas* (Paper read to the Royal Society of Health Congress, Eastbourne, 1958), *Journal of the Royal Society for the Promotion of Health*, July/August 1958

Date of Survey	Area	Numbers interviewed	References
1957	Orkney	233 people of pensionable age	Richardson, I. M., Brodie, A. S. and Wilson, S. (1959), 'Social and Medical Needs of Old People in Orkney: Report of a Social Survey', *Health Bulletin, Scotland*, Vol. 17, No. 4
1957	Woodford	210 persons of pensionable age	Willmott, P. and Young, M. (1960), *Family and Class in a London Suburb*, London, Routledge & Kegan Paul
1958–60	Aberdeen	474 people aged 60 and over	Richardson, I. M. (1964), *Age and Need*, E. and S. Livingstone, Edinburgh
1958	Great Britain	853 people receiving meals in areas with a meals service; 1,317 people of pensionable age living in private households	Harris, A. I., *Meals on Wheels for Old People: A Report of an Inquiry by the Government Social Survey*, London, The National Corporation for the Care of Old People, 1960
1958–59	Rural area in Shropshire	328 people of pensionable age	Miller, M. C. (1963), *The Ageing Countryman: A Socio-Medical Report on Old Age in a Country Practice*, London, National Corporation for the Care of Old People

Date of Survey	Area	Numbers interviewed	References
1958–60	England and Wales	489 residents of Homes and Institutions who were of pensionable age (other information also about 8,000 persons of pensionable age in a random sample of 173 Homes)	Townsend, P. (1962), *The Last Refuge: A Survey of Residential Institutions and Homes for the Aged in England and Wales*, London, Routledge & Kegan Paul
1959–60	Seven Areas: Salisbury, Leicester, Hexham Rural District, Seaton Valley, Glasgow, Wimbledon and East Ham	1,078 'units' consisting of one person or a married couple of pensionable age	Cole Wedderburn, D. with Utting, J. (1962), *The Economic Circumstances of Old People*, Occasional Papers on Social Administration, No. 4, Welwyn, Herts, The Codicote Press
1960	Lewisham	1,370 people aged 65 and over	Harris, A. I. assisted by Woolf, M., *Health and Welfare of Older People in Lewisham*, The Social Survey, Central Office of Information, June 1962
1960	Swansea	1,962 individuals of all ages, including about 200 aged 65 and over	(Preliminary) Rosser, C. and Harris, C. C. (1961), 'Relationships through Marriage in a Welsh Urban Area', *The Sociological Review*, Vol. 9, No. 3, pp. 293–321

Date of Survey	Area	Numbers interviewed	References
1960–61	Newcastle-upon-Tyne	123 people aged 65 and over in geriatric wards of hospitals and in Residential Homes (together with other information)	Kay, D. W. K., Beamish, P. and Roth, M. (1962), 'Some Medical and Social Characteristics of Elderly People under State Care' in Halmos, P. (ed.), *The Sociological Review*, Monograph, No. 5
1962	Barrow	829 old people living at home (and other information about elderly hospital patients)	Edge, J. R. and Nelson, I. D. M. (1963 and 1964), 'Survey of Arrangements for the Elderly in Barrow-in-Furness. 1 and 2', *Medical Care*, 1964, Vol. 2, No. 1, p. 7.
1962	West Hartlepool	320 people aged 75 and over living alone	Bamlett, R. and Milligan, H. C. (1963), 'Health and Welfare Services and the Over 75's', *The Medical Officer*, CIX, No. 25
1962–63	Edinburgh	200 people aged 65 and over	Williamson, J. *et al.*, 'Old People at Home: Their Unreported Needs' (May 25th, 1964), *The Lancet*

From: Townsend, P. and Wedderburn, D., *The Aged in the Welfare State*, G. Bell and Sons, 1965, App. 1, pp. 140–3.
Details of some major national social surveys of old people published since 1964 have been added by the author.

Some major national social surveys of old people published since 1964 compiled by Anthea Tinker

Date of Survey	Area	Numbers interviewed	Purpose	References
1961–62	A stratified sample of local authorities in Great Britain	4,209 people aged 65 and over	A study to find out how effective social services were in meeting the needs of the aged, to find out whether it was true that certain functions formerly performed by the family had been taken over by the social services and to examine new needs. This is the British part of a cross national survey	Townsend, P. and Wedderburn, D. (1965), The Aged in the Welfare State, G. Bell and Sons
1962–4	Harrow Northampton Oldham S Norfolk	195 people aged 65 and over. This followed an initial screening of 538 people of this age	A study of old people who are isolated. It is concerned with those who live alone, are socially isolated, lonely or have a sense of anomie	Tunstall, J. (1966), Old and Alone, Routledge and Kegan Paul
1962	A stratified sample of local authorities in Great Britain	4,209 people aged 65 and over	A cross national study of old people in Great Britain, Denmark and the United States of America to describe the present capacities of the elderly including their economic and social circumstances	Shanas, E. et al. (1968), Old People in Three Industrial Societies, Routledge and Kegan Paul

283

Date of Survey	Area	Numbers interviewed	Purpose	References
1965–66	Worthing Oakham (RD and UD) Salisbury Holyhead Sheffield Preston Maidenhead Kidderminster Gosport Dundee Coatbridge Buckie	9,866 people over retirement age in their own homes and residential care	The NCCOP sponsored this survey to try to measure need for given services. They had observed that local authority 10 year community care plans showed wide differences in planned provision	Harris, A. (1968), *Social Welfare for the Elderly*, HMSO
1966	A London Borough south of the river	300 people aged 70 and over referred to the welfare department	An attempt to measure the effectiveness of social work by comparing 2 groups of old people half of whom were allocated to trained case workers and half to untrained	Goldberg, E. M. (1970), *Helping the Aged*, Allen and Unwin
1968	Clacton Bexhill	1,000 people aged 55 and over	The main aim was to find out more about the process of retirement to the coast from the point of view of the retired persons themselves	Karn, V. (1977), *Retiring to the Seaside*, Routledge & Kegan Paul

Date of Survey	Area	Numbers interviewed	Purpose	References
1976	Stratified random sample of 90 parliamentary constituencies	2,622 elderly people: 1,354 under 75 and 1,268 75 and over	To investigate the social circumstances of elderly people living in private households in the community. To enable health and social services to be deployed to the best effect and also to provide information which may make it possible to devise new forms of assistance. Comparisons are made between the under 75s and those over 75	Hunt, A. (1978), *The Elderly at Home*, HMSO
1977	Hove Merton Moss Side Northampton	1,646 elderly people: 802 under 75 and 844 75 and over	To discover more about the needs, conditions and resources of elderly people over 75 so that policies may be developed to enable the 75 and overs in the next 2 decades to lead satisfying lives. Comparisons are made between the under 75s and those over 75	Abrams, M. (1978), *Beyond Three Score and Ten*, Age Concern

Document ten
A DEFINITION OF RETIREMENT

Dr Alex Comfort considers the effect of retirement:

RETIREMENT. We can only alter the manipulative cost-accountancy concept of retirement, which kicks people out of society when they can't be milked further, by changing society. On the other hand, from the standpoint of self-defence, retirement has to be met, unless you are wholly self-employed, a housewife, an intellectual of a certain kind or a peasant – these people never retire or don't notice that they have.

Ideally, retirement isn't the occasion for leisure, unless the work you did was incredibly arduous and not even then, for 'leisure', as packaged by golden-age promotions, is Dead Sea fruit; you can read and play shuffle-board just so long. However much he grumbled about the hassle of daily work, the man who without knowing it had all his friends and most of his significance at work usually enjoys about a week of staying at home, although breaking habits and lowering tempo are disorientating even then. If his wife isn't working outside the home he gets under her feet. If he tries to do all the jobs he has put off until retirement he commonly finds that his strength or his heart, if his work was sedentary, protest. A man who had been doing heavy work will quite often go on doing it at home.

Women in the conventional order, who if they worked were in reality expected to hold down two full-time jobs, are in fact protected from some of this because there is no retirement from 'homemaking'. But the more the sex roles come to resemble each other, the more the problems of men and women are becoming similar.

Sad things happen to retirement fantasies – the couple who withdraw to a mountain cottage they'd seen in summer, and find that in winter they get snowed in and there are no food or postal deliveries; or there is simply the fact that when the fantasy home, or trip, comes it's unreal and not a part of living, however tiresome living was. Nest eggs which looked huge when laid may prove good for only a couple of bites after twenty years of inflation. Only two kinds of folk are really happy conventionally retired – those who were always lazy, and those who have waited a lifetime to get around to a consuming, non-fantasy interest for which they have studied, prepared and planned, lacking only the time to do it the way they wanted.

From: Comfort, A., *A Good Age*, Mitchell Beazley, 1977, pp. 181–83.

Document eleven
RESEARCH ON GERONTOLOGY

Professor D. Bromley, a psychologist, gives an overview of research on gerontology:

1. AN OVERVIEW

We have come a long way. We have sampled an extensive scientific literature, finding many causes for dismay, a few for satisfaction and hope. Possibly the most striking aspects of gerontology are the sheer scale of the subject and its fantastic complexity. The notion that gerontology is a *multidisciplinary* study should now be abundantly clear.

There seems to be no escaping the fact that the primary cause of human ageing is to be found in the degenerative physical changes that take place in the body over time;[1] and if biologists uncover the mechanism(s) of ageing within cells or tissues and continue to find preventive or remedial measures, then many, perhaps most, of the concomitant psychological and social changes that have been described will no longer take place. What has been lacking, perhaps, in the social and behavioural sciences is a sustained attempt to test out ideas about the beneficial effects of different kinds of preventive or remedial measures upon longevity, personal adjustment and human performance.

In many ways, the prospects for research on ageing are similar to what they were ten or fifteen years ago.[2,3] The main change has been a remarkable proliferation of research work – so massive and often so technical that no one individual can hope to master more than a small portion of it. The early psychological and biological findings pointed, almost without exception, to serious adverse effects in old age. Attempts to discover the natural advantages and compensations of ageing have yielded little of value. Research findings, fully documented in the scientific literature, provide the evidence for this point of view. Unfortunately much of what we know about the social and psychological aspects of human ageing consists of masses of detailed, low-level, empirical observations, lacking system and explanation. It is not sufficient merely to observe that certain age-changes take place; we need to know *why* they take place. Explanations, however, are not entirely lacking – age-differences in skilled performance are explained in terms of compen-

287

satory reactions to, or effects of, less efficient central and peripheral mechanisms; age-changes in intellectual creativity are explained as inevitable consequences of mental slowing and loss of sustained variation in problem-solving behaviour; age-changes in social adjustment and personality are explained in terms of alterations in the complex pattern of role-relationships binding the individual to society.

The least developed area of human gerontology, possibly, concerns motivation and personality. Everyday experience frequently illustrates the way in which personal qualities, such as patience, confidence, humour and sociability, which give people their distinctiveness, also help to determine the way they cope with the problems of maturity and old age. Personality and adjustment in later life depend to some extent on the individual's conception of himself built up during the years of development and early maturity. People see their lives in terms of periods or phases associated with definite events and circumstances. Today's patterns of adjustment sometimes repeat or are analogous to those of yesterday and establish important continuities in personality and identity. It seems likely that the normal effects of ageing are to delineate the character more sharply, simplify its structure and dynamics, and bring about a kind of ultra-stable relationship between the person and his circumstances. The importance of 'personal dispositions' does not diminish with age; on the contrary, they are likely to play an even more important part during maturity and old age when the person may be under greater stress. However, there is surprisingly little *scientific* evidence relevant to this opinion. The results obtained from the usual methods of assessing personality are not very satisfactory, but this is partly a reflection of the current state of personality-study in psychology. The investigation of age-changes in personal qualities which are *critical* for adjustment and performance is an important future task in the psychological study of ageing.

1. COMFORT, A., *The Process of Ageing*. London, Weidenfeld & Nicolson, 1965.
2. BROMLEY, D. B., 'Research prospects in the psychology of ageing'. *J. ment. Sci.*, 102, 272–9, 1956.
3. See pp. 114–47 in *Age with a Future*. Ed. by P. From Hansen.

From: Bromley, D., *The Psychology of Human Ageing*, Penguin, 1966, pp. 284–6.

Document twelve
SOME CONCLUSIONS OF THE BEVERIDGE COMMITTEE

The Beveridge Committee in their report on social insurance and allied services concluded that there were three special problems. One of these was age and they discussed alternative proposals for pensions.

CONCLUSION

254.   There is no valid objection, either on the ground of equity or on the ground that a means test may discourage thrift, to postponing introduction of adequate contributory pensions for a substantial period of transition, during which needs are met by pensions subject to means test. As regards equity, the people who reach pensionable age during the transition period will not have paid contributions at the new rates for any substantial time. As regards thrift, only those who are now so old that they may expect to require pensions before the transition period ends can be affected at all, and of these only a small proportion can be affected substantially. The rising scale of contributory pensions will make it possible for everyone except people who are already close to pension age, by a very moderate additional provision of their own, to secure income adequate for subsistence and have no need for any means pension. There is all the difference in the world between a permanent system of pensions subject to means test and a transitional system of supplementation of rising contributory pensions, such as is suggested here. The first must be rejected; the second is not open to serious objection.

255.   There is no reason also to doubt the power of large numbers of people to go on working with advantage to the community and happiness to themselves after reaching the minimum pensionable age of 65 for men or 60 for women. The numbers of people past the pensionable age who, at each census, described themselves as still occupied rather than retired is very great. So is the number of those working as exempt persons after this age under the present schemes of health and unemployment insurance. There is no statistical evidence that industrial development is making it harder for people to continue at work later in life than it used to be; such evidence as there is points in the opposite direction. The natural presumption from the increasing length of total life is that the length of years during which working capacity lasts will also rise, as health improves, as by freedom from want in

childhood and by freedom from want and idleness in working years the physique and the courage of the citizens are maintained. A people ageing in years need not be old in spirit, and British youth will rise again.

From: Beveridge, Sir W., *Social Insurance and Allied Services* (The Beveridge Report), HMSO, 1942, p. 99.

Document thirteen
PREVENTIVE POLICIES AND THEIR EFFECT ON THE HEALTH OF THE ELDERLY

In *Prevention and Health: everybody's business* the DHSS consider the health problems of the aged.

It is self evident that the scope for reducing overall mortality among the elderly is limited and some have questioned the morality of devoting large resources to seeking to extend their lives for what must inevitably be relatively short periods of time, especially when the quality of that extended life may sometimes be open to question not least by those affected. By comparison, even small reductions in mortality among the young are clearly worth striving for since more years of life will be saved than by reductions, even large ones, at older ages. It has been calculated that, for England and Wales, if all deaths during the productive years (15 to 64) were avoided the added years of life would amount to 592 years for very 10,000 men and 350 years for every 10,000 women.

We do not have comprehensive data on the amount of disability among the aged, but defects of sight, hearing, and mobility become increasingly common with advancing years. Registration is known to be incomplete, but about 14,000 new cases of blindness are registered every year in Great Britain, the most important causes being senile degenerative disorders, cataract, and glaucoma. It is estimated that a quarter of all people of 65 and over suffer from a significant degree of deafness and about a million people of all ages in this country use a hearing aid. To maintain their mobility, and in many cases their independence, large numbers of people of 65 and over need chiropody treatment (more than a million people of 65 and over receive National Health Service chiropody treatment every year).

Another problem liable to arise among the isolated elderly is nutritional deficiency. The reasons include immobility, inadequate management of money or the co-existence of other serious diseases and obviously a proportion of these cases are preventable. Since there are about 2.7 million people aged 75 and over in Britain, including 1.75 million single or widowed, if even a small proportion of them are affected, this would represent a large number of cases of preventable disease.

Thinning of the bones (osteoporosis) is a common finding in old people, affecting particularly old women, and may explain the high frequency of fracture of the wrist, the hip, and the spine among them. Research is at present being pursued to test various theories; one has it that the condition is caused by lack of vitamin D, another by reduced secretion of sex hormones after the menopause. Should it be possible to unravel the cause or causes and prevent this condition, the benefits in terms of releasing hospital beds could be substantial.

From: DHSS, *Prevention and Health: everybody's business*, 1976, HMSO, pp. 37–8.

Document fourteen
THE GUIDING PRINCIPLES OF THE BEVERIDGE REPORT

The Beveridge Committee lay down the three guiding principles behind their recommendations for social insurance and allied services.

THREE GUIDING PRINCIPLES OF RECOMMENDATIONS
6.   In proceeding from this first comprehensive survey of social insurance to the next task – of making recommendations – three guiding principles may be laid down at the outset.

7.   The first principle is that any proposals for the future, while they should use to the full the experience gathered in the past, should not be restricted by consideration of sectional interests established in the obtaining of that experience. Now, when the war is abolishing landmarks of every kind, is the opportunity for using experience in a clear field. A revolutionary moment in the world's history is a time for revolutions, not for patching.

8.   The second principle is that organisation of social insurance should be treated as one part only of a comprehensive policy of social progress. Social insurance fully developed may provide income security; it is an attack upon Want. But Want is one only of five giants on the road of reconstruction and in some ways the easiest to attack. The others are Disease, Ignorance, Squalor and Idleness.

9.   The third principle is that social security must be achieved by co-operation between the State and the individual. The State should offer security for service and contribution. The State in organising security should not stifle incentive, opportunity, responsibility; in establishing a national minimum, it should leave room and encouragement for voluntary action by each individual to provide more than that minimum for himself and his family.

10.   The Plan for Social Security set out in this Report is built upon these principles. It uses experience but is not tied by experience. It is put forward as a limited contribution to a wider social policy, though as something that could be achieved now without waiting for the whole of that policy. It is, first and foremost, a plan of insurance – of giving in return for contributions

benefits up to subsistence level, as of right and without means test, so that individuals may build freely upon it.

From: Beveridge, Sir W., *Social Insurance and Allied Services* (The Beveridge Report), HMSO, 1942, pp. 6–7.

Document fifteen
THE END OF THE POOR LAW

The National Assistance Act 1948 set up the NAB with a duty to assist persons in need and gave local authorities powers.

An Act to terminate the existing poor law and to provide in lieu thereof for the assistance of persons in need by the National Assistance Board and by local authorities; to make further provision for the welfare of disabled, sick, aged and other persons and for regulating homes for disabled and aged persons and charities for disabled persons; to amend the law relating to non-contributory old age pensions; to make provision as to the burial or cremation of deceased persons; and for purposes connected with the matters aforesaid.

[13th May 1948.]

PART I. INTRODUCTORY

1. The existing poor law shall cease to have effect, and shall be replaced by the provisions of Part II of this Act as to the rendering, out of moneys provided by Parliament, of assistance to persons in need, the provisions of Part III of this Act as to accommodation and other services to be provided by local authorities, and the related provisions of Part IV of this Act.

From: National Assistance Act 1948, p. 1.

Document sixteen
PENSION CHANGES

The Social Security Act 1973 provided for all employed people to be covered by a second, and earnings-related, pension on top of the basic state pension. For those who did not come under an approved occupational scheme a state scheme was to be established.

1973 CHAPTER 38

An Act to establish a basic scheme of social security contributions and benefits replacing the National Insurance Acts, to assimilate to it the operation of the Industrial Injuries Acts and the Old Cases Acts; to make further provision with respect to occupational pension schemes (including schemes financed from public funds), to establish an Occupational Pensions Board with functions in respect of such schemes (including in particular functions with respect to the recognition of schemes, the preservation of benefits and the modification of schemes for the purpose of obtaining recognition and other purposes); to establish a contributory reserve pension scheme under a Reserve Pension Board providing pensions in respect of service in employment which is not recognised pensionable employment; and for purposes connected with those matters.   [18th July, 1973.]

From: Social Security Act 1973, p. 1.

Document seventeen
MORE PENSION CHANGES

The Social Security Pensions Act 1975 made some changes to the earnings-related scheme including linking pensions with the rise in prices or earnings, whichever was greater.

1975 CHAPTER 60

An Act to provide for relating the rates of social security retirement pensions and certain other benefits to the earnings on which contributions have been paid; to enable employed earners to be contracted-out of full social security contributions and benefits where the requisite benefits are provided by an occupational pension scheme; to make provision for securing that men and women are afforded equal access to occupational pension schemes; and to make other amendments in the law relating to social security (including an amendment of Part II of the Social Security Act 1975 introducing a new non-contributory benefit called 'mobility allowance'); and to make other provision about occupational pensions.   [7th August 1975.]

From: Social Security Pensions Act 1975, p. 1.

SUGGESTIONS BY ELDERLY PEOPLE IN 1976 ABOUT HOW
THEY COULD BE HELPED

In 1976 a sample of 2,622 elderly people were asked for suggestions
about forms of help. Visits from voluntary helpers, regular medical
and welfare visits and help with fuel bills or free coal topped the list.

Table 15.7.1. Suggestions for ways in which elderly people could be helped

	Grand total
All elderly persons WEIGHTED	(3,869)
(unweighted figures)	(2,622)
	%
Suggested forms of help	
Increase old age pensions	8.5
Don't tax pensions	3.5
Provide free, cheap phones, phone calls	7.9
Help with fuel bills, free coal	10.1
Help with TV licence, free licence	2.6
Introduce, extend, free, cheap travel	7.0
Other financial help	3.8
Voluntary helpers to assist with tasks	6.8
Voluntary helpers to chat, provide company	11.1
Regular medical, welfare visits	10.8
Provision of suitable housing	4.6
Provision of aids for handicapped	1.8
Provision of better public transport	3.2
Provision of recreational facilities	4.2
Provision of other local facilities (e.g. library, post office, shops, pub)	2.5
Other forms of assistance	5.3
No suggestions	40.6
Proxy interviews	2.8

Some people made more than one suggestion so percentages add to more than
100 per cent.

From: Hunt, A., *The Elderly at Home*, OPCS, 1978, HMSO, p. 132.

Document nineteen
THE ELDERLY PEOPLE WHO ARE OLD AND COLD

A survey in 1972 of over 1,000 old people disclosed disquieting information about their conditions.

HOW GREAT A PROBLEM?

The starting point for our enquiries was that relatively little was known about the size of the problem of hypothermia or the cold elderly. Indeed there were wildly conflicting estimates and many assertions, but few hard facts. We can now summarize our results and discuss them in relation to other findings. Does a clear picture emerge?

From all the reliable evidence now available it is possible to demonstrate that:

(1) large proportions of the elderly have cold living conditions;
(2) while most of them maintain reasonable inner body temperatures, a significant minority fail to do so and are at risk of developing hypothermia;
(3) of those at risk a small proportion have inner body temperatures below the hypothermic level;
(4) a small (but significant) proportion of elderly hospital admissions are hypothermic; and
(5) an unknown number die from hypothermia in hospitals, in their own homes and elsewhere.

The above conclusions can be discussed with reference to our own and other evidence.

From: Wicks, M., *Old and Cold*, Heinemann, 1978, p. 158.

Document twenty
THE ELDERLY WHO ARE FOUND DEAD

A survey of 203 people who had been found dead or dying in their homes at least 18 hours after they had last been seen took place in York in 1972. Most (143) were over retirement age. The authors conclude that there is no certain way of ensuring that people do not die alone.

The danger of active interventionist policies to ensure that aid is brought quickly to those who collapse is that such policies may interfere with the lives and deaths of those who prefer to remain at home. This is not intended to imply that no action should be taken, but rather that social policy should aim to provide a valid choice. The elderly should be free to choose whether or not to live alone. If they have been bereaved of relatives and friends they should be enabled to develop new social contacts if they so desire. If they are at risk of sudden collapse they should be informed of this, and if they wish to they should be provided with the opportunity to make use of good neighbour schemes, alarm systems or telephone schemes. These services and facilities should be made available to old people so that they can make a reasoned choice. For such a choice to be meaningful, it must be based on accurate information as to what services are available, and on a wide range of alternatives, ranging from shared living schemes to telephone checks.

The evidence of this research suggests that there is no major demand on the part of those who were found dead for considerably greater resources to be provided for their scrutiny. However, many old people living alone must worry about what will happen if they collapse and are unable to get assistance. Perhaps if a wider range of preventative services were made available, and if they were more widely known about, they would be used. However, there is no evidence from this research that there is a dramatic case for the development of services to prevent found deaths.

From: Bradshaw, J., Clifton, M. and Kennedy, J., *Found Dead*, Age Concern, 1978, pp. 23–4.

THE ELDERLY MENTALLY HANDICAPPED IN INSTITUTIONAL CARE

In a report to the Secretary of State for Social Services by the National Development Group for the Mentally Handicapped entitled *Helping Mentally Handicapped People in Hospital* special recommendations were made about the elderly.

6.7 ELDERLY RESIDENTS

6.7.1. Most elderly hospital residents are only mildly intellectually handicapped. Many of them were admitted over 20 years ago, and some have even lived in hospital since early childhood, having been admitted under Poor Law and similar legislation at a time when society relied on mental handicap hospitals to provide care and shelter for people who would under no circumstances be admitted today.

6.7.2. For this group more than for any other the mental handicap hospital is their home. They have not known any other home, and may not wish to be 'rehabilitated'. On the other hand, they should not have decisions on such matters made for them by others who take it on themselves to announce that it would be 'cruel' or 'unkind' for them to live outside hospital. Many of them are quite capable of thinking for themselves, and should be given the opportunity to consider alternatives to hospital if these can be made available.

6.7.3. A number of authorities have followed a policy of opening old people's homes specifically for people who have lived in hospitals for many years. These homes enable friends to stay together and to use the home as a base from which to use local facilities. A few live in ordinary old people's homes, and others, while remaining in hospital, live in accommodation very like an old people's home – sometimes a converted nursing home or a large house formerly belonging to the medical superintendent. Hospital authorities have also purchased or made use of larger houses in the community for elderly mentally handicapped people.

6.7.4. Particular care must always be taken in moving any elderly person from one environment to another. The transition should be very carefully planned and should be effected very slowly and by small degrees. The

resident should be able to change his mind if he decides that he would rather stay in hospital after all, and should be allowed to return to hospital if his new life in a hostel or an old people's home does not suit him. Every effort must be made to involve the resident himself in the determination of his needs and, like all residents, the elderly should be individually reviewed as part of the process of assessment and meeting of needs that we discuss in Chapter 5.
6.7.5. The BGS/RCN Report referred to above identified four main categories of problems as regards the care of the elderly:

  i. The lack of consideration of feelings and of maintenance of dignity, privacy and personal identity.
  ii. Failure to maintain independence and mobility.
  iii. Shortcomings related to personal hygiene and physiological needs.
  iv. Lack of social, remedial and recreational stimulation.

These problems apply just as forcefully to the elderly residents of mental handicap hospitals.

From: DHSS, The National Development Group for the Mentally Handi-capped, *Helping Mentally Handicapped People in Hospital*, HMSO, 1978, pp. 67–8.

LOCAL AUTHORITY PLANS FOR HEALTH AND
WELFARE SERVICES IN 1966

Local authorities were asked in 1962 to prepare plans for the
long-term development of their health and welfare services. In a
review of these plans the MOH commented on the differences in
provision.

100.   It will, however, be apparent from the foregoing paragraphs and from
the plans of individual authorities that the level of particular services
provided by a small minority of them falls below what is acceptable, and that
some of these authorities do not appear to be planning to improve unsatisfactory services to an acceptable standard over the next ten years. In some
areas the figures may well obscure the true position – for example where a
satisfactory service is being provided by a voluntary body, or where facilities
provided by one authority are meeting the needs of an adjoining area. But
where the provision of a service appears to be substantially below an adequate
level and likely to remain so over the whole period of the present plans, the
Minister proposes to arrange for his officers to discuss the position with the
authority concerned with a view to action to remedy any deficiency. It is his
strong wish to work as rapidly as possible towards a situation in which an
acceptable standard of service is provided throughout England and Wales;
and he is confident that all authorities will share that wish, and will be ready
to co-operate in reaching that objective.

From: MOH, Health and Welfare, *The Development of Community Care*,
Cmnd 3022 (1966), HMSO, p. 26.

Document twenty-three
VIEWS ABOUT SERVICES FOR THE ELDERLY FROM THE ROYAL COMMISSION ON THE NATIONAL HEALTH SERVICE

The Royal Commission on the National Health Service felt that the health needs of the elderly were one of the major problems facing the NHS.

6.33.   Services for the elderly demonstrate very clearly the requirements for community care already discussed. Everything possible should be done to assist old people to remain independent, healthy and in their own homes. It is important to detect stress and practical problems, and to ward off breakdown, for example by regular visiting of those who are identified through GP case registers as being at risk, by providing physical aids or adapted or sheltered housing, and by assistance from home helps, chiropodists, or meals on wheels. Planned short-term admissions to residential care play an increasing part in helping the elderly remain in their own homes or with relatives. The supporting role of relatives is of great importance and their needs for relief from time to time must be met. Voluntary bodies and volunteers can often help in numerous understanding ways.[1] Where there is illness the full resources of the primary care team have often to be deployed, and a heavy load of work and responsibility falls on the district nurses and the home help services. Day centres are helpful, and day hospitals have been widely developed: their place in a comprehensive service urgently requires critical evaluation and this is being studied by the DHSS. When independence at home is no longer possible, care in a nursing home or local authority residential home may be appropriate.

6.34.   Illness in old age commonly has both physical and mental aspects. A deterioration in an old person's faculties may or may not be accompanied by disturbances of behaviour, and may or may not be due to or worsened by physical illness. Detailed assessment is often necessary and the skill of geriatricians, psychiatrists, nurses and social workers may be jointly called upon. We recommend that all professions concerned with the care of the elderly should receive more training in understanding their needs.

[1] Personal Social Services Research Unit, University of Kent, *Kent Community Care Project: an interim report*, 1979.

6.35. Many elderly patients admitted to district general hospitals do not need the technology which that type of hospital can provide. They frequently remain in hospital long after any investigations or active treatment have been completed because they are not fit to go home and there is nowhere else for them to go. Residential homes cannot care for those who are physically very dependent and need nursing care, or whose behaviour is more than mildly disturbed.

From: *Royal Commission on the NHS, Report* (the Merrison Committee), Cmnd 7615 (1979), pp. 62–3.

A VARIETY OF HOUSING FOR THE ELDERLY RECOMMENDED IN 1944

In 1944 the Ministry of Health, which was responsible for housing, published a *Housing Manual* giving guidance to local authorities on the types of provision that were needed. The section on the elderly started with some general considerations:

OLD PEOPLE

The type of accommodation required for old people will vary according to their age and disabilities. For the very old who may require a certain amount of care, the accommodation can take the form of small self-contained dwellings grouped together with a common day-room, a room for laundry work, a spare room for visitors, and quarters for a nurse or warden, as shown in Fig. 8. Consideration should be given to the possibility of providing hot water to the bathrooms from a common source and a small amount of central heating to give 'background' warmth. [73

For able-bodied old people who can look after themselves, accommodation might be provided in self-contained dwellings, either one or two storey cottages or cottage flats or on the lower floors of blocks of flats. Where there are lifts, the flats could even be on the higher floors. [74

All dwellings for old people should be sited within easy distance of churches and shops and in a position which will give an interesting outlook from the living room window. So far as possible the dwellings should not be segregated, as old people like to have contact with younger generations. (An interesting example of the setting of old people's dwellings among other houses is shown in Figs. 44 and 45.) To assist in keeping the dwelling warm a sheltered site should be chosen. [75

From: MOH, *Housing Manual 1944*, HMSO, p. 22.

CO-ORDINATION OF SERVICES FOR OLD PEOPLE

Advice was given to local authorities in 1961 about services for old people. The need for co-operation was highlighted as is shown below. Later sections dealt with specific services and the role of voluntary organisations.

SERVICES FOR OLD PEOPLE

Co-operation between housing, local health and welfare authorities and voluntary organisations

1.   The Minister of Housing and Local Government and the Minister of Health have been considering together how to improve the provision made for the well-being of old people.

2.   Housing, health and welfare authorities are concerned. So are voluntary organisations. All these must work in the closest co-operation if all the varying needs of old people are to be covered. The several services should be regarded as parts of a whole, the authorities and organisations responsible each making their contribution to the whole. This means that all concerned (including in a county borough the different committees) should make it a regular feature of their administration to meet together from time to time to review the provision made in their area, and to decide where and how it needs to be supplemented.

3.   It is widely recognised today that old people want to lead an independent life in their own homes for as long as they can, and that to do so gives them the best chance of an active and contented old age. To make this possible, housing authorities must provide, in adequate numbers, a full range of small bungalows, flats and flatlets designed for old people: some in which they can be fully independent (though with neighbours at hand in case help is wanted): others in which some friendly help is available in the person of a warden: others still in which provision can be made for some communal services in addition to a warden. The changes in subsidy proposed in the Housing Bill now before Parliament should enable every housing authority, the less well-off as well as those with adequate resources, to meet, in time, all

the demands of their area. With a fully adequate range of housing designed to meet the different tastes and needs of the old, hospital and welfare accommodation can be used by those who really require it.

From: MHLG Circular 10/61; MOH Circular 12/61, *Services for Old People*, 1961, HMSO, p. 1.

GUIDANCE ON DESIGNING OLD PEOPLE'S HOUSING

A circular in 1969 gave advice to local authorities on both the principles of housing for elderly people and detailed design guidance which had to be adhered to if a subsidy was required.

APPENDIX VI
This check list is offered as a guide to the special aspects of designing for old people's dwellings.

Introduction to the check list
The mandatory requirements for accommodation specially designed for old people are set out in Appendix I to Circular 82/69 (Welsh Office Circular 84/69), and the yardstick additions in Appendix II to that Circular are based on those standards.

The purpose which underlies the design of housing for the elderly is the provision of accommodation which will enable them to maintain an independent way of life for as long as possible. With improved health services more people may be expected to remain in a home of their own for the rest of their lives. If they are to do this in comfort, they will need housing designed with the special requirements of the elderly in mind, coupled with the availability, as far as possible, of a balanced range of different types of accommodation to meet their varying needs and preferences. It has to be remembered too that most old people for whom housing is being provided will eventually be living alone and all housing for old people needs to be planned for sociability so as to avoid loneliness and isolation. This is particularly desirable where rehousing involves moving to a new area and, though the subject is outside the scope of this circular, good housing management practice can assist by keeping together groups of friends and neighbours as far as practicable.

Of the different types of housing which can be provided for the elderly, bungalows – traditionally regarded by old people themselves as the ideal form of housing – are best suited to couples who are able to maintain a greater degree of independence, who can manage rather more housework and who may want a small garden.

Two storey flats are more economical of land than bungalows, can provide a more compact layout, fit in well with family housing and can be used on infill sites. Many people over the age of 65 can still manage one flight of stairs and an upper flat may be preferred by those who dislike sleeping on the ground floor. Taller blocks with lifts can provide acceptable accommodation for old people, if suitably designed and sited, in those places where the density justifies their use.

For less active old people, often living alone, who need smaller and labour-saving accommodation, grouped flatlets as described in Circular 36/67 (Welsh Office Circular 28/67) and the two publications 'Flatlets for Old People' and 'More Flatlets for Old People' are the most suitable. The tenants of these flatlets will have the services of a warden and also communal facilities such as a common-room and laundry; and possibly a guest room as well. Bathrooms may be shared for one-person flatlets (in a ratio of one bathroom to four flatlets) or private in the case of two-person flatlets but every flatlet will contain a w.c. and hand basin. Additional facilities such as a call-bell system will also be needed.

From MHLG, *Housing Standards and Costs: accommodation specially designed for old people*, Circular 82/69, 1969, HMSO, p. 14.

HOUSING POLICY FOR THE ELDERLY IN 1977

A Consultative Document, *Housing Policy*, was published in 1977, which outlined the policies of the Labour government. In a section on the elderly previous policies were endorsed, but the proposed abolition of local authority residential qualifications was stressed as was the need for co-operation between authorities.

12.40.   The proposed abolition of local authority residential qualifications – discussed in Chapter 9 – will help elderly people who have to move and would benefit from local authority accommodation – for example those who have had to give up homes on going into hospital, or who have previously lived in tied houses, or those who wish to move to live near relatives, perhaps in 'granny annexes'. Housing associations are supplementing the work of many local authorities in helping the elderly to move out of large property by providing them with alternative accommodation. This can often release housing which is itself suitable for conversion into smaller units for old people.

12.41.   The implementation of Government policy on the care of the elderly depends upon local housing authorities being fully involved with health and social service authorities in establishing effective methods of assessing need, planning provision, providing facilities and allocating resources. There is considerable scope for fuller co-operation in planning service developments in the three fields and for co-ordination of administrative policies – for example admission and discharge procedures in hospital and residential homes, and tenancy allocation procedures for housing. Local decisions have to be taken on the balance between the various forms of special and sheltered housing provision and residential accommodation, on the type of facilities and on staffing to be provided in sheltered housing, and on the support to be provided by domiciliary services.

From: DOE, *Housing Policy*, A Consultative Document, Cmnd 6851 (1977), HMSO, p. 115.

COMPARATIVE TYPES OF HOUSING

David Plank, in *Caring for the Elderly: report of a study of various means of caring for dependent elderly people in eight London boroughs* for the GLC made some personal observations about the problems involved in this sort of exercise.

2.59.   The deleterious effects of institutionalization on individuals are undoubtedly real (though often exaggerated and in many instances avoidable by good and well-informed practice). However, they must be seen in their proper perspective if the current unhappy situation is to be improved. There has been an over-reaction to the findings of Professor Townsend and others concerning institutionalization. They have provided a basis for much righteous indignation and bogus emotion on the part of people who should know better. Many interested and caring people seem unwilling to acknowledge the necessary consequence of this over-reaction for many dependent elderly people, viz. their condemnation to a woefully inadequate level of care in their own homes in situations of high personal risk, distress and miserable environment or to relatively permanent placement in surroundings inappropriate to their needs. The related failure to define the role of sheltered housing and its relationship with residential homes and domiciliary care, may have led to a situation where some tenants are receiving levels of care well in excess of their needs relative to those of others and may be leading to a situation where wardens will find it increasingly difficult to cope adequately with the needs of their ageing tenants.

2.60.   Frequent incantation of the words 'domiciliary care' does not mean that such a thing really exists for many highly dependent old people. It tends to be cheaper than other forms of service simply because it often stands for desperately poor levels of care. This is not so widely known, perhaps because the recipients are not as readily accessible as residents in homes who can be seen in a few specific places. It is time to dispose of the negative/positive myths associated with residential/domiciliary care and to stop thinking of provision for the elderly in the sterile, blind alley terms of residential versus domiciliary care. There is need for many forms of care for elderly people, including various forms of communal living. The issue is not residential versus domiciliary services but how to ensure that people get the care most appropriate to their needs. Some of the questions we have yet to answer are: what are the services most appropriate to those needs – including residential care, new forms of communal living, various degrees of sheltered housing and varying levels of domiciliary support? what are the relative costs and benefits associated with existing and new forms of care for elderly people and their families? how do we ensure that administrative rigidities are removed so that people can get the services they need no matter which agency happens to provide them? how best can we cope with the fact that forms of communal living such as residential homes and grouped sheltered housing schemes are dynamic rather than static, i.e. their populations age and become more dependent over time? and how do we improve the quality of life associated with the various forms of care by means of good professional practice? If this study makes some contribution to the answering of these questions, then it will have been worthwhile.

From: Plank, D., *Caring for the Elderly: report of a study of various means of caring for dependent elderly people in eight London boroughs*, GLC Research Memorandum, 1977, pp. 21–2.

RETIRING TO THE SEASIDE

Retirement migration has been studied by a number of researchers. Dr Valerie Karn, in research involving over 1,000 elderly people who had moved to Bexhill and Clacton found that the majority were pleased with the move but there were problems for the health and social services.

Thus while it is tempting and attractive to dwell on the comments of the few who mentioned the exclusion of the retired and elderly from the social life of the cities, and to see the move to retirement resorts as a conscious reaction to the attitude of society to the old, the fact is that the retired people themselves rarely mentioned this. They were concerned with the environmental advantages of the seaside compared with the cities. Their reasons for moving were to do with the desire for a better climate, clearer air, the sea and better health.

True, after they had been there some years, they had become conscious of the social advantages of living in a mainly retired community, and this figured prominently in their reasons for liking the town and for finding it easier to make friends. But, whatever the reasons for the success of the move, improvement of environment and health had been the initial motive.

The link with a previous holiday area is clear. It was an area with a pleasant environment with which they were familiar and which was, very often, not too far from the area in which they had spent their working life. It fitted in, too, with the image they had of retirement as being a period of rest and quiet without the strain and rush of town life.

So these were the ideas with which people retired to the seaside. But how did it work out in practice?

The answer must be, I believe, 'Remarkably well', according to the evidence of this survey. Social surveys are certainly very fallible instruments but one cannot select which parts of them to disbelieve just because they contradict one's original expectations. It is a fact that 84 per cent of the people interviewed in Bexhill and 79 per cent in Clacton said they would, with hindsight, and given their time again, make the same decision to move. In addition 26 per cent of the retired people in Bexhill had actually persuaded friends or relations to join them in the town and so had 18 per cent in Clacton, a notable vote of confidence.

There were some, of course, for whom the move was not so successful. Widows were particularly likely to regret moving, 24 per cent of them in Clacton did so, and so did 12 per cent in Bexhill. In addition, there was considerable evidence that, whether or not they regretted their move, many men and women moved away when they were widowed. By no means all went back to the cities. They might go to other resorts, perhaps to join friends living there, or with some hope of finding a place which did not remind them of the time before they were widowed. There was a small minority of people who moved rapidly from one resort to another constantly searching for the perfect retirement home.

Such wanderings were unhappy but unusual. It was common, however, for retired people to have two or more homes after retirement. The first retirement home was frequently over-ambitious for later old age when the upkeep of the house and garden became too much. If this stage were reached, the fortunate moved into a more suitable flat, small bungalow or sheltered housing scheme. The less fortunate, or less affluent, were forced to stay on in their house or to move into even more unsuitable property, such as a converted flat up many stairs and with a high rent and little security of tenure. Others moved into hotels or private homes.

THE HEALTH AND SOCIAL SERVICES

It is the situation of such old people, in acute need of better health and social services, that worries the local authorities in the resort areas. Many feel that continued migration of old people to their towns will end in complete breakdown of the services. Certainly the review of the services in this study showed that most services were well below the national average in the proportion of elderly residents covered by them. In addition one can argue that, in areas where such a large proportion of old people have no children or relatives near and where even the neighbours are also predominantly elderly, the services need even greater coverage than the average.

There are three main problems in improving the services. One is national, namely to achieve adequate health planning and to give the necessary priority to geriatric services which are so often neglected. The second is to overcome the financial handicaps which the resorts experience because of their lack of non-residential rateable value and the low incomes of the majority of their residents. The third problem is that of recruitment of staff for the health and social services in the resorts and constitutes possibly the biggest question-mark concerning the viability of the resorts.

From: Karn, V., *Retiring to the Seaside*, Routledge and Kegan Paul, 1977, pp. 242–4.

RESIDENTIAL QUALIFICATIONS AND THE ELDERLY

Elderly people in local authority accommodation who want to move to another area may face problems because they lack a residential qualification in the latter. The Cullingworth Committee identified a number of groups of elderly people who may be debarred from council accommodation by residential rules:

297. The evidence we received suggests that there are at least six ways in which elderly people may be debarred from council houses by residential rules:

   i. Elderly people who, for one reason or another, give up their houses on moving into hospital.

   ii. Elderly people who, because of the nature of their employment, have been highly mobile.

   iii. Those who wish to move from an isolated rural area to a less isolated location which happens to be in the district of another local authority.

   iv. Those retiring from employment to which their housing was 'tied' and which is in an area with little or no council accommodation, or who again wish to settle in another area.

   v. Elderly people who wish to move to be near younger relatives living in other parts of the country.

   vi. Those who break their residence connection by moving to live with relatives in another area, but who for various social reasons wish to return to the area which they have left.

From: MHLG, WO, *Council Housing Purposes, Procedures and Priorities* (the Cullingworth Committee), 1969, HMSO, p. 99.

Document thirty-one
POWERS TO PROVIDE HOME HELPS AND OTHER SERVICES

Under the National Health Service Act 1946 local authorities were given powers to provide home helps and certain preventive services.

PREVENTION OF ILLNESS, CARE AND AFTER-CARE

28. – (1) A local health authority may with the approval of the Minister, and to such extent as the Minister may direct, shall make arrangements for the purpose of the prevention of illness, the care of persons suffering from illness or mental defectiveness, or the after-care of such persons, but no such arrangements shall provide for the payment of money to such persons, except in so far as they may provide for the remuneration of such persons engaged in suitable work in accordance with the arrangements.

(2) A local health authority may, with the approval of the Minister, recover from persons availing themselves of the services provided under this section such charges (if any) as the authority consider reasonable, having regard to the means of those persons.

(3) A local health authority may, with the approval of the Minister, contribute to any voluntary organisation formed for any such purpose as aforesaid.

DOMESTIC HELP

29. – (1) A local health authority may make such arrangements as the Minister may approve for providing domestic help for households where such help is required owing to the presence of any person who is ill, lying-in, an expectant mother, mentally defective, aged, or a child not over compulsory school age within the meaning of the Education Act, 1944.

(2) A local health authority may, with the approval of the Minister, recover from persons availing themselves of the domestic help so provided such charges (if any) as the authority consider reasonable, having regard to the means of those persons.

From: National Health Service Act 1946, paras 28–9.

Document thirty-two
POWERS TO PROMOTE WELFARE

Under the National Assistance Act 1948 local authorities were empowered to promote the welfare of certain disadvantaged groups. Elderly people who came into any of these categories benefited from this legislation.

WELFARE SERVICES
29. – (1)   A local authority shall have power to make arrangements for promoting the welfare of persons to whom this section applies, that is to say persons who are blind, deaf or dumb, and other persons who are substantially and permanently handicapped by illness, injury, or congenital deformity or such other disabilities as may be prescribed by the Minister.
(2)   In relation to persons ordinarily resident in the area of a local authority the authority shall, to such extent as the Minister may direct, be under a duty to exercise their powers under this section.

Local authorities were also empowered to make contributions to voluntary organisations.

31.   A local authority may make contributions to the funds of any voluntary organisation whose activities consist in or include the provision of recreation or meals for old people.

From: National Assistance Act 1948, Section 29 (1), (2) and 31.

Note: Consolidating legislation relating to the provision of meals and recreation for old people was given in the Health and Social Services and Social Security Adjudications Act 1983.

Document thirty-three
A DUTY TO PROVIDE RESIDENTIAL ACCOMMODATION

The National Assistance Act 1948 laid a duty on local authorities to provide residential accommodation for needy old people.

LOCAL AUTHORITY SERVICES

Provision of accommodation
21. – (1)   It shall be the duty of every local authority, subject to and in accordance with the provisions of this Part of this Act, to provide –
(*a*) residential accommodation for persons who by reason of age, infirmity or any other circumstances are in need of care and attention which is not otherwise available to them;
(*b*) temporary accommodation for persons who are in urgent need thereof, being need arising in circumstances which could not reasonably have been foreseen or in such other circumstances as the authority may in any particular case determine.
(2)   In the exercise of their said duty a local authority shall have regard to the welfare of all persons for whom accommodation is provided, and in particular to the need for providing accommodation of different descriptions suited to different descriptions of such persons as are mentioned in the last foregoing subsection.

From: National Assistance Act 1948, Part III, Section 21 (1) and (2).

POWER TO PROVIDE WELFARE SERVICES FOR THE ELDERLY

The general power for a local authority to provide welfare services for the elderly, either itself or through a voluntary organisation, was given in the Health Services and Public Health Act 1968.

PROMOTION BY LOCAL AUTHORITIES OF THE WELFARE OF OLD PEOPLE

45. – (1)   A local authority may with the approval of the Minister of Health, and to such extent as he may direct shall, make arrangements for promoting the welfare of old people.

(2)   A local authority may recover from persons availing themselves of any service provided in pursuance of arrangements made under this section such charges (if any) as, having regard to the cost of the service, the authority may determine, whether generally or in the circumstances of any particular case.

(3)   A local authority may employ as their agent for the purposes of this section any voluntary organisation having for its sole or principal object, or among its principal objects, the promotion of the welfare of old people.

From: The Health Services and Public Health Act 1968, Section 45 (1), (2) and (3).

THE SEEBOHM COMMITTEE AND THE ELDERLY

The Committee on *Local Authority and Allied Personal Social Services* (the Seebohm Report) 1968, recommended the creation of a new social service department which would have a co-ordinated approach to people's problems. Comments were made about the need for the development of domiciliary services, as well as a comprehensive approach, for the elderly.

THE DEVELOPMENT OF THE DOMICILIARY SERVICES

309.   Although for many years it has been part of national policy to enable as many old people as possible to stay in their own homes, the development of the domiciliary services which are necessary if this is to be achieved has been slow. There are certain services of home care, such as home nursing and domestic help, which are provided by all local authorities. Neither service is specially for the old though both are used largely by them. There is also a wide variety of other help for old people, like meals on wheels, chiropody, and laundry service, which is provided by local authorities or voluntary committees or sometimes jointly, but the extent of their cover differs considerably from place to place and nowhere do they assist more than a very small proportion of the old. Furthermore it appears that individual services have been started without sufficient thought for priorities or evidence of need over the whole area to be served. This piecemeal and haphazard development is unlikely to use scarce resources to the best advantage even though some assistance may be given to a fortunate few.

310.   A unified social service department will be able to take a more comprehensive view of the development of such services, but to do so it will have to know the extent and pattern of need in its area and be aware of all the local resources likely to be available. It will have to discover from local voluntary organisations what part they can play in providing a comprehensive service to the maximum number of old people. It will have to investigate fully the contribution which relatives, neighbours and the wider community can make and how the social service department can best enable such potential assistance to be realised. In this sense a considerable develop-

ment of community care for the old may be achieved, even in the near future, by enlisting such help.

311.   In particular, of course, services for old people in their own homes will not be adequately developed unless greater attention is paid to supporting their families who in turn support them. The problems of old people living alone have attracted much attention, but many of those who are most dependent live with younger relatives who often are themselves getting on in years. Just as we emphasised the need for shared responsibility between the family and the personal social services where there were problems in the social care of children (Chapter VIII) so we wish to stress it in the case of the old. If old people are to remain in the community, support and assistance must often be directed to the whole family of which they are members. This is one of the reasons which convinced us that services for the elderly should become an integral part of the social services department.

From: Home Office *et al.*, *Local Authority and Allied Personal Social Services* (the Seebohm Committee), HMSO, 1968, p. 96.

THE BRITISH ASSOCIATION OF SOCIAL WORKERS LAYS DOWN GUIDELINES FOR SOCIAL WORK WITH THE ELDERLY

In 1977 BASW pointed out that many agencies seemed to give work with the elderly a low priority and often workers with little experience or training were expected to undertake all, or a large proportion of, the work with this group. They suggested certain guidelines which they summarised as:

1.   These guidelines have illustrated the same need for expertise in social work with the elderly as with other vulnerable groups. Those who are most vulnerable amongst the elderly are those whose identity is damaged by retirement, those who are bereaved and who suffer loss of any kind and the mentally and physically frail, many of whom will be over 75.

2.   Many agencies seem to give work with the elderly a low priority and often workers with little experience or training are expected to undertake all, or a large proportion of, work with this group. The enormous contribution made by volunteers, social work assistants, relatives, neighbours and *all* others concerned with the social and emotional care of the elderly is neither denied nor minimised by emphasising those areas which are seen to be most appropriately dealt with by the qualified social worker. These can be summarised as follows:

(*a*) Assessing need in deciding the help required and by whom it should be given. This should, where possible, be multidisciplinary in nature, the social worker operating as a member of a caring team.

(*b*) Providing skilled social work help with problems of relationship, problems arising from crises, loss, change or other social, emotional or medical condition. The complex nature of many problems in old age arising from medical, social or psychological sources should be continuously borne in mind.

(*c*) Providing the skill in helping to overcome psychological problems related to receiving practical, financial and advocatory help. More skill is required to enable the elderly to make the best use of the practical resources than is often appreciated.

(*d*) Providing group and community work, where the social worker has received training in appropriate skills. Group work with the elderly offers a further dimension to social work with the elderly. Both the elderly and their relatives gain mutual strength and ability to cope with their problems through group discussions.

(e) Understanding and accepting the degree of risk which the client is prepared to take, and balancing this with the sometimes over-anxious reaction of society. Enabling relatives and neighbours to tolerate these dilemmas.

(f) Enabling and supporting others in caring, such as relatives, 'good neighbours' and volunteers.

(g) Participating in planning and policymaking related to elderly people. This is not the exclusive terrain of the qualified social worker, though her knowledge of areas of social need will give her an important role in this process.

3. Another conclusion which must be drawn from these guidelines is that social work courses should include more teaching on the process of ageing and work with the elderly, and more placements for students in this field.

4. Social work with elderly people is as demanding and rewarding as work with and other client group. It can succeed in making life positive and meaningful for those with whom we have been most concerned in these guidelines.

From: *Social Work Today*, 12.4.77, p. 13.

Document thirty-seven
THE LAST REFUGE

In a survey of residential institutions and homes for the elderly Professor P. Townsend presented disquieting evidence about their conditions:

So far as it is possible to express in a few words the general conclusion of this book it is that communal Homes of the kind which exist in England and Wales today do not adequately meet the physical, psychological and social needs of the elderly people living in them, and that alternative services and living arrangements should quickly take their place.

and about the lack of alternative accommodation:

In investigating the physical and mental capacities of elderly residents, the events and circumstances leading to their admission and the life they follow in Homes, we reached certain important conclusions. The majority are not so handicapped by infirmity that they could not, given a small amount of support from the domiciliary social services, live in homes of their own in an ordinary community. A large number enter Homes for reasons of poverty, lack of housing, social isolation and absence of secondary sources of help among relatives and friends, and they do so unwillingly. Few of them take the initiative themselves and rarely are they offered practicable alternatives – such as housing, emergency grants and services or permanent help from the domiciliary services. Nearly all, once admitted, are expected to stay permanently, although the great majority, so it seems, would prefer not to do so.

From: Townsend, P., *The Last Refuge*, Routledge and Kegan Paul, 1964, pp. 222 and 226.

Document thirty-eight
THE STRENGTH OF FAMILY TIES

In a paper on research problems and priorities in community care Professor P. Abrams discusses the strength of family ties.

Perhaps surprisingly, in view of all the talk there has been of the death of the family, kinship remains the strongest basis of attachment and the most reliable basis of care that we have. This is especially true among women. Between mothers and daughters, and between sisters to a lesser degree, almost any call for help is legitimate and will, if at all possible, be satisfied. In these relationships a productive balance of trust, dependency and reciprocation is most easily struck. Hence, socially significant transfer payments between the generations are readily arranged. The bulk of the helping that is reported as community care turns out on closer scrutiny to be kin care of this sort.[1] And our next strongest basis of social involvement is that of the non-located 'moral communities' associated with churches, races, friendship nets and certain kinds of occupations. Neighbours, or more broadly local communities, come a very poor third and the relationships within them provide at best a means of mediating larger processes of social care – they are the means of contact and communication rather than of care as such. Perhaps, then, we should be paying more attention to kinship ties and to the moral communities of religion, race and occupation as possible contexts for basic social care, and less to the supposed communities of locality. It seems to be within the former relationship that the mix of certainty, trust and relative lack of resources most conducive to long-range reciprocity is most likely to occur 'naturally'.

From: Abrams, P., in Barnes, J. and Connelly, N. (eds), *Social Care Research*, Bedford Square Press, 1978, p. 87.

---

[1] 'If I'm ill I knock on the wall and they go and get my sister.' The 'classic' English community study is of course almost exclusively a study of care among kin – although it is hardly ever read that way: YOUNG and WILLMOTT (1957).

Document thirty-nine
HELP RECEIVED BY THE ELDERLY

For most domestic tasks for which the elderly need help relatives are the main source. Audrey Hunt's survey, *The Elderly at Home*, provided evidence to reinforce previous surveys. Sources of help for certain selected types of task are given below:

Table 10.9.2. Help given with bathing

	Bath only with help	Cannot bath at all
Elderly persons WEIGHTED	(254)	(320)
(unweighted figures)	(205)	(268)
	%	%
Help received from:		
Person(s) in household	61.0	7.5
Relative(s) outside*	18.5	1.2
Friend(s) outside	4.7	0.9
District nurse, health visitor	8.7	9.1
Home help	1.6	—
Other person outside	3.5	3.1
No one	2.0	81.2
Not stated	2.4	0.6
Whether help is enough		
Yes	89.0	17.2
No	2.8	0.3
Not stated	3.9	0.6
None received, not stated whether any received	4.4	81.8
Total	100.0	100.0

* Usually daughters/in law or sons/in law.

Table 10.9.8. Help given in going out of doors

	Unable to go out on own
Elderly persons WEIGHTED	(307)
(unweighted figures)	(243)
	%
Help received from:	
Other person in household	57.0
Daughter/in law outside household	15.3
Son/in law outside household	7.8
Other relatives outside household	4.6
Friend outside household	10.7
Home help	2.0
Other person outside household	5.2
None received	8.1
Not stated	6.5
Whether help is enough	
Yes	73.0
No	6.8
Not stated	5.5
None received, not stated whether any received	14.7
Total	100.0

Table 10.12.1. Help given with domestic tasks (based on all informants)

Job	Informant	Other informant	Both jointly	Home help (LA)	Paid help	Person(s) in h'hold	Outside household			Job done by:	
							Relative	Friend	Other	Not done	Not stated
Open screw top bottles	% 90.3	4.3	0.2	0.5	0.2	2.3	0.9	0.9	1.0	0.4	–
Do little sewing jobs	% 85.1	6.6	0.1	0.4	0.1	3.4	1.9	1.1	0.3	0.9	0.1
Jobs involving climbing	% 57.0	9.2	1.0	4.0	4.1	9.0	11.8	3.5	1.0	3.0	0.4
Using a frying pan	% 94.6	2.5	–	0.1	–	2.0	0.4	–	0.1	0.2	0.2
Make a cup of tea	% 97.4	1.1	–	–	–	1.2	0.2	–	–	–	0.1
Cook a main meal	% 91.2	4.1	–	0.2	–	3.2	0.9	0.1	0.6*	0.1	0.1
Cut the lawn†	% 44.5	6.6	–	–	3.6	7.0	4.3	2.1	0.1	2.3	0.2
Heavy jobs in garden†	% 30.1	7.6	0.2	–	7.0	10.0	10.8	3.3	0.6	9.3	0.9
Light jobs in garden†	% 61.6	2.2	–	–	2.3	4.8	2.7	1.1	0.3	2.4	0.3
Sweep floors	% 88.7	4.3	–	2.3	0.8	2.9	0.5	0.1	–	0.2	0.2
Wash floors	% 78.3	6.2	–	4.7	1.5	5.2	2.1	0.2	2.1	1.5	0.4
Make fires, carry fuel†	% 38.2	2.4	–	0.5	0.2	2.2	0.4	0.2	–	0.1	0.2
Wash clothes	% 85.5	4.3	–	1.3	1.1	3.3	3.3	0.5	0.8	0.1	0.2
Clean windows inside	% 76.4	6.2	0.2	5.1	2.4	5.4	2.8	0.5	0.1	0.9	0.3
Clean windows outside†	% 44.1	7.0	–	2.1	29.6	5.4	2.9	0.6	0.2	5.2	0.5
Wash paintwork	% 76.1	5.3	0.2	3.7	1.9	5.6	3.3	0.3	0.4	3.3	0.3
Minor repairs (e.g. fuses)	% 50.2	10.7	0.1	0.6	8.1	9.2	13.7	6.6	2.8	0.5	0.6
Repairs & redecoration inside	% 39.5	6.2	0.1	–	24.6	9.3	12.9	1.4	5.6‡	3.8	0.5
Repairs & redecoration outside	% 14.2	3.5	–	–	29.6	5.6	4.7	0.6	3.2	2.5	0.6

* Meals on Wheels.
† Cases where these do not apply are not shown, so percentages total to less than 100.
‡ Includes 4.3 per cent naming local authority.

From: Hunt, A., *The Elderly at Home*, OPCS, DHSS, HMSO, 1978, pp. 75, 78 and 82.

Document forty
FAMILY SUPPORT AND THE ELDERLY

Some views about community care are based on links between the generations. A researcher argues that the solution for each family may be different.

The problem selected is a specialised one but I would maintain that the same sorts of pressures and social sanctions apply to create stereotyping to all similar inter-generational issues where the old person is in the unaccustomed position of seeking assistance. However, it is not the assumption of a gift relationship between kin which is under attack, but the very indiscriminacy and rigidity of its application. It is still taken for granted that all families are somehow the same and can bear equal burdens. There is a failure to understand the way in which each family unit must tease out a unique working relationship which serves to meet differing needs and appetites. Clearly some family types (and the earlier analysis would suggest it was those with loose-knit networks) and families constrained by certain types of situational factors will be incapable of taking additional needs into their midst. In cases where the elderly are forced or obligated onto strained families, there is likely to be a negative result for both parties.

The point at issue is not only that society has not openly accepted a more diverse view of the family and that some types are less robust than others, but that there is a complete failure to see family life as an ever-active on-going process, rather than a series of stages in the well-known cycle. Families, like organisms, are constantly negotiating new positions of equilibrium. Old people too need to be involved in a negotiated settlement before their fate is determined. The relationship of parent-in-law to their sibling's family is openly acknowledged as a negotiated settlement, but once the gift relationship is reversed the rules are suddenly suspended in favour of traditional and frequently damaging solutions.

From: Johnson, M., *Old and Young in the Family: a negotiated arrangement*, paper given to the British Society of Gerontology, University of Keele, March 1973, pp. 9–10.

THE EFFECTIVENESS OF VISITING THE ELDERLY

Some criteria for assessing the quality of visiting the elderly were suggested in one research study.

EFFECTIVENESS OF VISITING
From interviews with both visitors and old people, an attempt was made to judge the impact of the visiting process on the old person's situation and from this to judge the quality of the visiting taking place. Since each set of circumstances was unique the main criterion was how appropriate were the visitors' efforts to the old person's need. The closeness of match between what was being offered and what the old person indicated as unmet needs had to be judged within the context of what could be reasonably expected of voluntary visitors. Thus judging the effectiveness of the visiting in helping to meet the old person's needs is not necessarily a measure of praise or criticism for the visitors. Regular arrangements to undertake house cleaning or nursing, or arranging for alternative housing are not normally to be expected from a voluntary friendly visitor (though cases can be found where just these things had been undertaken *faute de mieux*). Where visitors were offering a service, e.g. a regular friendly call which seemed to be making no impact at all on the old person's circumstances (and this might be either because these were very satisfactory or very unsatisfactory), it might not have been the visitor who was at fault. Rather it was the organisation which sent her and which had made no attempt, directly or through a referring agency, to assess what the old person needed, and what kind of contribution, if any, could be made by a voluntary visitor.

On this basis, visitors were rated on five counts, viz. relevant knowledge of the old person's personal circumstances, significance of services rendered, regularity and frequency of contacts, availability in case of emergency and general quality of relationships established. It must again be emphasised that some old people interviewed would not necessarily have welcomed as close or frequent a relationship as some others enjoyed with their visitors, and that some old people because of family and neighbourly support had not the same demand for visits or for personal services as the more isolated. A visitor who does no more than give pleasure by regular friendly calls and other tokens of continuous and sincere interest in an old person may be a very successful visitor if *such friendly calls are appropriate to the situation*. If friendly calls are all that is offered in a situation where simple practical services are urgently needed, the visits may make little useful impact and may even create resentment because of their irrelevance to the old person's pressing needs. Of course, even where a need cannot be met, for example, re-housing or daily personal care, friendly calls may be supportive and thus helpful, but only if the visitor is sensitive to the unresolved problems and observant of any ways in which he or she is able to mitigate hardships.

From: Shenfield, B., *The Organisation of Voluntary Service*, PEP, 1972, pp. 33–4.

GOOD NEIGHBOUR SCHEMES

A study by the Volunteer Centre of some good neighbour schemes pointed out both the advantages and some problems. It concluded:

CONCLUSION

The attraction of encouraging neighbourhood care often seems to be taken for granted. This discussion has attempted to examine some of the potential advantages and disadvantages of such a policy. It has been suggested that there is not one best form of caring; neighbourhood care may be good or bad, from the different viewpoints of different participants with different needs and problems.

In view of the fact that the policy scales seem to be heavily weighted in favour of neighbourhood care (both for ideological reasons – the return to community – and because of its assumed cheapness and preventive efficiency) two further potential disadvantages should perhaps be noted. Firstly, it may be suggested that a policy of encouraging neighbourhood care may serve to formalise (and 'professionalise') what is essentially an informal relationship, thus destroying or radically transforming what it seeks to promote. Secondly, it may be argued that for a variety of reasons (both economic and historical) neighbourhoods vary in their resources for caring. If reliance upon neighbourhood care is not to perpetuate and exacerbate the existing inequalities in caring provision, its encouragement may require increased resources and a more integrated planning approach between health, social and housing services.

From: Leat, D., *Limited Liability?* A report on some good neighbour schemes, The Volunteer Centre, 1979, p. 35.

Document forty-three
THE INFORMAL SYSTEM OF MEETING SOCIAL NEED

The Wolfenden Committee on *The Future of Voluntary Organisations* suggested that there were four systems of meeting social need: the informal, the commercial, the statutory and the voluntary. Details of the first system are given below:

FOUR SYSTEMS OF MEETING SOCIAL NEED
1. The informal system of social helping
The help and support that family, friends and neighbours give to each other is so much taken for granted that it often hardly enters into the discussion of the provision of social services. The relative neglect of this field by sociologists and social administrators means that we have very little exact knowledge about factors which affect the weakness or the strength of informal support networks in different sectors of our society.

Such studies as have been made[1] suggest that the volume of informal help is very substantial, and imply that if for any reason such help ceased to be available an enormous burden would be placed on other systems of provision. The contribution of the informal system today would seem to be of three main kinds: (a) in the provision of care for the young and the weak, especially the sick, the handicapped and the elderly; (b) in the transfer of material resources, particularly between members of a family, from those with a surplus to those with a deficit, as with parental help to a newly married son or daughter in house purchase, or in the purchase of furniture; (c) in the provision of advice and psychological support as from the experienced to the inexperienced in matters such as child rearing, coping with crises such as desertion, divorce and widowhood.[2]

But there are important limits to what the informal system can do. First, it is not equipped to provide services which involve professional expertise and expensive plant and equipment. So while it might, for example, provide successfully in many instances for the care of the chronic sick, it cannot provide the necessary treatment for many acute complaints. Or again, while it may provide invaluable advice on how to handle the in-laws, it may not be able to produce the necessary information on social security regulations, rent acts, and the like. Second, while financial and material help may be transferred within the system, only in the richest strata of society will such transfers be adequate to meet all the heavy financial demands of long-term unemployment, sickness, homelessness and old age. Finally, the system by its very nature varies in its strength from time to time and from place to place.

1. MORRIS, MARY, *Voluntary Work in the Welfare State*, Appendix III: Voluntary Work in Bradford; AVES, GERALDINE, *The Voluntary Worker in the Social Services*, Appendix 3; BAYLEY, M., *Mental Handicap and Community Care*, 1973; SHANAS, E. *et al.*, *Old People in Three Industrial Societies*, 1968, ch. 5; SAINSBURY, S., *Measuring Disability*, 1974.
2. COLLINS, A. H. and PANCOAST, D. L., *Natural Helping Networks: A Strategy for Prevention*, National Association of Social Workers (US), 1976.

From: Wolfenden, Lord, *The Future of Voluntary Organisations*, Croom Helm, 1978, pp. 22–3.

OLD AGE AND THE GIFT RELATIONSHIP

In his book *The Gift Relationship* Titmuss claimed that this relationship binds people together in complex societies. The example given was blood donorship where the gift is usually given to and received from strangers. Malcolm Johnson argues that many old people are excluded from the gift relationship:

It is from the gift relationship that many of the retired and old are excluded in western society. They are expected to receive forms of support which are well-meaningly offered. But they are no longer accorded the privilege of reciprocation. They are almost entirely excluded from the economic structure (mainly at the behest of the trade unions). Only 19 per cent of men and 12 per cent of women over retirement age have jobs of any kind, and often these are very menial. I do not suggest that old people should have to extend their working lives against their will. Many of them have no further desire to work in the way they did previously. A lifetime of work has broken them; worn them out. But there are those who want to continue in employment because they are fit, vital, and have much still to give; yet are prevented.

The economic sphere has an overawing influence on all that takes place in developed societies. Exclusion from active participation in it is exclusion from a vital part of the elaborate gift exchange which is the modern economy. If we are to rehabilitate the elderly into the network of social exchange, we must give them better access to this economic sphere.

It is too simple, however, to suggest that all should be allowed to continue in their lifework until an age of their choosing. One of the interesting aspects of the growth of leisure in recent years is that a man goes home from work to do for pleasure what is another man's job. The specialist demands of our way of life leave potentialities and talents unused and undervalued, sometimes undiscovered. Among the elderly there is a rich seam of such skills and aptitudes locked away, and thus squandered, because of the restricted recipient role we impose on the old. If we could offer new possibilities for taking a place in the economic sphere (and this might mean not only paid work but also unpaid – which could save public, and private, money) many older people would be enthusiastic.

From: Johnson, M., 'Old age and the gift relationship', *New Society*, 15.3.75, pp. 639–40.

Document forty-five
THE ELDERLY AS COUNCILLORS

The Maud Committee on *Management of Local Government* saw value in the contribution of wisdom and experience which older councillors brought to local government but were anxious about the high average age of members.

513.   In one respect we can be more precise. We are anxious about the high average age of members. The contribution of members is not necessarily diminished with age, but the presence of too many elderly members may deter young people from standing for election. The research report stresses the deference shown to the aged in some local authorities.[1] Age may well bring maturity of judgment and the weight of experience; but the elderly are less likely to introduce innovation and to understand new techniques or be able to respond to social and economic changes.

514.   The emphasis should, we believe, be on encouraging the younger members of society to stand for election and on encouraging them to stay in local government. **We recommend that there should be legal provision that a person aged 70 or over is disqualified from standing for election to a local authority.**

From: MHLG, *Management of Local Government* (the Maud Committee), Vol. 1, Report of the Committee, HMSO, 1967, p. 144.

[1] Volume 5. Chapter 3. The council members: paragraph 9.

MEASURING NEED IN OLD PEOPLE

One of the most difficult problems in social policy is how to assess need. In a study of old people in Scotland two researchers, Professor Isaacs and Mrs Yvonne Neville, summarise some of the different approaches.

Different surveys of old people have employed different concepts of 'need' and different scales classifying medical and social disability. The fundamental problem of how need is to be measured has not found a generally acceptable solution.

Following a review of the literature the authors conclude:

While much effort has been made to classify the physical and mental capacity of the respondents of surveys, there have been fewer attempts to classify them socially, other than by the criteria of age, sex, marital status, living arrangements and social class. The need for a comprehensive index of social support does not seem to have been widely recognized. However, all surveys have demonstrated the striking differences between the needs of different groups as identified by the social factors referred to above, and by other measures such as their distance from close relatives and their frequency of contact with relatives and neighbours. An example is the comparison made by TOWNSEND and WEDDERBURN (1965) of disabled subjects at home and in institutions, where the two groups were shown to differ less in respect of physical disability than they did in terms of marital status, location of children, and similar social indices.

There are in the literature few attempts to characterize old people on a combined scale of physical and social disability, despite numerous demonstrations that it is the conjunction of these two aspects which determines the need for services. Exceptions are the use by TOWNSEND (1968), and by HARRIS (1968), of an index of the need for Home Helps which took account of the number of people who were both unable to perform housework and who had no one to help them. The development of combined indices will have a part to play in measuring the differences between areas, the changes with time, and the influence of services on the elderly community.

From: Isaacs, B. and Neville, Y., *The Measurement of Need in Old People*, Scottish Home and Health Department, HMSO, 1976, pp. 134–36.

Document forty-seven
AIMS AND OBJECTIVES OF SERVICES FOR THE ELDERLY

A House of Commons Public Expenditure Committee examined the relationship of expenditure to needs in 1972. A memorandum was submitted by the DHSS which examined the aims and objectives of services for the elderly.

AIMS AND OBJECTIVES – GENERAL DISCUSSION

11.   Aims and objectives might ideally be expressed in terms of the type and quality of life which old people should lead, the help, support or care which they need to enable them to do so, and the appropriate contribution of public authorities. However difficulties arise. Professional views differ on the best form of help or care in particular circumstances and there are rising professional and community expectations about the amount and quality of services which old people should receive. These changes in expectations arise partly from changes in views about which should be provided by public services or at public expense as opposed to by the family or the community at large (including voluntary bodies). Some of the *variations in local Authorities' services* may in part be accounted for by differences in view about the proper contribution of public services. Another factor is that as standards in the social services rise, the services are increasingly being asked to cater for people who previously made their own provision, or relied on help from relatives or neighbours. The concept of need is therefore a subjective one varying between individuals and over time.

12.   A clear distinction must be drawn between need and demand. Apparently similar levels of need can give rise to quite different demands for services, and it is not always the need which is apparently greatest which is reflected in demand. The level and pattern of demand are also considerably affected by local circumstances and historical factors, particularly since demand for health and personal social services tends to reflect supply. There are other obvious objections to formulating objectives in terms of demand. Nevertheless the pressure of unsatisfied demand is in practice one of the main determinants of the development for services.

13.   A further important point is that practical objectives must be set within resource constraints. Given that expectations and demand are partly

conditioned by supply, and at least in qualitative terms are open-ended, the resource constraint must necessarily be in part arbitrary. Even if resources were unlimited it would be difficult if not impossible to establish a 'right' level by objective means.

14. General aims for the services can be formulated in terms such as 'to enable the elderly to maintain their independence and self-respect'; 'to enable them, so far as they are able and willing, to take part in and contribute to the normal range of social life of their community'; 'to enable them to live in their own homes as long as they wish and are reasonably able to do so'; 'to provide for essential needs which the elderly, with the support of their friends and families, cannot meet for themselves'; 'to provide treatment and care of an appropriate standard for those suffering from chronic disabilities'; 'to restore patients with illness or disability to as healthy a state as possible', etc. Even at this level of generality the possibility arises of conflicts between the ideals embodied in different aims. Thus a chronically sick old person may wish to stay in his own home though he could be looked after better (in the technical sense) and more economically in a residential home or hospital. It is necessary also to have regard to the welfare of the old person's family when setting aims, and this can be in conflict with what is best for, or desired by, the old person himself.

15. Perhaps more important is the lack of means of measuring the extent to which such general aims are achieved and the extent to which the health and personal social services contribute. Independence, for example, can never be complete and it is difficult to define criteria by which to judge it. Maintenance in one's own home poses the question of whether the resulting quality of life is in fact satisfactory. In each case the goal, if achieved, depends on many factors besides the services provided.

From: House of Commons, Expenditure Committee (Public Expenditure (General) Sub-Committee), Session 1971–72, *Relationship of Expenditure to Needs*, minutes of evidence 23.5.72 by DHSS, pp. 3–4.

Document forty-eight
DIFFERENT INTERPRETATIONS OF NEED

In a survey of local social services Amelia Harris found that local authorities interpreted need in varying ways over home helps.

1.1. WHAT IS 'NEED'?

The first problem one meets is how to define 'need'. The legislation is rather loosely worded; 'those needing care and attention not otherwise available to them' or 'provide domestic help for households where such help is required . . .', leaving it to the providing Authorities to determine in what circumstances assistance may be given. This is not necessarily a bad thing, as it allows generous Authorities to act generously. On the other hand, it allows frugal Authorities to provide less liberally.

If, for example, we consider the provision of home helps. All Authorities provide this service. But the circumstances in which this help is given, and the duties performed, vary between the Authority which says that elderly people should be given, as far as possible, as much help as they need to keep their homes the way they would have kept them themselves had they been able, and the Authority which rules that home helps should spend the minimum amount of time necessary to ensure that the rooms used exclusively by old people are kept in a sanitary condition. The first of these Authorities would argue that seeing their homes sparkling and polished, with their knick-knacks dusted, has a big psychological effect – that their duty is not merely to try to keep old people going in their own homes for as long as possible, but to keep them happy in their homes. The second of these Authorities argues that as the service is subsidised by public money, it should be kept to the bare essentials to prevent deterioration.

Again, some Authorities rule that a home help can be provided for elderly people who are living with a working daughter; others say that even if the daughter is working full-time, no home help may be provided. Some Authorities will 'compensate' a daughter who has to curtail her working hours because she needs to look after an aged parent by employing her as a home help for that number of hours. The duties might vary. One Authority will say the home help can keep all rooms clean, including the working daughter's if necessary, as this will help to keep the daughter from feeling the care of the parent is too much for her, and asking for a residential place. Others will say that only rooms used by the old person should be cleaned, including communally used rooms, while others still insist on only cleaning rooms used exclusively by the old person.

The same differences of interpretation of 'need' occur in other fields such as Residential Homes, housing and meals-on-wheels. It must be emphasised that these differences are not necessarily due to practical difficulties in meeting a need, but in policy as to the circumstances which justify help being given.

It would have been impossible so to define the circumstances in which assistance is necessary so that the criteria would be acceptable to all National and Local Authorities. It was therefore decided that what had to be done was to establish the criteria used by individual Authorities, and base need on these criteria.

From: Harris, A., *Social Welfare for the Elderly*, HMSO, 1968, pp. 2–3.

UNDERCLAIMING OF BENEFITS BY THE ELDERLY

In a wide-ranging book on *The State, Administration and the Individual* Michael Hill devotes a chapter to access to benefits in the welfare state. He presents some evidence about underclaiming of benefits and cites the elderly as an example.

Underclaiming of benefits by pensioners is a subject that has been given wider attention in recent years than the examples considered so far. Politicians and the public are more willing to treat this as a matter of key social concern and more effective steps have been taken to overcome it. Perhaps the most important evidence of underclaiming of national assistance by old people was provided in Cole and Utting's *The Economic Circumstances of Old People*, published in 1962. As a check on this evidence the government carried out their own survey. This study, *Financial and other circumstances of Retirement Pensioners*, published in 1966, showed that over 850,000 were failing to obtain national assistance to which they were entitled. It was with a view to correcting this situation that the government replaced national assistance by supplementary pensions, giving pensioners' rights, to a prescribed minimum, statutory force. At the same time the Ministry of Social Security set out to find the 'missing' pensioners, with an advertising campaign and instructions to staff to try to improve the 'take-up' rate. To try to deal with reluctance to acknowledge dependence upon a means-tested benefit national insurance and supplementary pensions were paid on a single book order, thus eliminating the recognizable book. Yet, Atkinson, in *Poverty in Britain and the Reform of Social Security*, estimated that despite all this the increase in the number of pensioners receiving supplementary pensions between 1965 and 1968 was very largely attributable to the changes that were made by the 1966 Act and subsequent regulations in the basic rates of benefits and the rules about the calculation of resources. He suggested that the increase in recipients 'not explained by the higher assistance scale amounts only to some 100,000–200,000'.

From: Hill, M., *The State, Administration and the Individual*, Fontana, 1976, pp. 63–4.

NEIGHBOURHOOD CARE AND OLD PEOPLE

An experiment in neighbourhood care took place in Nottingham and was evaluated. The researchers summarise the aims and conclusion of the project.

COMMUNITY WORK AND COMMUNITY CARE

The basic aim of the project was to discover whether it was possible to foster and support local community initiatives in caring for the elderly, using community development methods. This was undertaken with two background assumptions in mind:

1. that to be fully effective a service must be responsive to the individual and that this means helping him in his own situation locally;
2. that the local community contained resources for helping people which could only be tapped at local level.

Later they conclude:

WHAT THE COMMUNITY OFFERS

The key point about this approach to community care is to seize on what the community can offer, and this is a great deal. There is plenty of evidence that, far from having left everything to the welfare state, vast numbers of people care for their relatives, their neighbours, and other people in their locality. Local people can provide immediate help, continuous service, companionship and, for want of a better term, keeping an eye on things, in a way that the official services can never hope to match. They can also, because they are so close to the situation, provide feed-back about people's real needs which is essential if services are to be effective.

WHAT THE COMMUNITY NEEDS

If the community is to fulfil this role, however, it needs support. Individuals need help or advice from trained social workers when a situation is too much for them to manage alone. Community groups need advice, stimulation, encouragement; they also need straightforward administrative and financial help at times. All these may be made more possible as local authority social service departments decentralise their activities to area offices, and the social workers, for their part, will find many allies, as well as invaluable two-way channels of communication.

It should be stressed that a policy of neighbourhood involvement in community care will not provide services on the cheap. It will bring to light many needs of which the social services were not previously aware; it will make more demands both on specialised services such as mental health and on the regular domiciliary services such as home helps, and it will involve social workers in attending meetings of care groups and supporting their members. The social services and the local community are not substitutes for one another; they are both indispensable parts of a humane provision for those members of our society who need help.

From: Cheeseman, D., Lansley, J. and Wilson, J., *Neighbourhood Care and Old People*, Bedford Square Press, 1972, pp. 81–2.

THE EFFECT OF INFLATION ON PENSIONERS AND OTHER GROUPS

Professor Rudolf Klein considers the changes in Britain's economic situation and the effect on social policies. The need for priorities in a time of inflation is a theme and the position of pensioners and other groups discussed.

The other fundamental change in the context of social policy is that Britain now has a rate of inflation quite unprecedented in recent experience. No one has yet begun to draw up a balance sheet of what this means in social terms, or even to decide what should be included in any such exercise in social accounting. But it hardly needs arguing that inflation will affect, and may change, the social landscape.

In theory, inflation could be socially neutral, at least in a closed economy. If all prices and earnings were to change in step, and if the relationship between them were to remain the same, there would be no need to worry greatly about the social effects. In practice, inflation does not work like that.[1] It is one of the most powerful instruments of income redistribution yet invented. It shifts purchasing power from those who are weakly organised to those who are strategically situated and militantly led. It discriminates in favour of those who have the skill and the know-how required to protect their money, as against those who do not. It helps those who already own their own homes, as against those who want to buy one. It makes budgeting and planning, both public and private, that much more difficult: one of the costs of inflation is the confusion caused about what is really happening, and the consequent difficulty of controlling spending – a theme which emerges strongly from the subsequent chapters. It may, additionally, cause a general sense of disorientation and disorganisation, so undermining the traditional civic values which implicitly underly most social policies.

To some extent, social policy can anticipate the consequences of inflation and deal with them. This is the case, for example, with cash benefits. In effect, pensions, supplementary benefits and other social security payments have for long been indexed: after a time lag (and of course the length of that time lag becomes crucially important when inflation accelerates), their value has always been adjusted so as roughly to maintain their purchasing power.

But it is much less easy to be sure about the additional demands for help which will flow from inflation.

For example, private savings and occupational pensions have hitherto allowed many elderly people to manage on their own resources rather than seeking supplementary benefits. But inflation, by eroding the value of the savings and undermining the ability of pension funds to keep pace, may be creating a new class of poor. This is all the more so since pensioners tend to rely on Government-backed forms of saving: one survey[2] found that 'national savings certificates, defence bonds etc. were the type of assets most frequently held, followed by deposits with banks and building societies'. Inflation is consequently re-distributing resources from the small saver – who is getting a negative return on what is therefore a dwindling amount of capital in real terms – to the Government and the financial institutions. This situation will, to a very limited extent, be improved by the introduction of index-linked bonds. Even so, a great deal of additional poverty may well be generated.

So not only has economic growth stopped, and with it the hope that rising public expenditure on community services and social benefits could be painlessly financed without any re-assessment of society's basic priorities. At the same time, inflation is creating extra demands for those services and benefits. To compound the problems of social policy in this new era of perplexity and stringency, the costs of dealing *with* inflation have to be added to the costs imposed *by* inflation.

From: Klein, R., *Inflation and Priorities*, Centre for Studies in Social Policy, 1975, pp. 2–3.

[1] ROBERT M. SOLOW. *The intelligent citizen's guide to inflation*, The Public Interest, Winter 1975, no. 38, pp. 30–36.

[2] MINISTRY OF PENSIONS AND NATIONAL INSURANCE. *Financial and other circumstances of retirement pensioners*, HMSO, 1966.

A SATISFYING OLD AGE

The results of a survey of old people by Dr Mark Abrams show that for those aged 75 and over the greatest emphasis in life satisfaction is on primary social relationships – family, friends and neighbours.

What is perhaps most striking about the replies is that most of the circumstances which very elderly people see as the basis for a happy and satisfying life are not immediately susceptible to improvement by public policy based on more public expenditure in the form of cash benefits. If we accept the criteria put forward by the elderly themselves then such an improvement calls for an increase in the resources devoted to their health care and to the provision of acceptable surrogates for 'good neighbours and good friends' and for devoted kin. Both are particularly important for the well-being of those who live alone, and if adopted are likely to be slow processes.

From: Abrams, M., *Beyond Three Score and Ten*, Age Concern, 1978, p. 50.

PERSONAL MOBILITY, SELF-CARE, AND SOME DOMESTIC TASKS

A comparison between 1976 and 1980 of those unable to manage on their own.

Table 10.44 Personal mobility, self-care, and some domestic tasks: percentages unable to manage on their own: GHS 1980 compared with *The Elderly at Home* 1976 *Persons aged 65 and over*

	GHS: 1980	1976	'The Elderly at Home'*
Percentage unable on own to:			
walk out of doors	12	13	go out of doors
get up and down stairs and steps	8	6	get up and down stairs and steps
get around the house (on the level)	2	2	get around the house or flat
get to the toilet	2	2	get to the lavatory
get in and out of bed	2	2	get in and out of bed
cut toenails	28	25	cut toenails
bath, shower, wash all over	9	16	bath
brush hair (females), shave (males)	2	2	brush hair (females), shave (males)
wash face and hands	1	2	wash
feed	0	1	feed
wash paintwork	18	24	wash paintwork
clean windows inside	17	24	clean windows inside
sweep or clean floors	10	11	sweep floors
do jobs involving climbing	33	43	do jobs involving climbing
wash small amounts of clothing by hand	7	15	wash clothes
open screw top bottles or jars	10	10	open screw top bottles or jars
cook a main meal	7	9	cook a main meal
use a frying pan	4	5	use a frying pan
make a cup of tea	2	3	make a cup of tea

* Hunt, A. *The Elderly at Home*, OPCS, 1978 DHSS, HMSO.
From: OPCS, *The General Household Survey 1980*, HMSO, 1982, Table 10.44, p. 214.

TABLE OF STATUTES AND COMMISSIONS

STATUTES

1908 Old Age Pension Act
1925 Widows, Orphans and Old Age Contributory Pensions Act
1929 Local Government Act
1946 National Health Service Act
1946 National Insurance Act
1948 National Assistance Act
1957 National Insurance Act
1962 National Assistance Act 1948 (Amendment) Act
1965 Redundancy Payments Act
1966 National Insurance Act
1968 Health Services and Public Health Act
1970 Chronically Sick and Disabled Persons Act
1970 Local Authority Social Services Act
1970 National Insurance Act
1971 National Insurance Act
1972 Local Government Act
1972 Pensioners and Family Income Supplement Payments Act
1973 National Health Service Reorganisation Act
1973 Social Security Act
1974 Housing Act
1974 Rent Act
1975 Social Security Act
1977 Housing (Homeless Persons) Act
1978 Domestic Proceedings and Magistrates' Courts Act
1978 Homes Insulation Act
1980 Health Services Act
1980 Residential Homes Act
1980 Housing Act
1981 Social Security Act
1982 Social Security and Housing Benefits Act

1983 Health and Social Services and Social Security Adjudications
Act

COMMISSIONS

1895 Royal Commission on the Aged Poor
1909 Royal Commission on the Poor Laws
1968 Royal Commission on Local Government
1979 Royal Commission on the National Health Service

SELECT BIBLIOGRAPHY

THE ELDERLY

ABEL-SMITH, C. and TOWNSEND, P., *The Poor and the Poorest*, G. Bell and Sons, 1965.

ABRAMS, M., *Beyond Three Score and Ten*, First and Second Reports, Age Concern, 1978 and 1980.

AGE CONCERN, *The Attitudes of the Retired and Elderly*, Age Concern England, Bernard Sunley House, 60 Pitcairn Road, Mitcham, Surrey, 1974.

AGE CONCERN, *Manifesto – On the Place of the Retired and the Elderly in Modern Society*, Age Concern, 1975.

AGE CONCERN, *Profiles of the Elderly*, Vols. 1–3, 1977, Vol. 4, 1978, Vol. 5, 1980, Vol. 6, 1981. Age Concern.

AGE CONCERN (Greater London), *Housing Advice for the Elderly*, Age Concern, 1975

ALLEN, I., *Short Stay Residential Care for the Elderly*, Policy Studies Institute, 1983.

ANDERSON, W. FERGUSON (ed.), and JUDGE, T. G., *Geriatric Medicine*, Academic Press, 1974.

ARIE, T., *Health Care of the Elderly*, Croom Helm, 1981.

BOSANQUET, N., *A Future for Old Age*, Temple Smith and New Society, 1978.

BOWLING, A., and CARTWRIGHT, A., *Life after a Death*, Tavistock, 1982.

BRADSHAW, J., CLIFTON, M. and KENNEDY, J., *Found Dead*, Age Concern, 1978.

BREARLEY, C. P., *Social Work, Ageing and Society*, Routledge and Kegan Paul, 1975.

BREARLEY, C. P., JENNINGS, R., JEFFREYS, P. and PRITCHARD, S., *Risk and Ageing*, Routledge and Kegan Paul, 1982.

BROMLEY, D. B., *Psychology of Human Ageing*, Penguin, 1966.

BUTLER, A., OLDMAN, C. and WRIGHT, R., *Sheltered Housing for the Elderly: a critical review*, University of Leeds, Department of Social Policy and Administration, Research Monograph, 1979.

BUTLER, A., OLDMAN, C. and GREVE J., *Sheltered Housing for the Elderly: Policy, Practice and the Consumer*, Allen and Unwin, 1983.

CARVER, V. and LIDDIARD, P. (ed.), *An Ageing Population – a reader and sourcebook*, Hodder and Stoughton in association with the Open University Press, 1978.

CHANCELLOR OF THE EXCHEQUER, *Report of the Committee on the Economic and Financial Problems of the Provision for Old Age*, Cmnd 9333, HMSO, 1954.

COLE, D. and UTTING, J., *The Economic Circumstances of Old People*, Codicote Press, 1962.

COMFORT, A., *The Process of Ageing*, Weidenfeld and Nicolson, 1965.

COMFORT, A., *A Good Age*, Mitchell Beazley, 1977.

DAVIES, B., BARTON, A., MCMILLAN, I. and WILLIAMSON, V., *Variations in Services for the Aged*, Bell and Sons, 1971.

DAVIES, L., *Three Score Years . . . and then?*, Heinemann, 1981.

DHSS, *A Nutrition Survey of the Elderly*. Report by the Panel on Nutrition of the Elderly, HMSO, 1972.

DHSS, *Priorities for Health and Personal Social Services in England*, A Consultative Document, HMSO, 1976.

DHSS, *Priorities in the Health and Social Services. The Way Forward*, HMSO, 1977.

DHSS, *A Happier Old Age*. A Discussion Document, HMSO, 1978.

DHSS, *Growing Older*, Cmnd. 8173, HMSO, 1981.

DHSS, *Care in Action*, HMSO, 1981.

DHSS, *Report of a Study on Community Care*, DHSS, 1981.

DHSS, *The respective roles of the general acute and geriatric sectors in the care of the elderly patient*, DHSS, 1981.

DHSS, *Care in the Community*, DHSS, 1981.

DHSS, *Report of a study of the acute hospital sector*, DHSS, 1981.

DHSS, *Ageing in the United Kingdom*, DHSS, 1982.

DHSS, *Elderly People in the Community: their service needs. Research contributions to the development of policy and practice*, HMSO, 1983.

ELDER, G., *The Alienated*, Writers and Readers Publishing Co-operative, 1977.

EOC, *The Experience of caring for Elderly and Handicapped Dependents*,

EOC, 1980.

EOC, *Caring for the Elderly and Handicapped: Community Care Policies and Women's Lives*, EOC, 1982.

EOC, *Who Cares for the Carers?*, EOC, 1982.

FOGARTY, M., *Retirement Age and Retirement Costs*, Policy Studies Institute, 1980.

GOLDBERG, E. M., *Helping the Aged: a field experiment in social work*, Allen and Unwin, 1970.

GOLDBERG, E. M. and CONNELLY, N., *The Effectiveness of Social Care for the Elderly*, Heinemann, 1982.

GRAY, J., MUIR, A. and MCKENZIE, H., *Take Care of Your Elderly Relative*, Allen and Unwin, 1986.

GREGORY, P., *Telephones for the Elderly*, G. Bell and Sons, 1973

HADLEY, R., WEBB, A. and FARRELL, C., *Across the Generations. Old People and Young Volunteers*, Allen and Unwin, 1975.

HARRIS, A., *Handicapped and Impaired in Great Britain*, OPCS, Social Survey Division, HMSO, 1971.

HEALTH ADVISORY SERVICE, *The Rising Tide*, NHS, Health Advisory Service, 1982.

HEDLEY, R. and NORMAN, A., *Home Help: key issues in service provision*, CPA, 1982.

HOBMAN, D., *The Social Challenge of Ageing*, Croom Helm, 1978.

HOBMAN, D. (ed.), *The Impact of Ageing*, Croom Helm, 1981.

HODKINSON, H. M., *An Outline of Geriatrics*, Academic Press, 1975.

HOLME, A. and MAIZELS, J., *Social Workers and Volunteers*, BASW, 1978.

HOME OFFICE, DES, MHLG and MOH, *The Report of the Committee on Local Authority and Allied Personal Social Services* (the Seebohm Committee), HMSO, 1968.

HUNT, A. assisted by FOX, J., *The Home Help Service in England and Wales*, the Government Social Survey, HMSO, 1970.

HUNT, A., *The Elderly at Home*, OPCS, Social Survey Division, HMSO, 1978.

ISAACS, B., LIVINGSTONE, M. and NEVILLE, Y., *Survival of Unfittest*, Routledge and Kegan Paul, 1972.

ISSACS, B. and NEVILLE, Y., *The Measure of Need in Old People*, Scottish Home and Health Department, HMSO, 1976.

JOHNSON, M., with DI GREGORIO, S. and HARRISON, B., *Ageing, Needs and Nutrition*, Policy Studies Institute, 1981.

JONES, S. (ed.), *Liberation of the Elders*, Beth Foundation Publications and Department of Adult Education University of Keele, 1976.

KARN, V., *Retiring to the Seaside*, Routledge and Kegan Paul, 1977.

LEAT, D. and DARVILL G., *Voluntary Visiting of the Elderly*, The Volunteer Centre, 1977.

MARSHALL, M., *Social Work with Old People*, Macmillan, 1983.

MEACHER, M., *Taken for a ride*, Longman, 1972.

MOH, *Survey of Services Available to the Chronic Sick and Elderly, 1954–55*. Summary report prepared by Boucher, C. A., HMSO, 1957.

MHLG and WO, *Housing Standards and Costs: accommodation specially designed for old people*. MHLG Circular 82/69, WO Circular 84/69, HMSO, 1969.

MPNI, *Reasons Given for Retiring or Continuing at Work*, HMSO, 1954.

MPNI, *Financial and Other Circumstances of Retire Pensioners*, HMSO, 1966.

MORONEY, R., *The Family and the State*, Longman, 1976.

NCSS and NATIONAL INSTITUTE FOR SOCIAL WORK TRAINING, *The Voluntary Worker in the Social Services* (the Aves Committee), Bedford Square Press, 1969.

NORMAN, A., *Transport and the Elderly*, NCCOP, 1977.

NISSEL, M. and BONNERJEA, L., *Family Care of the Handicapped Elderly: who pays?*, Policy Studies Institute, 1982.

NORMAN, A., *Rights and Risk*, NCCOP, 1980.

NORMAN, A., *Mental Illness in old age: Meeting the Challenge*, CPA, 1982.

PARKER, S., *Work and Retirement*, Allen and Unwin, 1982.

PEACE, S., KELLAHER, L. and WILLCOCKS, D., *A Balanced Life*, Survey Research Unit, School of Applied Social Studies and Sociology, Polytechnic of North London, 1982.

ROBB, B., *Sans Everything*, Nelson, 1967.

ROBERTS, N., *Our Future Selves*, Allen and Unwin, 1970.

ROWLINGS, C., *Social Work with Elderly People*, Allen and Unwin, 1981.

ROWNTREE, B., SEEBOHM, *Old People*. Report of a survey committee on the problems of ageing and the care of old people, The Nuffield Foundation, Oxford University Press, 1947.

SHANAS, E., TOWNSEND, P., WEDDERBURN, D., HENNING, F., MILHØF, P. and STEHOUWER, J., *Old People in Three Industrial Societies*, Routledge and Kegan Paul, 1968.

SHELDON, J. H., *The Social Medicine of Old Age*, The Nuffield Foundation, 1948.

SHENFIELD, B. E., *Social Policies for Old Age*, Routledge and

Kegan Paul, 1957.

STOTT, M., *Ageing for Beginners*, Blackwell, 1981.

SUMNER, G. and SMITH, R., *Planning Local Authority Services for the Elderly*, Allen and Unwin, 1969.

TAYLOR, R., FORD, G. and BARBER, H., *The Elderly at Risk*, Age Concern, 1983.

TINKER, A., *Housing the Elderly: how successful are granny annexes?*, DOE, Housing Development Directorate, Occasional Paper 1/76, 1976 (HMSO 1980).

TINKER, A., *Housing the Elderly near Relatives: moving and other options*, Housing Development Directorate, Occasional Paper 1/80, HMSO, 1980.

TODD, H. (ed.), *Old Age: a register of social research*, CPA, annually.

TOWNSEND, P., *The Family Life of Old People*, Penguin, 1963.

TOWNSEND, P., *The Last Refuge*, Routledge and Kegan Paul, 1964.

TOWNSEND, P. and WEDDERBURN, D., *The Aged in the Welfare State*, G. Bell and Sons, 1965.

TOWNSEND, P., *Poverty in the United Kingdom*, Penguin, 1979.

TUNSTALL, J., *Old and Alone*, Routledge and Kegan Paul, 1966.

WAGER, R., *Care of the Elderly*. An exercise in cost benefit analysis, Institute of Municipal Treasurers and Accountants, 1972.

WALKER, A. (ed.), *Community Care*, Blackwell and Robertson, 1982.

WARNES, A. *Geographical Perspectives on the Elderly*, Wiley, 1982.

WICKS, M., *Old and Cold*, Heinemann, 1978.

WILLIAMS, I., *The Care of the Elderly in the Community*, Croom Helm, 1979.

INDEX

Abbey National, 210
Abbeyfield Society, 87,88
Abel-Smith, Brian, 69, 126
Abel-Smith, Brian and Townsend,
    Peter, 44, 46
Abrams, Mark, 20, 24, 119, 125, 126,
    159, 163, 191–2, 249, doc 1, doc 52
Abrams, Mark and O'Brien, John, 236
Abrams, Phillip, 231–32, doc 38
abuse, 52, 205
adaptations, see Housing – adaptations
advice, 8, 23–4, 95, 107, 137, 143, 180
Agate, J., 228
Age Action Year, 139–40
Age Concern, 24, 31, 54, 64, 87, 91, 95,
    113, 125, 130, 134, 136, 137, 139,
    143, 146, 149, 156, 157, 160, 166,
    167, 184, 188, 189, 192, 194, 218,
    232, 234,
    Director of, 6, doc 2; see also
    Hobman, David
ageing, 4, 7–9, 19, 22, 23, 31, 43, 55,
    58, 114, 168, 191, 195, 205, 230,
    234, 245, 250, 251, doc 2, doc 7, doc
    11
aids, 102, 104, 221, 224
alarm systems, 108–9, 115, 210, 221,
    doc 20
Allen, Isobel, 224, 227
Allon-Smith, Roderick, 242
Anchor Housing Association, 84, 87
Anchor Housing Trust, 210
Anderson, W. Ferguson, 59, 65
Anderson, W. Ferguson (ed.) and
    Judge, T.G., 21
anomie, 163

architects/architecture, 11, 23
Arie, Tom, 204, 205
Association of Directors of Social
    Services, 213, 216, 222
attendance allowance, 49, 103, 222
Aves Committee, 137, 141, 142, 143,
    144, 145, 147, 166–7

Barclay report, 217
Barker, Jonathan, 218
Bayley, Michael, 184, 188, 230
Bebbington, Andrew and Davies,
    Bleddyn, 242
bed blocking, 75
bedfast, 59–60, 149
Bell, Colin R., 128, 165
benefits, 4, 41–2, 44, 45, 49, 51,
    179–80, 187, 189, 195–97, 212,
    218, 225, 228, doc 49
bereaved, 64
Bergmann, Klaus and Jacoby, Robin,
    204
Beveridge, Lord, Report, 32, 41, 42,
    50, 135, doc 12, doc 14
Beyer, Glenn H. and Nierstrasz,
    F. H. J., 24, 121
Birch report, 114
Birren, James E., 22
Black report, 203
Blythe, Ronald, 247
boarding house, 223
boarding out, 109–10, 221–22
Boldy, Duncan, Abel, Pat and Carter,
    Kenneth, 86
Booth, Tim, 215
Bosanquet, Nicholas, 25, 49

Boucher Report, 32
Bow Group, 24
Bowling, Ann and Cartwright, Ann, 205, 227
Bracey, H. E., 19, 128, 165, 184
Bradshaw, Jonathan, 174–6
Bradshaw, Jonathan, Clifton, Margaret, and Judith Kennedy, 22, 32, doc 20
Brandon, Ruth, 23, 122
Brearley, C. Paul, 22, 111, 115, 247
Brearley, C. Paul, Jennings, R., Jeffreys, P., and Pitchard, S., 250
Bristow, Anna, 218
British Association of Social Workers (BASW), 8, 64, 110, 111, 163, doc 36
British Medical Association (BMA), 21, 62
Britton, Rachel, 125
Brockington, F. and Lempert, S. M., 21, 165
Brocklehurst, John, 8, 112
Bromley, Denis, 21, doc 11
Brooke, Rosalind, 180,
Buckle, Judith, 94
Butler, Alan, 87, 210
Butler, Alan and Oldman, Christine, 92
Butler, Alan, Oldman, Christine and Greve, John, 210
Bytheway, William and James, Lana, 86, 87

Carers, 219, 221, 224, 225–234, 244, 250, 251
Carers, Association of, 227
Carter, Jan, 221
Cartwright, Ann, Hockey, Lisbeth and Anderson, John, 21, 63
Carver, Vida and Liddiard, Penny, (eds), 22
census, 16–17, 195
Central Council for Education and Training in Social Work, 114
Central Policy Review Staff (CPRS), 11, 188
Centre for Policy on Ageing (CPA), 23, 31, 218, 232
Challis, David, 244
Challis, David and Davies, Bleddyn, 215

Challis, Linda, 241
Chambers, Rosalind, 235
charities, 133, 134, 139, 140, 218
Cheeseman, David, Lansley, John and Wilson, Judy, 148, doc 50
chiropody, 36, 73, 99, 100, 103, 107, 136, 196, doc 13, doc 23
Christmas bonus, 43
Chronically Sick and Disabled Persons Act 1970, 94, 102, 108, 217–18
churches, 134, 148, 149, 231
Citizens Advice Bureau (CAB), 2, 137, 143
Clarke, Raymond and Stone, Molly, 223
class, social, 6, 156, 159, 165, 199, 203, 247, 248
Clegg, Joan, 38, 133
Clough, Roger, 250
clubs, 100, 106, 107, 148, 163, 180, 191, 196, 221
Cole, Dorothy and Utting, J., 44, doc 49
Comfort, Alex, 8, 22, 192, doc 3, doc 7, doc 10
compulsory removal, 112, 206
community, 38–9, 119, 131, 133, 159, 160, 166–7, 183, 185, 193–95, 199, 210, 217, 221, 230, 234, 237, 244
community care, 21, 22, 36, 37–9, 65–6, 69, 77, 105, 115, 119–31, 133–50, 182–5, 195, 200–2, 204, 212–16, 218–22, 225–34, 237, 239, 244, 250, 251, doc 22, doc 23, doc 40, doc 41, doc 50
confusion, 22, 65, 112, 113, 115, 206, 224
Conservative Political Centre, 24
constant attendance allowance, 183, 228
Consumers' Association, 23
Contact, 145
continuing care projects, 206
co-ordination of service, 66, 75–7, 96, 101, 116, 188, 190, 230, doc 25
Cost benefits, 25, 181, 206
costs, 68, 89, 104, 202, 213, 214, 238–39, 242, 244
Councillors *see* Local Authority Councillors
crime, 249
Crossroads Care Attendant Scheme, 102, 115, 218, 228, 233
Cullingworth, Barry, 121, 124

Cullingworth Report, 31, 82, 89, 93, 94, doc 30

Davies, Bleddyn, 116, 215, 233
Davies, Bleddyn, Andrew Barton, Ian McMillan and Valerie Williamson, 25, 178
Davies, Louise, 206
Davis, Norman, doc 6
day care centres, 77, 100, 104, 106, 107, 115, 116, 143, 146, 180, 196, 213, 214, 215, 221, 225, 233, 244, doc 23
day hospitals, 69, 74, 107, doc 23
de Beauvoir, Simone, 22
dementia, 65, 203–4, 246, 251
demography, *see* elderly – numbers
dental treatment/dentures, 48, 73–4, 77
Department of Health and Social Security (DHSS), 23, 26, 31, 32, 33, 36, 37, 45, 50, 52, 61, 62, 65, 66, 68, 69, 71, 74, 76, 101, 102, 103, 105, 106, 107, 108, 110, 111, 113, 114, 116, 129, 130, 131, 150, 168, 176, 178, 180, 188, 190, 195, 197, 200, 202, 216, 219, 221, 226, 232, 238, 246, 250, doc 13, doc 21, doc 23, doc 39, doc 47
Department of the Environment (DOE), 32, 62, 63, 82, 83, 84, 85, 86, 90, 94, 178, 208, doc 27
dependency, 13–14, 16, 87, 107, 135, 154, 156, 157, 174, 184, 189, 208, 239, 245, doc 6
diet, 46, 60–1, 177
Dignity in Death Alliance, 232
disability, 59–60, 67, 101, 103, 174 179, doc 13, doc 15, doc 32
Disability Alliance, 232
disabled, 3, 5, 20, 32, 63, 93–4, 99, 101–2, 113, 129, 130, 163, 173, 182, 183, 188, 190, 211, 217–18, 225, 227, 228, 234, 244, 246
discretionary payments, 50–1, 197
disengagement, 8, 191
doctor, *see* general practitioner
domestic help, 33, 100, 101, 226, 240
Domestic Proceedings and Magistrates Court Act 1978, 166
domiciliary services, 32, 33, 36, 38–9, 66, 68, 77, 87, 88, 89, 92, 100, 101, 102, 103–12, 115, 183, 196,

200–06, 208, 212–22, 240, 243, 246, doc 28, doc 35
domiciliary services, intensive, 206, 210, 219
Donnison, David, 52
Donnison, David and Chapman, Valerie, 2
dying, the, 63–4, 204–5, doc 20

earnings rule, 52
Eastmann, Mervyn, 205
economic aspects/problems, 25, 32, 44, 194–99, 200, 213–15, 217, 237–40
education, 22, 23, 42, 107, 159, 199, 218, 228, 235, 251
effectiveness, 181, 215–6, 221, 244
Elder, Gladys, 8, 25, 33
elderly, contribution of, 154–70, 184, 234–37, doc 44
  financial position of, 32–3, 41–52, 116, 191–2, 195–97, 218, 241, 248, 249
  found dead, 22, 32, 64, 191, doc 20
  in residential care, *see* Residential care/homes
  living alone, 15–17, 20, 63, 89, 108,162, 248, 249
  near relatives, 93, 183
  numbers, 8, 9–17, 167, 189, 246, 251, doc 1, doc 4, doc 6
  very old/frail, 6, 12–13, 14, 16, 21, 42, 59–60, 67, 74, 87, 106, 112, 115, 167, 182, 189, 193, 200, 203, 206, 212, 215, 222–23, 234, 237, 238, 246, 247, 248, doc 1
  workplaces for, 54
  young, 6, 12, 16, 170
employment 6, 52–6, 155, 156, 190, 198–99, 227, 228, 236, 245, 248
equal opportunities, 5, 50, 183, 189, 198, 228, 248
Equal Opportunities Commission, 198, 226, 227, 228
ethnic minorities, 5, 16, 173, 188, 218
euthanasia, 205
evaluation, 147, 180–2, 243–5
Evans, J. Grimley, 250
exceptional circumstances addition (ECA), 46, 50
exceptional needs payments (ENP), 46, 50

exchange relationship, 154–8
expectation of life, 12, 123
extra care, 87
Eyden, Joan, 35

Fabian Society, 24
family, 2, 3, 20, 25, 39, 61, 65, 74, 88,
    91, 93, 101, 102, 103, 109, 119–31,
    146, 148, 155, 156, 164–6, 169,
    182–4, 185, 187–8, 190, 192–3,
    201, 204, 212, 218, 225–29, 244,
    248, doc 20, doc 23, doc 38, doc 39,
    doc 40
  extended 25, 119, 120–2, 125, 127,
    188, 190
  expenditure surveys, 47
  practitioner services, 202, doc 5
Family Policy Group, 225
Family: Study Commission on, 129, 226
Faulkner, Hugh, 9, 156
Feather, Vic, 160
Ferndale Home Improvement Scheme,
    211
finance *see* elderly, financial position of
Finch, Janet and Groves, Dulcie, 228
Finsberg, Geoffrey, 236–37
fish scheme, 149
Fisher Committee, 52
Fleiss, Arthur, 210
Fletcher, Ronald, 120, 123, 165
Fogarty, Michael, 199
Forder, Anthony, 155, 157, 174, 175
Fox, Ronald, 62
friends, 3, 23–4, 119, 133, 147–50,
    163, 182, 184, 225, 229
fuel, 47, 48, 51, 62, 134
funeral expenses, 46

gate-keepers, 72, 179
General Household Survey, 83, 84, 91,
    122, 124, 144, 167, 195–96, 199,
    203, 209, 226, 233, 234, doc 53
general practitioner (GP), 11, 33, 35,
    61, 69–73, 75, 76, 77, 193, 196,
    206, 251, doc 23; *see also* Health
    Service
geriatrician, 6, 7, 74, 77, 187, doc 23
geriatrics, 7, 68–9, 74–5, 112, 144, 201
gerontology/gerontologists, 8, 23, 192,
    doc 11
Gilholme, Katia, 158

Gingerbread, 55
Goldberg, E. Matilda, 22, 174, 180
Goldberg, E. Matilda and Connelly,
    Naomi, 216, 221, 231, 235, 244
Goldberg, E. Matilda and Neill, June,
    72, 111
Goodman Committee, 136, 137, 139,
    140
good neighbour schemes, 108, 116, 136,
    149, 167, 185, 231, doc 42
grandparents, 7, 88, 121, 124, 166, 169
granny annexes, 88, 128, 156, 165, 166,
    175, 184, doc 27
granny battering, 205
Gray, Muir, 62, 205–06
Gray, J. A. Muir and McKenzie,
    Heather, 228
Gregory, Peter, 32, 108
Groombridge, Brian, 22
Grundy, Emily and Arie, Tom, 222
guidelines, 103–5, 106, 107, 111, 178,
    223
Guillebaud Report, 31, 68

Hadley, Roger and Webb, Adrian, 163
Hadley, Roger, Webb, Adrian and
    Farrell, Christine, 142, 147
Hall, Anthony, 179
handicapped, *see* disabled
Hanover Housing Association, 84, 163
Hardie, Melissa, 24
Harris, Amelia, 20, 32, 102, 105, 174,
    175, 176, 177, 182, doc 46, doc 48
Harris, Colin, 165
Hatch, Stephen, 142, 144
Hatch, Stephen and Mocroft, Ian, 139
health, 2, 20, 23, 24, 42, 53, 58–77, 99,
    199–206, 218, 248, 249, 251, doc 13
  Advisory Service (formerly Hospital)
    AS, 66, 67, 203–4
  authorities/departments, 23, 25,
    34–5, 70, 77, 86, 101, 108, 116
  authorities, regional, 76
  Care Evaluation Research Team, 21
  charges, 48
  districts, 70, 202, 241
health, continued
  ill, *see* ill health
  Services and Public Health Act 1968,
    54, 100, doc 34
  service, 12, 31, 33–5, 66, 67–77,

93, 100, 128, 178, 187, 188, 189, 192, 200–6, 223, 242, 246, 250, 251, doc 5, doc 22, doc 23, doc 29, doc 31

visitors, 71, 72, 76, 77, 174, 193, 196, doc 39

Health Services Act 1980, 69

Health and Social Services and Social Security Adjudications Act 1983, 202, 219, 222, 223, 232

heating, 46, 48, 50–1, 62, 177, 188, 210

Hedley, Rodney and Norman, Alison, 219, 243

Help the Aged, 24, 31, 107, 134, 136, 139, 140

Director of, 9; *see also* Faulkner, Hugh

Help the Aged Housing Trust, 211

Hill, Michael, 179, doc 49

Hinton, John, 63

Hinton, Nicholas, 230

Hobman, David, 8, 23, 25, 146, 156, 168, 190, 194, 223, 232, 249–50, 251, doc 2; *see also* Age Concern, Director of

Hodkinson, Malcolm, 6, 7, 21, 63

holidays, 35, 102, 109–10, 130, 221

Holme, Anthea and Maizels, Joan, 142, 143, 145, 147

home helps, 77, 99, 100, 101, 103, 104, 105–6, 115, 116, 130, 175, 177, 180, 196, 213, 214, 215, 218–19, doc 23, doc 31, doc 39, doc 50

organisers, 11, 32

home income plans, 210

homeless, 93, 95, 211

home nursing, 206

Home Office, 140, doc 35

Homes Insulation Act 1978, 48

Hooker, Susan, 7, 23

hospice, 204

hospital, 21, 24, 33, 65–6, 67–9, 73–7, 87, 100, 110, 111, 112, 113, 115, 135, 144, 181, 185, 200–6, 212, 238, 239, 241, 248, 250, doc 5, doc 7, doc 21, doc 23, doc 27; *see also* Health Service *and* day hospital

hostels, 35, 88, 99, 135

housebound, 59–60, 63, 149, 173

household, three-generation, 119, 120–2, 125

housing, 11, 21, 22, 32, 35, 42, 47, 51, 62, 76, 77, 80–96, 135, 173, 175, 188, 190, 207–12, 218, 251, doc 24, doc 25, doc 26, doc 27, doc 28, doc 29, doc 30

adaptations, 36, 61, 92, 100, 102, 104, 173, 207, 210, 211, 221

Advice Centres, 96, 137

amenities, 85, 90, 208–9

associations, 48, 81, 82, 83–5, 89, 92, 93, 95, 96, 134, 138, 202, 207–8, 210, 231

authorities/departments, 23, 25, 100, 102, 116, 189, 202, 210, 215

co-operatives, 93

co-ownership, 92

Corporation, 82, 84

equity sharing 92, 93, 242

film, 208

grants, 207, 211

granny annexes, *see* granny annexes

housebuilding, 208

location and design, 2, 92, 107, 113, 166, 188

mobility, *see* moving

mortgages, 210–11

near relatives, 93, 125, 183, doc 27

owner occupiers, 48, 52, 82, 83–5, 91, 92, 93–5, 138, 175, 207, 210–11

rented, 48, 83–5, 179

repairs, 46, 48, 94, 210–11

residential/old people's homes; *see* residential care

right to buy, 207

sheltered *see*, sheltered housing

tenure, 83–5, 92–3, 207

tied accomodation, 92–3, 95

types of accomodation, 85–9

under-occupation, 91

wheelchair, 94

Housing Act 1974, 82, 84, 94

Housing (Homeless Persons) Act 1977, 95

Housing Act 1980, 207

Housing benefit, *see* Unified Housing Benefit

Housing Services Advisory Group, 90, 94

Hunt, Audrey, 21, 32, 62, 73, 83, 85, 92, 93, 95, 103, 105, 106, 111, 122,

125, 126, 128, 130, 148, 156, 159, 162, 165, 167, 178, 179, 184, 191–2, 195–96, 247, 248, doc 18, doc 39, doc 53
hypothermia, 21, 32, 61–3, 191, 246, doc 19

ill health/illness, 44, 58–60, 67, 157, 203, 191, 251, doc 23
impairment, *see* disabled
incapacity, *see* disabled
income tax, 49
incontinence, 61, 130
informal care, 200, 212, 230–33, 239, 241, 245 *see* also family, community care, volunteers.
inner cities, 71, 206
institutional care, *see* residential care
insulation, 48, 62–3, 92, 207
integration, 190–1, 244
invalid care allowance, 228
Isaacs, Bernard, 128, 248
Isaacs, Bernard, Livingstone, M. and Neville, Yvonne, 20, 129, 179
Isaacs, Bernard and Neville, Yvonne, 174, doc 46
isolation, 8, 20, 157, 161–4, 173, 174, 182, 184, 219

Jefferys, Margot, 138, 139, 142
Jenkin, Patrick, 230
Johnson, Malcolm, 59, 130, 155, 212, 243, doc 40, doc 44
Johnson, Malcolm with Di Gregorio, Silvana and Harrison, Beverley, 220
joint care planning teams, 77
joint consultative committees, 76, 232
joint financing, 77, 201–2, 232, 240
Jones, Sidney (ed.), 158
Judge, Ken, 196

Karn, Valerie, 93, 137, 148, 249, doc 29
Keddie, Kenneth, 7, 23
Kent Community Care Project, 185, 215, 230, 233, 244, doc 23
Kettle, D. and Hart, L., 142
Klein, Rudolf, 189, doc 51
Knapp, Martin, 238

Land, Hilary, 130
Laundry, 46, 61, 99, 100, 107, 116

Le Gros Clark, F., 56, doc 7
Leat, Diana, 145, doc 42
Leat, Diana and Darvill, Giles, 142, 147
Leeds University, 86–7, 110, 208
leisure, 22, 158–9, 245
Levin, Enid, 204
Levin, Enid and Siddell, Moira, 228
lifeskills, 234
Link Scheme, 54, 134, 184
Livesley, Brian, 250
local authorities/government, 33–5, 177–8, 215, 216, 218, 219, 223, 230, 233, 243, doc 21, doc 22, doc 24, doc 25, doc 26, doc 27, doc 31, doc 32, doc 33, doc 47, doc 48
   Councillors,, 139, 168, 169, 178, doc 45
Local Authority Planning Statements (LAPS), 215
Local Authority Social Service Act 1970, 34, 101
Local Government Act 1929, 39
Local Government Act 1972, 34
local services, 33–5, 99–117, 242, doc 47
local studies, 23
loneliness, 20, 44, 59, 157, 162–4, 184, 191, 246, 248, 249
longitudinal studies, 25

Marshall, Mary, 217, 235
Maud Committee, 168, 178, doc 45
McKenzie, Heather, 228
Meacher, Michael, 22, 112
meals, 35, 99–100, 101, 102–3, 104, 106–7, 116, 196, 213, 214, 215, 220–21, 242, 243, doc 32
   on wheels, 36, 77, 103, 106–7, 108, 135, 136, 177, 180, 206, 220–21, doc 23
medical and allied prefessions, 2, 19, 64
   aspects, 16, 19, 21–2, 24, 32
   social work, 34, 76
Melville, Joy, 246
Members of Parliament, 168
mentally disordered, 21, 24, 64–6, 67, 101, 114, 129, 184, 188, 203–5, doc 21
mentally handicapped, *see* mentally disordered

mentally ill, *see* mentally disordered
Midwinter, Eric, 251
Millard, Peter, 129–30
Ministry of Health (MOH), 38, 68, 81, 100, 111, 141, doc 22, doc 24, doc 25
Ministry of Housing and Local Government (MHLG) and Welsh Office, 32, 81–2, doc 25, doc 26, doc 30, doc 45
Ministry of Pensions and National Insurance (MPNI), 32, 42, 45, 47, 53
mobility/mobile, 24, 59–60, 94, 102–3, 113, 123, 125, 162, 203, 208, doc 53
Moore, Sheila, 145
Morley, Dinah, 107
Moroney, Robert, 120, 130
Morris, Alf, 218
Morris, Mary, 144, 146
moving, 24, 92–3, 94, 125, 183, 211–12, 226
Murray, G. J., 135, 136

National Assistance Act 1948, 35, 42, 109, 112, 116, doc 15, doc 32, doc 33
National Assistance Act 1948 (Amendment) Act 1962, 100
National Assistance Board (NAB), 42–5, 95, doc 15
National Corporation for the Care of Old People (NCCOP), 21, 24, 31, 87, 111, 134, 137, 139, 140, 149
National Council for the Single Woman and Her Dependant, 130
National Council of Social Service (NCSS), 141
National Dwelling and Housing Survey (NDHS), 83, 85
National Fuel Poverty Forum, 232
National Health Service (NHS), *see* Health Service
National Health Service Act 1946, 33, 99, doc 31
National Health Service Reorganisation Act 1973, 188
National Institute for Social Work Training, 141
National Insurance, 42–3, 46, 50, 155, 198; *see also* Social Security

National Insurance Act 1946, 42, doc 16
National Insurance Act 1957, 42, doc 16
National Insurance Act 1966, 42 doc 16
National Insurance Act 1970, 42, doc 16
National Insurance Act 1971, 43, doc 16
National Mobility Scheme, 212
need, 89–91, 105–6, 119, 127–8, 173–6, 179, 181, 188, 189, 191, 237, 240, 242, 250, 251, doc 43, doc 46, doc 47, doc 48, doc 50, doc 51
neighbours, 3, 119, 133, 147–50, 164, 166, 167, 180, 182, 184, 200, 225, 229–34, doc 41, doc 42, doc 43
Nissel, Muriel and Bonnerjea, Lucy, 227
Norman, Alison, 113, 204, 232, 250
Norris, M. E., 25
Nuffield Foundation, 140, doc 7
nurses/nursing, 24, 33, 34, 61, 71, 72, 75, 76, 77, 87, 88, 100, 103, 115, 130, 135, 193, 196, 200, 206, 233, 241
nursing homes, 75, 194, 203, 206, 223–4, 241
nutrition, 32, 60–1, 106, 206–07, 220–21, doc 13

occupational therapy, 72, 102
Old Age Pension Act 1908, 32
old people's homes, *see* residential care/homes
Open University, 22
ophthalmic services, 73–4
Oriel, W., 236
owner occupiers, *see* housing, owner occupiers
Oxford Polytechnic, 86

Page, Dilys and Muir, Tom, 32, 86
Parker Morris Standards, 81–2, 208
Parker, Roy, 3, 198, 226
Parker, Stanley, 236
Parkes, C. Murray, 64
Part III Accomodation, *see* residential care/homes
Peace, Sheila, Kellaher, Leonie and Willcocks, Dianne, 224
Pensioners and Family Income Supplement Payments Act 1972, 43
pensions, 6, 32, 33, 35, 41–3, 44, 45, 46, 47, 48, 49, 50, 51, 52, 56, 89, 135, 156, 177, 187, 192, 195–99,

228, 240, doc 12, doc 15, doc 16, doc 51
  invalidity, 103
  occupational, 42–3, 45, 47, 50, doc 16, doc 17
  supplementary, 33, 42, 46, 47, 48, 50, 51, 156, 177, 196–97
people next door campaign, 149
Personal Social Services Council, 112
pharmaceutical services, 72–3
Phillips Report, 32, 44, 80
Phillipson, Chris., 199, 236
Physiotherapy, 23
Pincus, Lily, 64
Pinker, Robert, 126, 154, 155, 156, 157, 184, 217
Plank, David, 89, 91, doc 28
politics, 25, 129, 168–69, 178, 194, 235–36, 242
Poor Law, 30, 32, 33, 42, 43, doc 7, doc 15, doc 21
poverty, 43–6, 54, 59, 197
Power, Michael, 229, 247–49
Pre-retirement Association, 56, 161
prescriptions, 48, 189
prevention, 36–7, 67, 68, 72, 73, 76, 87, 99, 189, doc 13, doc 20
primary health care, 69–71, 76, 200–2, 206
primary health care team, 76
priorities, 67–8, 69, 189–90, 219, doc 51
private sector, 3, 83, 95, 111, 194, 210–11, 215, 220, 222, 223, 237, 240–42
Pruner, Morton, 22, 122, 130

quality of life, 246–49

Rapaport, Robert and Rapaport, Rhona, 229
rate rebates, 48, 197
Rattee, Anna, 109–10
recreation, 35, 99–100, 101, 107, doc 32
Red Cross, 135
redundancy, 53, 55
Redundancy Payments Act 1965, 53
rehabilitation, 67, 69, 72, 113, 115, 200
relatives, 15, 20, 23, 61, 65, 93, 102, 103, 107, 113, 115, 116, 119, 125,

126–31, 146, 148, 163, 165, 183, 204–226, doc 20, doc 23, doc 27, doc 38, doc 39, doc 40
removal expenses, 46
Rent Act 1974, 82
rent rebates/allowances, 48, 51, 197, 212
rented accommodation, *see* housing, rented
repairs, *see* housing, repairs
research, 5, 19–26, 31–2, 53, 55, 62, 85, 88, 90, 105, 106, 107, 110, 121, 122, 126, 128, 129, 136–7, 142, 147, 167, 178, 195, 199, 200, 204–5, 207, 211, 212, 216, 219, 221, 223, 226, 227, 228, 230, 233, 237, 238, 240, 242, 243, 244, 245, 247
researchers, 3, 58, 64, 89, 116, 147, 174, 181, 182
residential care/homes, 15, 16, 19, 24, 31, 33, 35, 37–8, 49, 64, 65–6, 75, 77, 80, 87, 88–9, 91, 96, 99, 100, 101, 103, 104, 107, 110, 111–13, 115, 116, 135, 143, 144, 146, 173, 181, 183, 185, 188, 192, 199, 200, 203–4, 210, 212–15, 217, 219–241, 233, 235, 238–42, 243, 247, 248, 250, 251, doc 21, doc 23, doc 27, doc 28, doc 30, doc 33, doc 37, doc 48
Residential Homes Act 1980, 223
Resource Allocation Working Party, 69, 178
retirement, 5, 6, 8, 9, 14, 15, 20, 22, 23, 25, 32, 42, 45, 46, 50, 51, 52–6, 89, 93, 95, 156, 158, 159, 160–1, 178, 182, 191, 193, 194, 197–99, 235, 236, 246, 251, doc 10, doc 29
risk, 250
Robb, Barbara, 21, 66
Rodgers, J. S., and Gray, J. A. Muir, 223
Rosser, Colin and Harris, Christopher, 121, 128
Rossi, Hugh, 217
Rowlings, Cherry 217, 224, 250
Rowntree, B. Seebohm, 43, 60, doc 8
Rowntree, Committee, 19, 43, 54, doc 8
Rowntree, Joseph, Memorial Trust, 133, 134
Royal Association for Disability and Rehabilitation (RADAR), 218

Royal Commission on Local
   Government, 178
Royal Commission on the National
   Health Service, 67, 69, 71, 72,
   73–7, 96, 189, 206, doc 23
Runcie, J., 206

Sainsbury, Sally, 102, 163, 188
Saunders, Cicely, 63
savings, personal, 41, 44, 45, 47
Seebohm Committee/Report, 31, 38,
   101, 110, 129, 135, 185, doc 35
segregation, 190–1
Select Committee on Social Services,
   198, 213–14, 216, 238–40
Shanas, Ethel, Townsend, P.,
   Wedderburn, D., Henning, F.,
   Milhof, P., Stenhouwer, J., 20, 103,
   120, 126, 128, 162, 164, 165, 174,
   190
Sheldon, J. H., 18, doc 7
Shelter, 211
sheltered housing, 16, 49, 61, 64, 75,
   80, 81, 84, 85, 86–9, 91, 92, 95, 96,
   112, 136, 163, 173, 178, 188,
   208–10, 224, 240, 241, 243, 247,
   doc 23, doc 24, doc 25, doc 26, doc
   27, doc 28
Sheltered housing, alternatives to,
   210–11
   private, 95, 210
   very, 88, 210, 222–23
Shenfield, Barbara, 22, doc 41
Shenfield, Barbara, with Allen, Isobel,
   142, 147
Short-stay residential care, 224–25
Sitting-in Services, 228
social administration, 2, 3, 173, 181
social policy, 4, 5, 7, 8, 10, 11, 15, 20,
   21, 24, 30, 37, 154, 167–8, 180,
   183, 184, 188, 190
social security *see* elderly, financial
   position of
Social Security Act 1973, 43, doc 16
Social Security Act 1975, 43, 195, doc
   17
Social Security Act 1979, 195–96
Social Security Act 1980, 195–97
Social Security Act 1981, 196
Social Security Advisory Committee,
   196

Social Security and Housing Benefits
   Act 1982, 196–97
social services, 3, 9, 12, 13, 16, 20,
   30–9, 65, 76, 93, 99–117, 120, 126,
   127–8, 129, 136, 141, 150, 154, 155,
   156, 157, 173–85, 187–8, 189,
   191–3, 200–6, 212–22, 229, 242,
   245, doc 5, doc 29, doc 35, doc 47,
   doc 50
social service departments, 23, 34, 63,
   76–7, 94, 96, 101–2, 108, 109, 110,
   114–16, 117, 129, 136, 139, 179,
   185, 210, 215–22, 230, 232–33
social surveys, 19–21, 179, doc 9
social work, 22, 37, 72, 100, 101,
   110–11, 114, 216–17, 244, 250, doc
   36
social workers, 2, 11, 19, 22, 37, 64, 71,
   91, 101, 104, 110–11, 114–16, 136,
   141, 142, 144, 146, 147, 157, 163,
   174, 177, 180, 192–3, 205, 215, 224,
   235, 251, doc 23, doc 36, doc 50
society, 3, 4, 5, 7, 8, 20, 120, 157, 158,
   160, 162, 183, 190–1, 193
spiritual life, 247
standards, 213–16, 223, 233, 240–41,
   250
Stevenson, Olive and Parsloe, Phyllida,
   110, 114
staff, 75, 114–15, 142–3, 145–6, 147,
   180, 192–3, 221, 223, 224,
   249–51
stigma, 36, 154, 157, 175, 179, 187, 190
Stone, Susan, 109
Stott, Mary, 251
Sumner, Greta and Smith, Randall, 25,
   90, 91, 100, 175
Supplementary Benefits/Commission
   (SBC), 42, 46, 48, 50–1, 52, 116,
   179, 189, 196–97

take-up, 36, 51, 179–80, 189, 207, 212,
   218, doc 49
Task Force, 134, 136, 144
tax credits, 194
Taylor, Hedley, 24, 204
Taylor, Rex, Ford, Graeme, and
   Barber, Hamish, 247–48
telephones, 32, 35, 102, 108, 161, 162,
   221, 235 doc 20
television licence, 221, 242–43

tending, 226
Tenants Exchange Scheme, 212
Thornton, Pat and Moore, Janette, 221
Tinker, Anthea, 88, 93, 125, 128, 130, 210, doc 9
Titmuss, Richard, 155, 158, 183, doc 44
town planners, 2, 11
Townsend , Peter, 20, 30, 31, 45, 46, 49, 111, 126–7, 162, 174, 182, 251, doc 9, doc 28, doc 37, doc 46
Townsend, Peter and Davidson, Nick, 203
Townsend, Peter and Wedderburn, Dorothy, 19, 20, 44, 45, 73, 103, 105, 122, 127–8, 165, 179, doc 7, doc 9, doc 46
transport/travel, 35, 46, 47, 49, 102, 107, 113, 146, 161, 162, 236, 242–43, 251
Trefgarne, Lord, 217
Tunstall, Jeremy, 20, 162, 164, 174, 182

unemployment, 32, 47, 54, 245
Unified Housing Benefit, 197, 212
University of the Third Age, 235

variations in services, 177–8, 242–3
visitor's charter, 24
voluntary organisations, consultation document on, 185
voluntary agencies/bodies, 2, 30, 35, 54, 99, 100, 102, 106, 107, 108, 109, 111, 114, 116, 119, 133–50, 166–7, 170, 182, 184–5, 194, 200, 217–18, 220, 222, 223, 229–32, 241, doc 23, doc 25, doc 32, doc 34, doc 41, doc 43
Voluntary Services Unit (Home Office), 140
voluntary social services, 3, 35, 38, 215
Volunteer Centre, 142, 144, 145, 147, doc 42
volunteers, 54, 108, 115, 119, 133, 136, 137, 141–7, 154, 166–7, 184–5, 192, 229, 233, 234–5, doc 18, doc 23, doc 41

Wade, Barbara, Sawyer, Lucianne and Bell, Judith, 223–24

Wager, R., 25, 88
Walker, Alan, 197–98, 230
Walker, Kenneth, 19
Wallis, John, 23
wardens, 82, 85, 86, 87, 88, 91, 100, 115, 167, 188, 243
Watson, Margaret and Albrow, Martin, 23
welfare authorities/services, 25, 34, 76, 100, 101, 128, doc 32, doc 34
Welfare State, 3, 119, 120, 125, 129, 157, 179, 184, 189
Welford, Alan, doc 7
Wenger, Clare, 230
Westland, Peter, 230
Wheeler, Rose, 211
Wicks, Malcolm, 22, 32, 62, 230, doc 19
widows, 42, 47, 53, 205, doc 29
Widows, Orphans and Old Age Contributory Pensions Act 1925, 32
Wilding, Paul, 251
Wilkin, David and Jolley, David, 224
Williams, Idris, 21
Williams Report, 115
Willmott, Peter, 127
Willmott, Peter and Young, Michael, 20, 122, 125, 126–7, 165
Wireless Telegraphy (Broadcasting Licence Charges and Exemption) Regulations 1970, 242–43
Wistow, Gerald and Webb, Adrian, 213–14
Wolfenden Committee/Report, 133, 135, 137, 138, 139, 140, 141, 142, 144, 145, 150, 185, doc 43
women, 15–16, 17, 47, 50, 53, 54, 58, 59, 64, 65, 95, 123–5, 127, 130, 144, 159, 162, 183, 189, 225–9, 247, 248
Women's Royal Voluntary Service, 106
World Assembly on Ageing, 195, 205, 234, 237
Wright, Ken, 238
Wright, Ken, Cairns, J. A., and Snell, M. C., 239

Young, Michael and Willmott, Peter, 119, 121, 124, 127, 130, 165
Younghusband Report, 110, 136, 141

Also from Longman

RESOURCES FOR THE WELFARE STATE
John F. Sleeman
First published 1979

This text sets out the economic implications of the welfare state
and pays particular attention to the means of raising the
resources needed to provide social services and the effects that
the use of these resources have on the working of the economy.
The author discusses the implications of the rapid expansion of
government spending in the early 1970s coupled with Britain's
relatively slow economic growth, inflation and balance of
payments.